Editor and Authors

Tim E. Taber - Editor

Tim E. Taber is the editor of, and contributor to, the KidneySteps Survival Guide. Dr. Taber practices nephrology and internal medicine at Indiana University Hospital in Indianapolis and is board certified by the American Board of Internal Medicine in the nephrology and internal medicine specialties. He is the Medical Director of Transplant Nephrology, and an Associate Professor of Clinical Medicine at Indiana University School of Medicine. Dr. Taber also serves as Chief Medical Officer for Indiana Organ Procurement Organization.

Victoria L. Hulett - Author with Kidney Disease

Victoria L. Hulett is an estate, business, and retirement planning attorney in Indianapolis who inherited a kidney disease that slowly progressed, destroying her kidney function. Her daughter, the other author, donated one of her kidneys to Vicki in 2008, resulting in a reversal of most of the ill effects of kidney failure. Vicki and her husband Bob spend much time on Seabrook Island, South Carolina.

Jennifer L. Waybright - Kidney Donor Author

Jennifer L. Waybright is a single mother of two young sons. After donating her kidney to save her mother, Jennifer left teaching and began nursing school. She will receive her degree in June 2011 and plans to work in a transplant center with kidney patients. Jennifer enjoys speaking on kidney donation and causes of kidney disease.

ACKNOWLEDGEMENTS

With our sincerest gratitude, we acknowledge the invaluable contributions the following individuals have made to the development and quality of the *KidneySteps Survival Guide* by way of their technical review of separate sections of the *Guide:*

Sara Blackburn, D.Sc., RD., Clinical Associate Professor, Dept. of Nutrition & Dietetics: IU School of Health & Rehabilitation Sciences.

Bonnie L. Blaser-Yost, Ph.D., Professor of Biology, School of Science, Purdue University School, Indianapolis, IN; with joint appointments in Cellular and Integrative Physiology, Anatomy and Cell Biology, IU School of Medicine.

David Bodle, J.D., Hackman Hulett & Cracraft, LLP, attorney for Indiana Organ Procurement Organization Inc.

Kathryn L. Carnes, RN., Transplant Coordinator, Indiana University Hospital, Indianapolis, Indiana.

Lynn Driver, President, Indiana Organ Procurement Organization Inc. (IOPO), Indianapolis, IN.

Jay Gaddy, M.D., Hematology, St. Vincent's Hospital, Indianapolis, IN.

Daniel Hubbard, M.Ed., Exercise Physiologist & Personal Trainer, Designer of the Hubbard Training System.

Martin L. Milgrom, M.D., Ph.D., Transplant Surgeon (TTS), Indiana University Hospital, Indianapolis, IN.

Chad Schulenburg, B.S., M.A., Nursing Faculty and Assistant Director of Education, Medtech College, Indianapolis, IN.

Mark Vojnovich, Technical Supervisor, Inpatient Dialysis Services (Home Therapies), Fresenius Medical Care, Indianapolis, IN.

Kelly M. White, RN., Dialysis Education Coordinator, Fresenius Medical Care, Indianapolis, IN.

Robert W. Yost, Senior Lecturer, Dept. of Biology, Indiana University/Purdue University, Indianapolis, IN. Adjunct Associate Professor School of Education Chair, Science Education Foundation of Indiana (SEFI) Executive Director, Celebrate Science Indiana Director, NABT-OBTA for Indiana.

A very special thanks for the much appreciated efforts of:

Deborah Carrithers, Legal Assistant. This *Guide* would not be possible without Deborah's endless patience and creative approach in transcribing and formatting all material in the *Guide.*

Sally R. Hubbard, J.D., M.Ed., School of Public Health at University of Illinois, and the Institute for Health Research & Policy. Sally's talented review and editing of each chapter as to style and consistency and her public health advice helped shape the *Guide.*

Thank you also to the many individuals who provided interviews, allowing us to enter their private worlds to give life to sections of this *Guide.*

TABLE OF CONTENTS

INTRODUCTION

AUTHORS' STORIES

Author with CKD

This is your author who has chronic kidney disease (CKD). CKD is the diagnostic label physicians are encouraged to use for those slowly losing kidney function; but my doctors more commonly told me I had kidney problems, damaged kidneys, renal issues, or some kidney failure. It all meant the same thing -- my body would face a serious survival challenge.

Numerous times over my life, family members proclaimed that our blood line had "bad kidneys and bad hearts." Annual reunions included listings of the relatives who had died from one or both of these conditions, followed by sighs of hopelessness. Genetics was just evolving, and no one had tied the recurring kidney and heart issues to anything other than fate.

My own mother died from heart failure precipitated by an undiagnosed form of CKD at age 49. By the time she learned she had kidney disease, she had minimal function left and was expected to die within days. However, she endured hemodialysis, rather poorly, for nearly three years. Mom had already given birth to two daughters (my sister and me); I had given birth to my two daughters; and, my sister was well on her way to having her three daughters.

Years after my mother's death and following a routine blood test, I received my CKD diagnosis. I had already lost over 60 percent of my kidney function but had no outward symptoms. Shortly after that, my sister was diagnosed with CKD. It was obvious that the family malfunctions resulted from faulty DNA. This was confirmed after I flew to Minneapolis for tissue testing for a hereditary condition called Alport's syndrome. I also learned that kidney disease and heart disease are interrelated, with the kidney disease often driving heart disease. My family's history reflects that nearly 50 percent of blood relatives inherited the genetic mishap and experienced kidney failure. Those family members also

1

had high blood pressure and often died from heart failure or stroke before complete loss of kidney function.

Genetics, being the random division of genes at conception that it is, resulted in neither of my daughters inheriting the defect, while all three of my sister's daughters have CKD. Alport's syndrome causes a defect in the collagen that helps form the basement membranes of major organs, including the kidneys. The filtering units of the kidneys slowly collapse over time. Both kidneys cease functioning at the same rate. In females, the process usually takes decades to become critical, if it ever does. Males often suffer kidney failure between adolescence and age 40. The condition can be relentless, currently is irreversible, and never goes into remission.

Medicine has progressed over the decades since my mother died. Newer drugs greatly relieve symptoms associated with CKD. Kidney dialysis has improved, and transplant surgery is miraculous. However, kidney disease itself remains under-diagnosed and undertreated, with no real progress in reversing the disease, even though CKD is widespread and becoming more prevalent. Over 27 million U.S. adults and thousands of children have the disease, and diabetes and hypertension lead its causes.

Our purpose in writing this book is to raise awareness of the prevalence and hardship of kidney disease and to provide a Guide for survival for anyone with compromised kidney function. Most people can take steps to slow progression and increase the odds of surviving the havoc CKD causes within our bodies.

I progressed to end stage. Not only did I have Alport's syndrome steadily destroying my kidneys, but also my left kidney was non-functional because of a childhood infection or a birth defect; the doctors never determined which. Even though I could not halt my CKD, I aggressively followed the principles set out in this Guide. The result was that I had few external symptoms, even as I reached end stage. The day before my transplant surgery, I worked ten hours at the office, lifted weights after work for 30 minutes, and briskly walked for 45 minutes. I ended the evening with a glass of red wine.

2

The next morning, I walked into the operating room at Indiana University Hospital. I left the hospital two days later and returned to work the second week following the surgery. Except for the CKD, I had kept myself in good health. Thus, recovery was easy and fast, with no complications. I continue to follow KidneySteps 3, 4 and 5 to protect the life-saving kidney my daughter gave me.

Author who Donated a Kidney

I am your author who "forced" my Mom to take my kidney. Actually, rather than forcing her, I helped her understand my motivation for wanting to give her a kidney, and I made it extremely difficult for her to refuse.

While Mom would deny it, she is a health nut, as am I. Growing up, my older sister and I were rarely permitted to have sugared anything, which eliminated candy and the well-advertised children's cereals--junk food that kids love but, according to Mom, would result in diseases such as diabetes, heart disease and obesity. Only when we had a sitter were we permitted to indulge in 100 percent-apple-juice popsicles, chips, and reduced-fat ice cream. Boy, did I beg for a sitter!

I also cannot forget the pile of vitamins and nutritional supplements sitting like jelly beans beside my breakfast bowl each morning! After ingesting these "appetizers," I had little room left for my oatmeal sprinkled with wheat germ. To satisfy Mom's concern about our health, I learned how to swallow these horse-sized pills before I could speak in complete sentences. This accomplishment was awe-inspiring to my fellow preschoolers when I had sleepovers.

I also learned the importance of exercise in one's daily life. Mom attended yoga and aerobics classes several days a week, dragging our young selves with her to sit at the rear of the class, probably to avoid the sitter cost and the accompanying junk-food indulgences. We walked two to three miles most days, swam, biked, skied, and hiked. We danced, performed gymnastics, and participated in track. Mom encouraged physical activity, and it remains an important habit in our lives.

Growing up, I often heard about the kidney problem in our family. It was a looming, incomprehensible cloud that family members referred to as "the kidney condition." I have a single memory of my maternal grandmother as she was hooked to the dialysis machine in her home. Naturally, I was curious about that stainless steel contraption drawing out Grandma's blood. The washing machine-sized vampire did not frighten me even though I was only three, but it did place special emphasis on the potential impact of the family's condition.

Over the years, I kept all of my doctors informed of the kidney condition, which we now know is Alport's syndrome. We didn't know about Alport's when I became pregnant with my first child. My obstetrician carefully monitored my blood pressure, blood chemistry, and urine for evidence of protein. My firstborn was a son. If males inherit Alport's syndrome, their early urine output may reveal blood. Ben's urine was clear and remains clear. If he had inherited the disease, he might well need dialysis by his current age of 9.

A few years after Ben's birth, we learned that my Mom's kidneys were dysfunctional and had been deteriorating for years, without obvious symptoms. Shortly after that news, my sister and I flew with Mom to Minneapolis to meet with Dr. Clifford Kashton, a leading research clinician on Alport's syndrome. He assured my sister and me that we had not inherited Alport's, because we did not evidence blood cells and protein in our urine. Mom's kidneys, on the other hand, would reach end stage (kidney failure) in four to five years, no matter what measures she took. Dr. Kashton advised Mom to stay as healthy as possible in all other respects. While I said nothing, I decided at that meeting I would donate a kidney to Mom when the time came.

For the next few years and as Mom's kidneys slowly died, she continued with her regular exercise and healthful eating habits. Mom's nephrologist told her these lifestyle disciplines allowed her to avoid cardiovascular disease, blood chemical imbalances, and loss of energy as she approached the need for dialysis. Most patients with progressive kidney disease will die from some other ailment that develops because of, and along with, the kidney disease. Mom avoided that result and remained in otherwise good health.

So, as Mom's kidney function tests revealed the end was near (despite her amazing appearance of good health), I watched her prepare for death. She never mentioned dying, but I could tell she was facing the possibility as she cleaned out closets and cabinets, gave items away, and redid her will.

In the meantime, I began the process that I describe in Chapter 12. Kidney donation felt right to me. Never at any point during my donation journey was I unsure or even fearful. I enjoyed all the pre-donation testing, as I met remarkable, dedicated nurses, doctors, radiology technicians, and transplant coordinators at Indiana University Medical Center. I learned much about my own body and its state of good health. I can thank the donation process for that (as well as the horse pills and exercise).

People tell me they are frightened to donate an organ. The information in Chapter 12 should calm them. Saving a life is an incredible thrill and can result in a change in the donor's life that is as significant as the result to the kidney recipient. After donating, I left my teaching career, and I am just finishing my accelerated nurses training. I intend to work in a transplant center, assisting donors and recipients.

My hope is that individuals at risk of or with kidney disease who read this Guide become well-informed, make the lifestyle changes necessary to keep their bodies as healthy as possible, and enjoy living.

Happy journey, and may the kidney force stay with you!

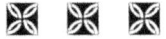

ABOUT KIDNEYSTEPS

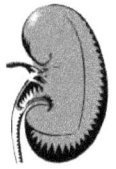

KidneySteps presents a 5-step program in the form of a Survival Guide to help you better your odds of avoiding and surviving kidney disease. The 5 steps are designed to increase your understanding of kidney disease and to provide clues in recognizing its causes, symptoms, and effects. **KidneySteps** tells you what you need to know so you can take charge of your health and partner with your physician to assure you have the best care. By following **KidneySteps**, you keep yourself your healthiest.

KidneySteps is for individuals who have:

- ❖ Diabetes
- ❖ High blood pressure
- ❖ An increased risk of developing chronic kidney disease (CKD)
- ❖ A diagnosis of CKD
- ❖ Dialysis
- ❖ A single kidney
- ❖ A transplanted kidney

KidneySteps provides current statistics so you can better evaluate your odds of survival.

KidneySteps cites recent research applicable to CKD.

KidneySteps outlines specific steps you can take to feel better and lead a healthy life despite your kidney issue.

KidneySteps incorporates the real-life experiences of someone with CKD and someone who donated a kidney.

FACE THE FACTS

The statistics relevant to chronic kidney disease (CKD), its causes and its results, are eye-opening. This silent killer has reached epidemic proportions in the U.S. and worldwide, and is developing in many of us without our awareness. We present a few of those statistics here. We also intersperse numerous statistics throughout this KidneySteps Guide.*

❖ Individuals with CKD develop cancer nearly twice as often as individuals without CKD.

❖ Those with CKD are nearly 50% more likely to be hospitalized with infections.

❖ Twenty-seven million U.S. adults evidence CKD—that is 1 in 8 adults.

❖ Up to 77% of those with CKD also have cardiovascular disease.

❖ Half of adults with CKD also have diabetes.

❖ On average, over 20% of dialysis patients die each year.

❖ Up to 92% of patients with CKD have high blood pressure, but only 20% manage it.

---

*Statistics in this Guide often come from the U.S. Renal Data System, USRDS, *2010 Annual Data Report: Atlas of Chronic Kidney Disease and End-Stage Renal Disease in the United States*, National Institutes of Health, National Institute of Diabetes and Digestive and Kidney Diseases, Bethesda, MD, 2010; or the Centers for Disease Control and Prevention (CDC); full citations in Reference sections of Chapters 6 through 22. These statistics are updated on our website at: www.KidneySteps.com

KidneyStep 1

Know Your Odds — the Quizzes

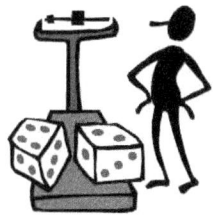

KidneyStep 1 of the KidneySteps Guide consists of five quizzes designed to:

❖ Increase awareness of risk factors commonly associated with chronic kidney disease (CKD) for earlier detection. Early detection of CKD raises your odds of slowing or halting kidney deterioration with appropriate treatment and lifestyle modifications.

❖ Provide a guide to the symptoms and factors you must control to increase your odds of surviving CKD.

❖ Encourage those with CKD to take an active role in addressing their serious health issues.

Quiz One -- Take Quiz One if you are unsure whether you have kidney disease or are at risk for kidney disease. The questions illustrate the factors most commonly associated with CKD.

Quiz Two -- Take Quiz Two if you have diagnosed CKD. The questions emphasize the health factors evident in the progression of CKD. Controlling those factors can delay the need for dialysis and transplantation and can decrease the odds of a cardiovascular event, a common CKD complication.

Quiz Three -- Take Quiz Three if you are on dialysis. Long-term survival with dialysis is a significant challenge. Quiz Three alerts you to the important factors requiring special attention for better survival odds.

Quiz Four -- Take Quiz Four if you were fortunate enough to receive a kidney transplant to treat your CKD. The quiz highlights the factors you can manage for your new kidney's survival.

Quiz Five -- Take Quiz Five if you only have a single kidney resulting from birth, accident, or purposeful kidney donation. (You kidney donors are heroes!) You are in a good survival position, but periodic blood and urine tests are reasonable precautions, as illustrated by the quiz.

1.

QUIZ ONE
YOUR ODDS OF KIDNEY DISEASE

(Take this Quiz if you do not know
whether you have kidney disease)

	YES	NO
Do you have diabetes?	___	___
Do you have high blood pressure, or are you taking blood pressure medication?	___	___
Do you have cardiovascular disease?	___	___
Has your grandparent, parent, uncle, aunt, child, or sibling had kidney disease?	___	___
Buy paper test strips for protein from the pharmacy, and hold a strip in your urine. Does the strip color change, indicating you have protein in your urine?	___	___
Do your hands, ankles, or feet swell?	___	___
Are you age 60 or older?	___	___
Are you African-American, Hispanic-American, Asian, or American Indian?	___	___
Do you use tobacco (smoke or chew)?	___	___
Do you take non-steroidal anti-inflammatory drugs (NSAIDs) such as ibuprofen, Advil®, etc., on a regular basis?	___	___
Are you obese (BMI greater than 30)?	___	___
Do you have an autoimmune disease? (*e.g.* lupus, hepatitis, chronic infection)	___	___

See next page for explanation and odds.

11

QUIZ ONE
EXPLANATION AND ODDS

Diabetes   Diabetes is the leading cause of chronic kidney disease (CKD).

> ❖ 50 percent of individuals with CKD also have diabetes.

> ❖ Diabetics comprise 54 percent of those who need dialysis or a transplant to survive.

High Blood Pressure   High blood pressure is the second leading cause of CKD. It also is a common CKD complication.

> ❖ Two-thirds of patients in the early stages of CKD and over 90 percent of patients in the later CKD stages have hypertension.

> ❖ Nearly 30 percent of U.S. adults currently on dialysis have kidney failure resulting from their hypertension.

> ❖ Less than 20 percent of people with high blood pressure adequately manage it, despite the damage it causes to the kidneys, heart, and vessels.

Cardio-vascular Disease   CKD accelerates cardiovascular disease and *vice versa*. About 76 percent of kidney patients also have cardiovascular disease. Odds of survival are reduced by more than half in patients who have cardiovascular disease when diagnosed with kidney disease.

Relative with CKD   Inherited kidney diseases are seen in up to 20 percent of individuals with end-stage renal disease. Kidney disease that is described as "cystic" often is inherited.

Protein in Urine Protein in the urine (proteinuria) is a sign of kidney disease, often the earliest sign. Protein is important to the body and normally is reabsorbed by the kidneys rather than lost in the urine. According to the National Kidney Foundation, if you have protein in the urine after two tests (a few weeks apart), you probably have CKD.

Swollen Ankles Swelling or puffiness in the ankles, legs, feet, hands, or around the eyes is a sign of potential kidney damage. However, not everyone with kidney disease experiences this swelling. The swelling indicates that the kidneys are not removing excess fluid and salts from the body. While you notice the water retention in your extremities, it is also occurring throughout the body, including in the heart muscle.

60 or Older Adults ages 60 and older are diagnosed with CKD at least four times as often as younger individuals--and die from it more readily.

Ethnic Differences CKD, diabetes and high blood pressure are disproportionately more common in African-Americans, Hispanics, Asians, and Native Indians. For example, the rate of CKD is 50 percent higher in African-Americans than in whites. Also, 30 percent of patients with end-stage renal disease are African-Americans, but African-Americans comprise only 15 percent of the U.S. population.

Tobacco Use Any form of tobacco use increases the odds of CKD and the odds of premature death. Smokers die twice as often from CKD as non-smokers.

Painkillers Extended use of common painkillers (NSAIDs) damages the kidneys.

Obesity   Obesity increases the risk of CKD and
diabetes--the leading cause of CKD. The
number of obese individuals, with a BMI of
30 kg/m^2 or over, has increased 35 percent
over the last 10 years. Diabetes and CKD also
have substantially increased over the same
time period.

Auto-   Autoimmune diseases and chronic infections
immune   can cause kidney disease, which results from
Disease   the body's immune responses to the infections.

YOUR ODDS:

If you answered "Yes" to any of the Quiz questions, you
should see your doctor for blood and urine tests to determine
if you have kidney disease. Early detection may allow you to
take steps to slow or halt progression of the disease. If you
are at an increased risk but do not have CKD, you should
follow the KidneySteps Program to reduce your odds of
developing CKD.

2.

Quiz Two
Your Odds of Surviving Chronic Kidney Disease

**(Take this Quiz if you have diagnosed CKD
but do not need dialysis/transplant)**

	Yes	No
Are you seeing a nephrologist (kidney specialist) on a regular basis to monitor your condition?	____	____
Do you have blood and urine tests **before** visiting the nephrologist so the results are available at your appointment?	____	____
Do you keep your blood pressure at 130/80 or less with an ACE inhibitor, ARB, or renin inhibitor (specific classes of anti-hypertensive drugs)?	____	____
If you have diabetes, is your hemoglobin A1c concentration less than 7%?	____	____
Is your total cholesterol less than 200 mg/dL?	____	____
Do you keep your blood potassium, calcium, and phosphorus levels within their normal ranges?	____	____
Do you have regular testing of your parathyroid hormone?	____	____
Is your doctor treating your anemia?	____	____
Do you take sodium bicarbonate?	____	____
Do you see a dietician for a special diet or eat primarily fruits, vegetables, whole grain foods, and low-fat dairy?	____	____
Are you physically active, exercising briskly at least 30 minutes most days each week?	____	____

See next page for explanation and odds.

QUIZ TWO
EXPLANATION AND ODDS

Those with CKD pose a challenge to healthcare providers. As CKD progresses, the patient has a high rate of adverse events and increased risk of death, particularly from cardiovascular disease. Addressing each factor highlighted in the Quiz is the best way to survive the havoc CKD imposes.

Nephrologist Less than 40 percent of people with diagnosed CKD see a nephrologist, a doctor who specializes in the diagnosis and treatment of the disease. General practitioners lack the significant specialty training to address adequately the numerous and deadly issues that arise as CKD progresses. Patients referred early to a nephrologist have a better chance of halting or slowing further deterioration of the kidneys.

Prior Tests The only way to monitor your health status properly is with regular blood and urine tests. As shown in KidneyStep 3, you will want a copy of your test results at the time of your appointment so you can review the results with your doctor as part of your "take control" efforts to improve your health.

Blood Pressure Controlling blood pressure is the primary treatment for many forms of CKD; yet, less than 20 percent of people with CKD effectively control pressure. ACE inhibitors, ARBs, and renin inhibitors are blood pressure medications that studies indicate may slow the progression of CKD in many patients, particularly those with diabetes.

Diabetes If you have diabetes and fail to control your blood glucose level, that excess glucose will combine with a hemoglobin component in your blood to form hemoglobin A1c. The higher the level of A1c in the blood, the greater the odds of further kidney damage.

Cholesterol	High levels of cholesterol, as well as triglycerides and certain other fats or lipids in the blood, lead to cardiovascular disease, which is an important and serious complication of CKD.
Potassium Calcium Phosphorus	Abnormal levels of any of these chemicals in the bloodstream are dangerous and frequently occur in patients with progressing CKD because the damaged kidneys cannot properly stabilize the levels. Excess potassium can cause sudden death from cardiac arrest. Too little calcium and too much phosphorus cause bone disease and even heart failure.
Parathyroid	As kidney function declines, the kidneys are unable to manufacture the active form of vitamin D necessary for bone health. This inadequacy results in over-activity of the parathyroid glands in their efforts to stimulate calcium preservation. Patients with CKD often require supplementation with a special vitamin D derivative.
Anemia	Anemia is an insufficient number of red blood cells or inadequate hemoglobin necessary to carry oxygen to all of the body's cells and is common in CKD. The failed kidneys become unable to make the hormone necessary to stimulate the bone marrow to produce red blood cells. Untreated anemia leads to fatigue, shortness of breath, and even heart failure.
Sodium Bicarbonate	A 2009 study found that taking sodium bicarbonate pills can slow the progression of CKD. The kidneys regulate the rate of acid excretion from the body. Those with CKD retain too much acid in the blood, creating a condition called acidosis. Acidosis causes fatigue and loss of too much protein from the blood. Sodium bicarbonate neutralizes the acidic blood.

Diet   Deteriorating kidneys cannot properly balance blood levels of chemicals existing in various foods, and your diet may need modification to accommodate the kidney inadequacy. Studies also indicate that eating excessive protein may accelerate kidney damage.

Exercise   Exercise reduces the odds of heart failure, stroke, bone loss, and a host of other conditions associated with kidney disease.

YOUR ODDS:

Every "No" answer in the Quiz lessens your odds of surviving CKD and increases your odds of dying from heart failure or stroke. Individuals with CKD are two to six times more likely to die from cardiovascular disease than CKD.

3.

QUIZ THREE
YOUR ODDS OF SURVIVING DIALYSIS

(Take this Quiz if you are on dialysis.)

	YES	NO
Did you begin hemodialysis with a healed AV fistula?	___	___
Have you survived the first 6 months of dialysis?	___	___
Do you see a nephrologist monthly?	___	___
Do you have blood tests at least monthly?	___	___
Do you have hemodialysis treatments more than 3 days per week or have lengthy night dialysis?	___	___
Have you avoided cardiovascular disease?	___	___
Have you avoided hospitalizations for blood clots, infections, or other complications of dialysis?	___	___
Are you currently an active listing on the transplant waiting list?	___	___
Do you regularly monitor your Kt/V number (measure of dialysis adequacy) and keep it higher than 1.25 (for hemodialysis) or 1.7 (for peritoneal dialysis)?	___	___
Is your anemia effectively treated?	___	___
If you have diabetes, do you control your blood glucose level properly?	___	___
Do you restrict your diet adequately to keep your potassium, calcium, and phosphorus levels in the normal blood serum ranges?	___	___
Do you exercise?	___	___

See next page for explanation and odds.

QUIZ THREE
EXPLANATION AND ODDS

AV Fistula   Patients who begin hemodialysis with a mature AV fistula in place have fewer infections and hospitalizations the first year of dialysis. The first year is particularly risky because of hemodialysis access and cardiovascular complications.

Survival 6 Months   Fifteen percent of dialysis patients die within the first 3 months of dialysis. Mortality on dialysis decreases somewhat after the first 6 months, with roughly 20 percent of dialysis patients dying each year thereafter. Only 39 percent of dialysis patients will live beyond 5 years. Patients who carefully manage their own condition and avoid infections and cardiovascular diseases can do well with dialysis.

Nephrologist   A nephrologist is trained to monitor your dialysis status and to recognize signs of concurrent diseases. Survival on dialysis requires careful and trained supervision to avoid or treat coexisting health issues.

Regular Blood Tests   The only way to know if you are receiving enough dialysis for optimum well-being is through blood tests. Blood tests are used to measure your Kt/V number, to determine your blood serum levels of toxins, as well as levels of critical elements like potassium, phosphorus, magnesium, and calcium. The tests identify anemia, inadequate vitamin D levels, and other risk factors for heart and bone disease common in dialysis patients.

Dialyze Often or Long   Studies show that patients who dialyze frequently or for long time periods survive longer and better than those dialyzing just 3 days each week for 3 to 5 hours. The more dialysis, the better for survival.

Cardio-vascular Disease Cardiovascular disease is the prominent cause of death for dialysis patients. You must be aggressive in avoiding additional cardiovascular disease risk factors. How you eat and exercise, even with dialysis, is important, as is strict control of anemia, blood glucose, and lipid levels.

Hospitali-zations The average dialysis patient is hospitalized twice a year for complications, many of which can be fatal.

Transplant Waiting List An active listing for a deceased donor kidney transplant means your health remains stable enough to survive the surgery and recovery.

Kt/V Monthly Kt/V blood tests measure dialysis effectiveness. A Kt/V level of at least 1.25 for hemodialysis and 1.7 for peritoneal dialysis indicates you are receiving adequate dialysis.

Anemia Anemia is extremely common in dialysis patients, causing fatigue and increasing the likelihood of cardiovascular events. Treating anemia is vital to long-term dialysis survival.

Diabetes Over half of dialysis patients have diabetes, which complicates overall survival and increases the likelihood of cardiovascular disease. Monitoring and properly controlling blood glucose lessens the risk of associated health issues.

Diet With dialysis, you quickly feel and see the effects of your food and fluid intake. The more you disregard food and fluid intake, the lousier you will feel. If failing to control your eating habits is what led to your CKD (which is the case for the half of dialysis patients with type 2 diabetes), the restrictive diet that dialysis patients must follow will present a substantial challenge. A poor diet provides almost immediate feedback with inferior dialysis results and associated overt ill effects.

Exercise Studies show that dialysis patients who exercise feel better, live longer, and are healthier.

YOUR ODDS:

If you answered "No" to any of the questions, your odds of surviving dialysis are lessened.

4.

QUIZ FOUR
YOUR ODDS OF SURVIVING AFTER TRANSPLANT

(Take this Quiz if you have a transplanted kidney)

	YES	NO
Did you receive a kidney from a living donor?	___	___
Did you receive a kidney from a deceased donor?	___	___
Were you on dialysis before your transplant?	___	___
Do you have diabetes?	___	___
Do you have cardiovascular disease?	___	___
Do you take all medications exactly as prescribed?	___	___
Do you drink a minimum of 3 to 4 quarts of non-alcoholic, non-sugary liquids every 24 hours?	___	___
Do you monitor your own blood pressure at least every other day and maintain it at less than 130/80 mmHg?	___	___
Do you have frequent blood tests?	___	___
Do you wash your hands often, avoid crowds and contagious diseases, and receive annual influenza vaccinations?	___	___
Do you follow a diet that focuses primarily on fruits, vegetables, whole grains, and modest amounts of meat and fish?	___	___
Do you exercise briskly at least 30 minutes most days each week?	___	___

See next page for explanation and odds.

QUIZ FOUR
EXPLANATION AND ODDS

Living Donor   The odds that a transplanted kidney from a living donor will survive are:

1 year	95%
3 years	88%
5 years	80%
10 years	58%

Deceased Donor   The odds that a transplanted kidney from a deceased donor will survive are:

1 year	89%
3 years	78%
5 years	67%
10 years	40%

Dialysis   Dialysis is a replacement for lost kidney function. It, however, is associated with other problems that may lower your life expectancy including cardiovascular disease. The longer you are on dialysis, the greater the toll on your overall health. This toll may not be reversed with kidney transplantation.

Diabetes   Diabetes increased your odds of CKD initially, and it continues to do so despite a transplanted kidney. Moreover, anti-rejection drugs can increase blood sugar levels. Control of blood sugar is critical to the survival of your new kidney.

Cardiovascular Disease (CVD)   CVD is the leading cause of death for transplant recipients, killing nearly half of them. If you have CVD, you must aggressively treat it with lifestyle changes. You literally must eat and exercise for your life (Kidney Steps 4 and 5).

Prescribed Drugs	Anti-rejection drugs help your body to avoid rejection of the grafted organ. Both the dosage and daily schedule for taking the drugs are critical. Taking too much, or too little, or skipping doses can lead to rejection of the kidney.
Liquids	Dehydration threatens the new kidney in several ways and may cause damage to your transplanted kidney.
Blood Pressure	High blood pressure is the second most common cause of CKD. It harms your transplanted kidney as it did your failed kidneys. Additionally, anti-rejection drugs may worsen high blood pressure. Careful monitoring and control of blood pressure is key to the survival of the new kidney and of you.
Regular Blood Tests	Lab tests are used to monitor your medication levels and the status of the kidney. Initially, you have blood tests 2 to 3 times per week. The frequency decreases over time. A medication level too high is toxic, and a level too low can lead to kidney rejection.
Infections	Because your immune system is compromised by the anti-rejection drugs, you are substantially more susceptible to infections and related diseases than normal. Over 1 out of 5 individuals with a transplant will die from infections.
Diet	Diet helps preserve your transplanted kidney by countering some of the side effects of your drugs, which may cause cholesterol and blood sugar increases. Healthful eating also helps correct some of the damage caused to your body when your old kidneys stopped functioning properly. (Such damage may include bone loss, chemical imbalances, increased lipid levels, anemia).

Exercise   You must exercise for your kidney's life and to counter the destruction to your body caused by your CKD. The exercises in KidneyStep 5 help you control high blood pressure and cholesterol; preserve bone density and muscle strength; and strengthen your cardiovascular system.

YOUR ODDS:

The odds your transplanted kidney will survive are set out in the explanation boxes to questions 1 and 2, above. If you answered "No" to quetions 2 through 5 and "Yes" to questions 6 through 12, your new kidney may well survive beyond the average reflected in the boxes.

5.

QUIZ FIVE
YOUR ODDS WITH ONE KIDNEY

(Take this Quiz if you have a single kidney)

	YES	NO
Can you answer "No" to all the questions on Quiz One?	____	____
Do you have blood tests annually to determine your kidney status?	____	____
Do you avoid high protein meals and diets?	____	____
Do you drink at least 3 quarts of non-alcoholic, non-sugary liquids each day?	____	____
Do you avoid high-impact activities such as football, soccer, wrestling, and boxing?	____	____
Do you follow an eating plan similar to that set out in KidneyStep 4--eating primarily whole grains, vegetables, fruits, low-fat dairy, and fish?	____	____
Do you follow an exercise routine similar to that set out in KidneyStep 5--exercising briskly at least 30 minutes most days of the week?	____	____

See next page for explanation and odds.

Quiz Five
Explanation and Odds

Quiz One Presumably, you could answer no to all Quiz One questions (except, perhaps, the question about relatives with CKD, age, or ethnic origin). Your screening in preparation for donation (if you are a kidney donor) would have eliminated concerns regarding the Quiz One questions.

Blood Tests All individuals should monitor kidney function (as well as heart, liver, and other organ functions) with annual exams, blood tests, and visits to their healthcare provider.

Protein The typical American eats significantly more protein than necessary for good health. Studies suggest that high protein diets may harm kidney function. Individuals with one kidney should avoid high protein diets.

Liquids Non-alcoholic, non-cola drinks are good for kidney function. The best liquids to drink are water, un-sweetened tea, and skim milk.

High Impact Your single kidney grows larger and heavier than normal to compensate for its sole status. This makes it more vulnerable to injury from the activities you perform. Thus, it is important to avoid activities that are more likely to result in a blow to the kidney.

Exercise and Diet As emphasized in KidneySteps 4 and 5, regular exercise and a diet that focuses primarily on vegetables, fruits, low-fat dairy, and whole grains are keys to good health and good kidney function.

Your Odds:

Your odds of surviving after donating one of your kidneys are statistically the same as if you had not made the donation. A reasonable person with a single kidney (for whatever reason), though, would take precautions to assure the single kidney remains fully functioning and that its status is monitored.

KIDNEYSTEP 2

KNOW YOUR STUFF

The purpose of KidneyStep 2 is to give you an advantage-- the edge you need to tip the survival odds in your favor. This edge applies whether you are at risk of chronic kidney disease (CKD) or whether you have already lost kidney function. We believe the old adage "knowledge is power," and KidneyStep 2 empowers you by supplying the facts, statistics, and current research you need to:

- Understand how your kidneys work.

- Know what causes kidney damage so you can, perhaps, avoid the damage.

- Recognize the common symptoms of CKD.

- Understand how CKD progresses and how you might slow or stop that progression.

- Prepare yourself for the hard choices surrounding dialysis or transplant, if your CKD approaches end-stage renal disease.

- Know the medical "lingo" used by your doctor so you can ask focused questions for better treatment.

- Take charge of your own condition, as you will learn to do in KidneyStep 3.

By familiarizing yourself with the information in Kidney Step 2, you will reduce your risks of kidney disease. Also, Kidney Steps will arm you with the relevant facts to secure aggressive treatment of kidney disease, if you already are impacted by it. Knowledgeable participation in your own care helps increase your survival odds.

6.

THE AMAZING KIDNEYS

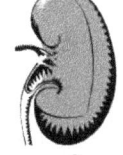

A. The Look of a Bean

1. The External View

Your kidneys are bean-shaped organs that produce urine and regulate important body functions. They are reddish-brown in color, like a kidney bean.

In an adult, each kidney is about 4½ to 5 inches long, 2½ inches wide, and 1 inch thick. Sometimes the kidneys are described as "fist-sized." Each kidney weighs about 6 ounces – not even half a pound.

> **Your kidneys are suspended in fat but will drop up to an inch when you move from supine to standing.**

The kidneys lie behind the abdominal cavity, near the muscles of your back, with one on each side of your spine. They are behind your bottom two ribs at about waist level. Your right kidney is slightly lower than your left, to make room for your liver. Typically, the left kidney is a little longer than the right.

The kidneys are organs in the **urinary system**. The urinary system is a simple system, with only four main parts:

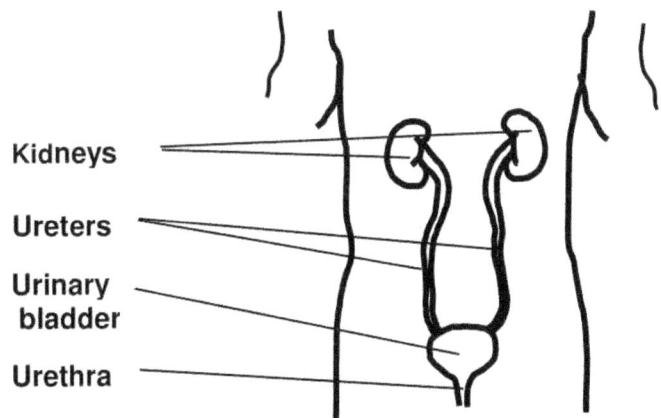

Kidneys

Ureters

Urinary bladder

Urethra

Some people have just one kidney. They may have been born with only one, lost one through an accident or disease, or donated one to another person who was dying of kidney failure. The body functions quite well with a single kidney. In fact, the single kidney grows larger than normal to compensate for the absence of the second kidney.

2. The Internal Kidney

The kidney is specifically designed to receive large quantities of blood, filter out toxins and extra water, and return to the blood useful substances needed by the body. The primary parts of the internal kidney are:

Renal Artery: A major branch of the aorta; brings unfiltered blood to the kidneys for filtering.

Renal Cortex: Under the capsule; contains blood vessels and urine tubes.

Renal Medulla: Fan-shaped and filled with blood vessels. The vessels fan out and become smaller and smaller. Nephrons are located across the renal cortex and in the renal medulla.

Capsule: Protective cover of the kidney, reddish brown in color.

Renal Pelvis: Innermost part of the kidney, where urine is collected.

Renal Vein: Takes filtered blood and remaining chemicals from the kidneys back to the body.

Ureter: The renal or kidney pelvis becomes the ureter, a tube that carries the urine to your bladder.

3. Introduction to the Filters (More Later)

While we are identifying the internal parts of the kidney, we will emphasize the filtering units within the kidneys. It is damage to these units that directly results in chronic kidney disease (CKD). You will want to know what these filtering units are called, how they work, and why they fail.

> **Important!**
> **Kidney disease is the result of damaged filtering units, called nephrons.**

Inside the renal cortex and renal medulla of each kidney are over 1 million **nephrons** (NEF-rons). Nephrons carry out nearly all of the kidneys' functions. They are microscopic units that filter unwanted chemicals from your blood **plasma** (the liquid part of your blood) to create urine.

In each nephron are clumps of the tiniest of blood vessels (capillaries). Each clump of capillaries is called a **glomerulus** (glo-MERR-you-luss; the plural is **glomeruli**). Blood plasma is cleansed as it filters through all the glomeruli of each nephron.

The covering of a glomerulus is semi-permeable. That is, it contains tiny holes that act like a coffee filter to allow small molecules (extra water and waste) to move out of the blood and into the nephron. The covering likewise prohibits larger, useful molecules (*e.g.,* blood cells and proteins) from leaving the blood.

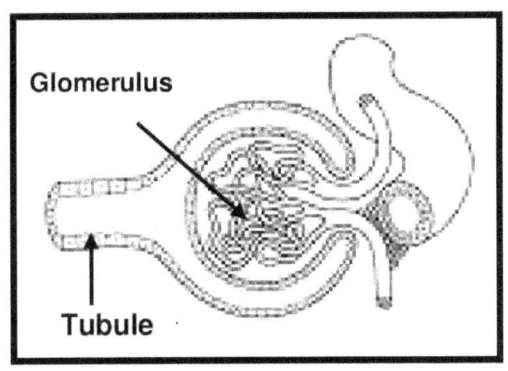

Glomerulus

Tubule

The blood flowing through the glomeruli also has a pressure 4 to 6 times higher than in other capillaries in the body. This higher blood pressure in the glomeruli helps push out the wastes dissolved in the blood. However, this higher blood pressure makes the kidneys particularly vulnerable to hypertension. If the blood pressure in the glomeruli remains too high for too long, the glomerular capillaries rupture, become scarred, and can no longer function. Over time, hypertension can lead to CKD.

Each glomerulus in the nephron is connected to a long **renal tubule** or duct. The renal tubule collects the fluids filtered through the glomerulus and further processes those fluids, resulting in the final product, urine.

B. The Important Functions of the Kidney

Your kidneys have three important functions. These functions are to:

1. **Filter wastes and extra water from your blood plasma, which:**
    * keeps blood volume stable
    * helps regulate blood pressure
    * eliminates harmful nitrogen-containing products and toxins
2. **Regulate the body's level of important chemicals to:**
    * maintain homeostasis
    * regulate acid-base balance in body
3. **Release critical hormones that:**
    * regulate the rate of red blood cell formation
    * regulate blood pressure
    * help regulate calcium by activating vitamin D

As kidney disease progresses, the ability of the kidneys to perform these three critical functions declines. This decline damages the body--particularly the heart--and death results without a kidney transplant or dialysis.

Function 1: Remove Wastes and Water

The little 5-inch kidneys are workhorses. Each day they filter nearly 200 quarts of blood through the nephrons and their glomeruli. No, you do not have that much blood in your body. The average person only has about 6 quarts of blood. This same blood repeatedly flows through the body to pick up new cell wastes and bring those wastes back through the kidneys for removal.

Normal kidneys will sift about 1½ to 2 quarts of waste products and extra water from the blood each day. This waste and water become urine, which leaves the kidneys through 10 to 12-inch-long tubes called **ureters** leading to your **bladder**. Your bladder expands to store the urine. When you urinate, the urine leaves the bladder through a tube called the **urethra**.

A. WHAT ARE THESE WASTES?

The waste products in your blood plasma are normal by-products of your body's cells as they metabolize, or change, food to energy. Each cell needs energy to perform its functions, whether the cell is a heart cell, brain cell, muscle cell or any other body cell. While your digestive tract removes waste from foods you eat, the kidneys remove metabolic waste produced by your cells.

Some of these waste products, particularly those with nitrogen, are lethal to your cells if they accumulate to excess. The primary waste product of cell metabolism is **urea**, a nitrogen-containing toxin. Urea is formed by the liver as the body's cells convert protein's amino acids into usable energy.

As blood flows throughout your body and around each of your cells, the blood picks up the urea and other harmful waste products and ships them to your kidneys for removal. If your kidneys fail to filter out the urea and other waste, they build up in the blood, causing damage to your cells, illness and death.

A blood test can measure the level of nitrogen-containing waste, like urea, in the blood. The level is expressed as **blood urea nitrogen (BUN)**. The nitrogen concentration in the blood is normally 10 to 20 mg/dL. If the level is higher, your kidneys may not be properly filtering the nitrogen-based toxins, a sign of kidney disease.

The BUN blood test is not the best test for early kidney disease detection. BUN may not be raised above normal range until about 60 percent of kidney function is lost. We will discuss tests more commonly used to measure kidney function and determine kidney disease in Chapter 8.

B. A LITTLE MORE ON FILTERING

Blood that needs filtering enters each kidney through the large renal artery. It then passes through progressively smaller arteries that eventually lead to the tiny capillaries (glomeruli) in the nephrons for filtering. In normal kidneys, blood cells, proteins, large particles and some water stay in the blood filtered through the glomeruli. Small particles, including a large amount of water, filter out of the blood and pass to the tubules of the glomeruli.

> Despite the kidneys' small size, they filter about 25% of your total blood every minute.

> The bladder can hold about 2½ cups (600 ml) of urine. Nerves in the bladder send "need to go" signals to the brain when the bladder contains about ¾ cup (200 ml) of urine, then "urgent" signals when the bladder has about 1½ cups (400 ml) of urine.

In the tubules, an important balancing process occurs to regulate what will be urine and what gets reabsorbed into the blood. The liquid filtered from your blood in the glomeruli contains not only wastes but also water, glucose, vitamins and other chemical electrolytes (like sodium, potassium, chloride, calcium, magnesium, and phosphate) that the body still can use to some extent. This mix of wastes and still-useful substances is sorted in the tubule structures within the nephrons. Excess salt, water, and other electrolytes stay in the tubules. Substances still needed by the body pass back into the blood through the tubule cells in precisely the amounts required by the body.

The filtered wastes leave the tubules and enter the kidney pelvis. Here your kidneys make final adjustments to allow additional reabsorption of the useful chemicals. The remaining waste liquid leaves the kidney pelvis and moves through the ureters into your bladder for eventual elimination.

The blood that leaves normal kidneys contains just the right amount of salts, water and other chemicals, as well as blood cells and protein. This freshened blood travels back through the body and to all of its cells to deliver balanced substances and to repeat its waste pickup.

C. URINE

Believe it or not, some people throughout history thought that drinking urine was healthful. Examples include ancient Siberian tribes, Romans and Buddhists, and even those in India in more recent years. In 2007, the Meng brothers drank their urine for six days when they were trapped in a collapsed coal mine in China without food or water. So, what is in this apparently drinkable concoction called urine?

❧ What makes up normal urine? ❧	
Excess Water	About 95 percent of urine is water.
Urea	The body's main waste produced when cells convert amino acids to energy. Urea is toxic and must be removed.
Excess Chemicals	Excess sodium chloride, potassium chloride, sulfates, magnesium, phosphates.
Uric Acid	Another waste created as cells break down.
Ammonia	Results when bacteria break down urea. Ammonia contributes to urine's smell.
Creatinine	Waste from muscle breakdown.
Hippuric Acid	Waste from digesting fruits and vegetables.
Ketone Bodies	Waste from digesting fats. Diabetics often have excess ketones in their urine from breaking down fats rather than glucose.

Urine also contains certain toxins you have ingested. For example, many prescription and over-the-counter drugs will contain harmful substances the kidneys help eliminate. The urine of individuals with diabetes will contain sugar.

Urine is yellow because it contains a pigment (urochrome) produced when the hemoglobin breaks down in retired red blood cells. The more dehydrated you are, the more yellow the urine is. You know you are drinking adequate water if your urine is a pale yellow.

Darker, red-tinged urine may be from blood, bile, drugs or simply eating beets. Urine that forms foam in the toilet bowl may mean protein is leaking into the urine, a sign of kidney damage.

As kidney function decreases, urine contains fewer and fewer waste products and becomes mostly water. Damaged kidneys are unable to filter the wastes from the blood, and those harmful chemicals stay in the body, slowly poisoning it.

Function 2: Regulate/Balance Chemicals

The principal function of the kidneys is to maintain **homeostasis,** or keep constant both the fluid volume in your body and the composition of critical chemicals in the fluid. The kidneys perform this balancing act to control just how much water, sodium (salt), potassium, calcium, acid and other elements remain in your blood or are removed from your blood. For numerous functions of the body to proceed properly, a perfect balance of body fluid volume and chemical composition is important. Excess levels are harmful and cause illness or death.

Consider water as an example of the importance of homeostasis, the balance that the kidneys help maintain. Every day, you take in water from foods and liquids. Your body's cells also produce water as they metabolize food to make energy. At the same time, you remove water from the body when you sweat, urinate, defecate, breathe out, and when it evaporates from your skin.

> **Homeostasis is the ongoing adjustments made within the body to keep the body "normal".**

The body must maintain a balance in the level of water entering and exiting. If the body holds too much water, the water collects in the cells and damages the organs, including the heart. Swollen ankles or puffiness in the hands or face are symptoms of this excess fluid retention. If the body loses too much water, you become dehydrated. The kidneys make these water level adjustments by filtering out more water if you have too much and retaining water if you have too little.

The kidneys also perform this same homeostasis function for other important chemicals in your body like potassium, phosphorus, salt, magnesium and calcium.

Function 3: Release Hormones

Your kidneys act as a gland, secreting hormones to control blood pressure, produce red blood cells, and stimulate bone growth. These important hormones include:

Renin (REE-nin). The nephrons in the kidneys secrete renin to help regulate blood pressure and water balance. Blood pressure inside the nephrons is higher than in other parts of the body to force wastes from the blood during the filtering process. This higher blood pressure results, in part, from the high volume of blood entering the kidneys.

The kidneys monitor blood volume and resulting blood pressure as the blood flows into them. If the pressure is too low for proper filtration, the kidneys release renin. As shown in the diagram below, the renin leads to the production of angiotensin II, which causes blood vessels to constrict to increase blood pressure. Angiotensin II also stimulates the release of another hormone, aldosterone, made in the adrenal glands. Aldosterone targets the kidneys' tubules, stimulating them to reabsorb sodium ions that were filtered from the blood. Chloride ions tag along (sodium and chloride equals salt). When salt moves into the blood, water moves with it. This increase in salt and water also causes blood pressure to increase.

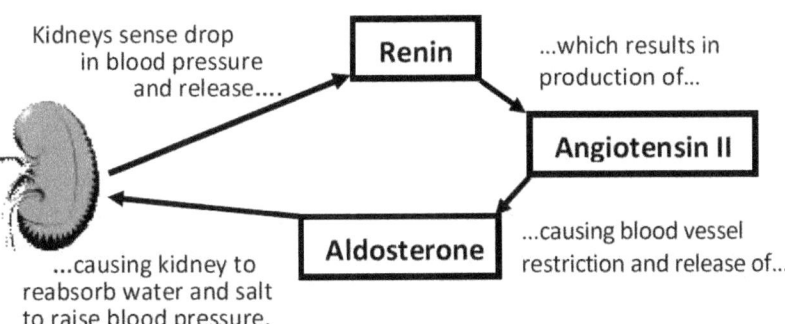

If the kidneys do not function properly, they often release too much renin. Too much renin leads to too much angio-tensin II and too much aldosterone, and blood pressure then increases. This explains why high blood pressure is a common feature of kidney disease.

Researchers find that environmental factors (*e.g.*, high-salt diet, protein deficiency) impact a pregnant mother and may increase the renin-gene expression in the child who later has a higher risk of high blood pressure.   *Current Hypertension Report, 2011*

Also, individuals with CKD often take blood pressure drugs, such as angiotensin-converting enzyme (ACE) inhibitors, angiotensin II reception blockers (ARBs), or renin inhibitors. These drugs block the formation of angiotensin II.

Erythropoietin (eh-RITH-ro-poy-eh-tin) or **EPO.** EPO is a hormone made by the kidneys that stimulates the bone marrow to produce more red blood cells as needed. EPO also helps prevent the premature death of red blood cells. If the kidneys are damaged, EPO production declines. This explains why anemia (not enough red blood cells) is a common feature of kidney disease.

Calcitriol (kal-si-TRYE-ol). Calcitriol is the active form of vitamin D, which helps maintain calcium for bones. Your skin cells synthesize vitamin D when exposed to the ultra-violet rays from the sun. You also ingest vitamin D from certain foods. This form of vitamin D travels through the blood first to the liver, where it is modified, and then to the kidneys. The tubules of the nephrons in the kidneys convert the modified vitamin D to calcitriol. Calcitriol then enters the blood-stream, stimulating the intestines to absorb calcium and phosphorus from food and also stimulating the kidneys themselves to reabsorb calcium for future bone growth.

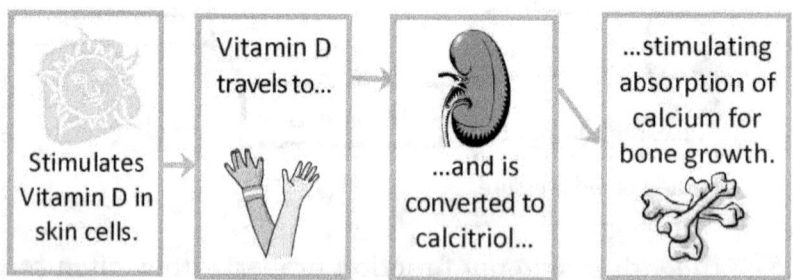

Stimulates Vitamin D in skin cells. → Vitamin D travels to... → ...and is converted to calcitriol... → ...stimulating absorption of calcium for bone growth.

When kidneys fail, they do not release sufficient calcitriol. This explains why vitamin D deficiency and weakened bones are prominent features of kidney disease.

Significant research is underway as to the importance of calcitriol. Calcitriol is earning prominence for its anti-inflammatory effects, impacting everything from bone health to heart and vessel health and disease resistance. Here is an example:

RESEARCH
➔
Researchers believe that calcitriol may slow the progressive decline in the ability to breathe in those with asthma and could be an effective therapy for those with COPD (chronic obstructive pulmonary disease).

British Journal of Pharmacology, November, 2009

The many functions of the kidneys are important for survival, and complete loss of kidney function causes death within a few days. While a person can survive (but not well) with only 10-15 percent of normal kidney function, when kidney function falls below that level, the person requires dialysis or a kidney transplant to survive.

7.

WHAT IS KIDNEY DISEASE?

Your kidney function (sometimes called renal function) is 100 percent if both kidneys are healthy. Small declines in kidney function usually will not cause any problems; such declines occur naturally as we age. However, many people with kidney disease have reduced kidney function that worsens over time.

> **1 out of 8 U.S. adults shows evidence of kidney disease.**

Function decreases when the nephrons (specifically, their glomeruli and tubules), the filtering units in the kidneys, become damaged. Damaged nephrons are unable to filter the excess fluid and waste in the blood to maintain the internal homeostasis (balance of important chemicals) necessary for good health.

If untreated, this buildup of waste products and fluid causes death. If kidney function is less than 25 percent, serious health problems begin. When kidney function drops below 10 percent, you have end-stage renal disease (ESRD) and will not live long without either dialysis or a kidney transplant.

Kidney damage can occur quickly because of trauma or injury; or, it can occur slowly over time because of disease, high blood pressure, or toxins.

A. Acute Kidney Injury

If severe kidney damage occurs abruptly (within 48 hours), you suffer from acute kidney injury (AKI), sometimes called acute kidney or renal failure.* Something has prompted the rapid breakdown of the glomeruli in both kidneys, and toxins accumulate quickly in the blood. Most often, AKI is accompanied by a severely decreased urine output.

---

* The term "acute kidney injury" is slowly replacing the term "acute renal failure," which is somewhat inaccurate because acute injury does not always result in renal failure.

Common causes of AKI include:

- Surgery or trauma accompanied by excessive blood loss, dehydration, or shock (causing very low blood pressure).

- Mismatched blood transfusion (causing an abnormal aggregation of the foreign red blood cells in the kidneys' glomeruli).

- An accident that injures the kidneys (such as blows to the lower back).

- Blockage of the renal artery leading to the kidney.

- Exposure to drugs or poisons that damage the kidneys, such as lead, mercury, certain antibiotics and antifungal agents, and some dyes used for x-rays.

Hospitalizations for AKI increased more than 200 percent between 2003 and 2008, the last 6 years surveyed by the U.S. Renal Data Service (USRDS).* About one percent of patients enter a hospital with AKI, and up to six percent develop AKI while hospitalized. The elderly, blacks, and men run an increased risk of an AKI episode. Likewise:

- People who already have kidney disease are 7 times more likely to have an episode of AKI and 4 times more likely to suffer ESRD because of it.

- Individuals with diabetes are 24 percent more likely to suffer ESRD because of AKI than are individuals without diabetes.

> **Up to 70% of people whose kidneys are injured while hospitalized die. Those surviving the injury are 3 times more likely to need future dialysis.**
>
> *Journal of the American Medical Association*
> **September, 2009**

- Up to 15 percent of patients develop AKI after cardiopulmonary bypass surgery.

---

* The USRDS is an arm of the National Institutes of Health, National Institute of Diabetes and Digestive and Kidney Diseases (NIDDK). Numerous statistics throughout this Guide come from the 2010 Annual Data Report of the USRDS.

- Up to 67 percent of intensive care patients develop AKI.

AKI is often not detected before it has seriously and irreversibly damaged kidney function. Consequently, mortality numbers for AKI are menacingly high:

- Over 28 percent of patients who survive an AKI hospitalization die within one year.

- If the AKI occurs in intensive care, the resulting death rate is up to 80 percent.

- Of those surviving AKI, nearly half develop chronic kidney disease, and up to 65 percent require long-term dialysis.

AKI can sometimes be reversed if the cause is identified and corrected early. Even if some of the nephrons are irreversibly destroyed, others may increase in capacity to compensate for the loss. Unfortunately, early injury is not usually evident, thus preventing proper intervention and correction. Immediately after a kidney injury, decreased urine output may be the only sign. In many cases of AKI, death or permanent loss of kidney function results too quickly.

Great interest exists among researchers to develop identifying markers for early detection of AKI. Currently, though, no identification marker is applied in real practice.

RESEARCH ➔ Scientists in Japan have identified a protein that the kidney secretes into the urine upon kidney injury. This bio-marker might be used to monitor AKI in its early stage.
American Journal of Pathology, 2009

As mentioned above, kidney stones can result in AKI if the stone is not removed.

A word about kidney stones.

Doctors call kidney stones **renal calculi**, and 10 percent of U.S. adults develop them. Kidney stones may result when urine is overly concentrated with uric acid, calcium, salts, cystine or other naturally-present wastes that crystallize to form hard mineral deposits the size of a pebble or larger. When a stone forms, it may block a ureter, thereby injuring the kidney. A blocked ureter causes the urine to back up into the kidney, damaging it. Often the stones can be removed, stopping further kidney deterioration.

Most Common Stones	Frequency
Calcium*	75 percent
Uric acid	6 percent
Cystine	2 percent
Struvite	15 percent
*with oxalate, phosphorus or carbonate	

RECENT RESEARCH →

Researchers found that people whose diets most closely matched the Dietary Approaches to Stop Hypertension (DASH) diet were 40 percent to 50 percent less likely to develop kidney stones than those not following the diet.

Journal of the American Society of Nephrology
October, 2009

Note: The DASH diet is the eating plan presented in Kidney Step 4.

B.   Chronic Kidney Disease

1. What is CKD?

Chronic kidney disease (CKD) is kidney deterioration that happens slowly and silently over time. CKD goes by several names, such as kidney failure, renal insufficiency, renal damage, or progressive renal disease.*

CKD is a serious and costly public health problem. Millions of people are at risk of developing this deadly disease and are not aware of their risk. The risk is particularly great for individuals with diabetes or hypertension.

_____

* In 2002, the National Kidney Foundation (NKF) developed clinical practice guidelines, the Kidney Disease Outcomes Quality Initiative (K/DOQI), for the definition, classification, evaluation and treatment of CKD. These Guidelines are applied not just in the U.S. but throughout the world. One purpose of the K/DOQI Guidelines was to create uniform terminology, but some clinicians remain tied to previous, imprecise labels for defining the disease. We will refer to the K/DOQI Guidelines in future chapters.

Most people with CKD will not know they have kidney dysfunction in the earlier stages, because they neither feel sick nor have noticeable symptoms as kidney function declines. Your author with CKD had lost over 60 percent of kidney function when she first learned she had kidney disease following a routine blood test. She suffered no outward symptoms until she had lost about 85 percent of kidney function.

> **CKD increased by 30% over the last 10 years and is expected to continue to increase. The USRDS estimates that over 27 million U.S. adults show signs of CKD.**

The common causes of CKD impact both kidneys simul-taneously by damaging the nephrons. As the nephrons die, kidney function is lost.

As a "silent killer," CKD is not reversible, although some causes of kidney destruction, if identified early, can be treated. CKD may worsen over time and may result in kidney failure, which is called end-stage renal disease (ESRD). A person can survive with only one-third of a single kidney, but people with ESRD have lost 90 percent of their kidney function and must undergo dialysis or receive a kidney transplant to live.

2. Who Gets CKD?

While anyone can develop CKD, certain groups are more vulnerable:

> **People weighing less than 5.5 lbs. at birth were found to be 70% more likely to develop CKD.**
> *Current Opinion in Pediatrics,* 2009

- ❖ African-Americans, Native Americans, Hispanics, Asians, and Pacific Islanders are more susceptible than whites to CKD.

- ❖ African-Americans are 4 times more likely to develop kidney disease than whites.

- ❖ Nearly 60 percent of African-Americans and 50 percent of whites with CKD also have diabetes.

47

❖ Up to 20 percent of those with CKD have a blood relative with the disease.

❖ Those over age 60 are nearly seven times more likely than people in their 30's or 40's to have CKD.

Patient Interview: Shirly has diabetes and high blood pressure, two risk factors for CKD. She also lost a kidney some years ago to cancer and suffers from repeated urinary tract infections. We asked Shirly about her kidney function. She told us, "My function was bad but is back to normal," [which is unlikely]. Shirly added, "I don't pay much attention to my diet or exercise." Shirly admitted that she does not know her level of kidney function. "I don't believe my doctor really checks it, and I don't ask."

Take Quiz 1 in Chapter 1 of this Guide to determine if you are at risk for CKD. Individuals at an increased risk should have annual urine and blood tests to monitor kidney function status. The key to delaying kidney disease progression is early detection and treatment. To encourage people to check for CKD, the NKF offers free screenings at locations around the country. Nearly 26 percent of people screened in 2009 discovered they have CKD, but only 2 percent had been aware of their risk. To find a screening location, check for the Kidney Early Evaluation Program at www.KEEPonline.org.

3. Stages of CKD

The NKF established criteria in 2002 for the diagnosis of CKD. A person is diagnosed with CKD if the person has:

1. Kidney damage for 3 months or longer, with or without decreased GFR, as evidenced by abnormalities revealed in appropriate tests; or,

2. GFR less than 60 for 3 months or longer, with or without kidney damage.

GFR means **estimated glomerular filtration rate** and is a measurement of the total filtering ability of all functioning nephrons in both kidneys. The fewer functioning nephrons, the lower the GFR. A blood test is used to measure and calculate GFR (we will discuss GFR in greater detail in

Chapter 9). Once a patient is diagnosed with CKD based on the NKF criteria, the CKD is defined by the stage of progression. Based on GFR, the 5 stages of CKD are:

Stage of CKD	Description	GFR (ml/min/1.73m²)
I	Normal, unless protein in urine	90 or above
II	Mild kidney disease	60-90
III	Moderate kidney disease	30-59
IV	Severe kidney disease	15-29
V	End-stage renal disease. Need dialysis/transplant to survive.	Less than 15

If you are at risk of or have CKD, you will want to memorize these stages to monitor your kidney function after blood tests.

The 5 stages of CKD are progressive. They move from the point where the person is healthy, but susceptible to CKD because of the presence of risk factors (Stage I), through later stages, where CKD is diagnosable (Stage III). The final stage is complete kidney failure (Stage V). The natural history of CKD is as follows:

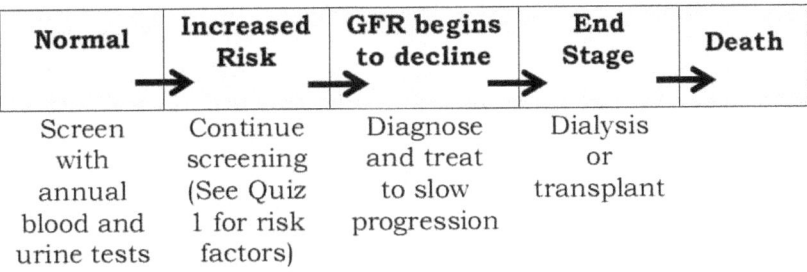

Normal	Increased Risk	GFR begins to decline	End Stage	Death
Screen with annual blood and urine tests	Continue screening (See Quiz 1 for risk factors)	Diagnose and treat to slow progression	Dialysis or transplant	

Each year, the USRDS reports updated data about patients with CKD. According to the 2010 USRDS Annual Data Report, about 27 million adults in the U.S. are currently diagnosed with Stages II through IV of CKD. Another 20 million adults are considered at risk of CKD or are in the early stages of CKD, but are undiagnosed because of the lack of obvious symptoms. Upon reaching Stage III of CKD, internal abnormalities such as high blood pressure, elevated triglycerides, chemical imbalances, anemia, bone loss, heart disease, and increased disease risks may develop as the unlucky patient remains unaware of the CKD.

Despite the high prevalence of CKD, its progression can take decades, with relatively few people reaching Stage V or end stage. Because kidney disease often begins late in life and progresses slowly, most people in the earlier stages of CKD die before they develop ESRD. Individuals most likely to reach end stage are those with diabetes, hypertension, and certain hereditary kidney diseases.

The real burden of CKD is the increased probability of developing cardiovascular disease. Having CKD in any stage directly increases the likelihood of developing heart and vessel disease. The NKF reports that individuals in the early stages of CKD are 5 times more likely to die from heart disease before progressing to end-stage kidney disease. In fact, heart disease is the number one killer of people with CKD (see more later in this chapter).

4. ESRD

When a patient reaches Stage V of CKD, the patient is said to have ESRD, also known as chronic renal failure or kidney failure. GFR has decreased to 15 ml/ min/1.73m^2 or less, and kidney function has dropped to 10 percent or less. The kidneys are unable to perform efficiently, and the body fills with extra fluid and nitrogen waste products (such as urea). This toxic condition is called **uremia** (yoo-REE-mee-uh). A patient with ESRD is very ill, and the uremia initially causes nausea, vomiting, hiccups, and lethargy. Without dialysis or a transplant, ESRD soon will lead to seizures, coma, heart failure, and death.

According to the 2010 Annual Report of the USRDS, 548,000 CKD patients in the U.S. suffer from ESRD. That number is expected to double over the next decade. The primary causes of ESRD in the patients who now have it are:

Cause of ESRD	%
Diabetes	44%
Hypertension	28%
Glomerular Nephritis (primary/secondary)	7%
Hereditary/congenital CKD	10%
Other (drugs, pain relievers, poisonings, obstructions, tumors, etc.)	11%

50

In the ESRD population, men slightly outnumber women, and about 30 percent are African-American. The prevalence of African-Americans with ESRD is three times the percentage in the general population.

Individuals most often reach ESRD between ages 46 and 65. Evidence links poverty and social deprivation to CKD, probably because both conditions impact overall kidney care during early stages. In many cases, ESRD would have been prevented had the patients known of the CKD earlier and received appropriate, aggressive treatment. We discuss detection and prevention in KidneyStep 3.

> **Effective January 1, 2010, Medicare pays for educational classes for patients in Stage IV of CKD, to help in decisions regarding dialysis/transplant.**

C. CKD and Being Older

The medical community debates whether older age is an actual cause of kidney disease. Certainly, the normal aging process leaves the kidneys vulnerable to disease, and the prevalence of CKD in those over age 65 is more prominent than in younger individuals. Plainly, getting older is difficult on the kidneys.

> **By age 60, we have only 75% of our former kidney function.**

1. Age-related Changes in the Kidney

Changes in kidney function and kidney structure during normal aging are quite dramatic. The deterioration of both function and structure begins during your 30's. The estimated glomerular filtration rate (the combined ability of all working nephrons of both kidneys to filter) begins to decline by as much as 7 percent per decade. By age 60, a normal person may have lost perhaps 25 percent of kidney function. This loss is accelerated in those who:

- have diabetes
- have high blood pressure
- smoke
- suffer from cardiovascular disease
- take certain drugs

Blood flow to the kidneys through the renal arteries also declines by about 10 percent per decade after the fourth decade. This reduces the filtration ability of the kidneys.

The size of the kidneys decreases by about 25 percent between ages 40 and 80, consistent with the natural shrinking of the aging body. Moreover, the glomeruli degenerate and become scarred as we age. As the number of these important filtering units decreases, the ability of the kidneys to filter the blood is reduced. As a result, the presence of protein in the urine also increases with advancing age and may not be evident in the normal urine test.

2. Kidney Disease as We Age

Age-related kidney deterioration generally poses little threat to our wellbeing, because even having half of normal kidney function is adequate to keep us in good health. However, the natural decline of kidney function with age makes the kidneys more susceptible to the impact of diabetes, high blood pressure, and other common causes of CKD. Consequently, CKD is more prevalent in the elderly as compared to the younger population. It is also accelerated if the elderly person has another risk factor for kidney disease. The following chart compares the rates of coexisting diseases in CKD patients both over and under age 65:

Percent of CKD Patients with Associated Diseases

Associated Disease	Age 65 or under	Over age 65
Diabetes	38 %	48.4 %
High blood pressure	66 %	94 %
Cardiovascular disease	30 %	77 %
Cancer	14 %	18.8 %
Lung disease (COPD)	8.3 %	25.6 %

2010 Annual Data Report, USRDS

About 40 percent of patients receiving regular dialysis are older than 65, and the mean age of those beginning treatment is greater than 60 years. These numbers are projected to increase through the next decade.

The elderly are more susceptible to acute kidney injury (AKI) than are younger individuals. Studies suggest that prominent causes of AKI in older Americans include: overuse of drugs such as pain relievers (NSAIDs) and blood pressure medication known as ACE inhibitors (66 percent of AKI cases); sepsis or infection (45.7 percent); and dehydration (45.7 percent). More than 80 percent of reported cases of pain reliever-induced AKI are in patients older than 60.

D. CKD and Its Sister: Cardiovascular Disease

CKD and cardiovascular disease (CVD) are closely linked, with one disease overwhelmingly increasing the odds of the other. As kidney function declines, the kidneys are unable to control blood pressure (because of decreased renin production), to maintain proper balances of blood chemicals (such as sodium, potassium, calcium), and to remove excess liquid from the blood. All of these deficiencies substantially increase CVD risk. Patients with CKD are 15 times more likely to have CVD than the general population. As kidney disease progresses, cardiovascular events rise dramatically, increasing to 20 times higher than normal in ESRD. CVD is the leading cause of death in most people with CKD.

Even in Stages I and II of CKD, when perhaps only micro-albuminuria is present, CVD risk is increased.

Likewise, a person with CVD has a substantially increased risk of kidney disease. The interplay between the heart and kidneys has received widespread attention in recent years, in part because of the disturbing number of patients evidencing both CKD and CVD.

As shown in the previous chart, up to 94 percent of individuals with CKD have high blood pressure and three-quarters of them have diagnosed heart disease. According to the National Kidney Foundation, those with Stage III CKD experience twice as many heart attacks and strokes as those without CKD and have over 5 times the number of CVD events.

Cardiovascular disease is particularly prevalent in CKD patients who have progressed to end stage. Only 15 percent of those with ESRD have a normal left heart ventricle. Dialysis patients have heart failure rates of up to 55 percent. A 20-yr-old on dialysis has the same chance of death from CVD as an 80-yr-old in the general population.

We can summarize this section by quoting the NKF's K/DOQI Clinical Practice Guideline 15, which states:

"All patients with chronic kidney disease should be considered in the highest risk group for cardiovascular disease...".

Both individuals at risk of kidney disease and those diagnosed with kidney disease require screening for CVD and aggressive treatment to modify CVD risk factors, such as hypertension, anemia, and salt and water retention.

8.

DETECTING KIDNEY DISEASE

A. Outward Signs

You probably will not know you have chronic kidney disease (CKD) until you have a urine or blood test. The early stages of CKD usually occur silently, without causing noticeable symptoms or pain. You are unlikely to see any change in the volume, color, or odor of your urine; and, you may continue to feel fine until your kidney function is seriously compromised.

As kidney disease worsens, your ailing kidneys may cause some of the following:

❖ Fatigue -- the earliest and most common symptom, fatigue can be constant or occur just at the end of the day. Generally, the fatigue results from the failing kidneys' inability to make EPO to trigger the production of red blood cells. (See Chapter 6). This results in anemia, not enough red blood cells to carry sufficient oxygen through the body.

❖ Changes in urination -- not a universal symptom, but urine may become foamy, contain blood, or change in frequency or amount.

> **Following KidneySteps 3, 4 and 5 can lessen symptoms and, perhaps, slow down or stop the progression of CKD.**

❖ Muscle cramps -- the second most common complaint, with cramping in the calf the likely location.

❖ Itching -- failing kidneys do not remove waste products from blood, resulting in itching.

❖ Loss of appetite -- even nausea, vomiting, and weight loss.

❖ Swelling, numbness or puffiness of the hands, feet, ankles, or around the eyes -- failing kidneys do not remove excess water and salt from the body.

- ❖ Hiccups
- ❖ Bruising easily
- ❖ Trouble sleeping
- ❖ Shortness of breath

Some people have no outward signs of kidney disease, even as the disease advances. These people often are surprised to learn that they have CKD and that it has progressed for years.

> **Staff Interview:** *Pat, a certified clinical transplant nurse who has worked with transplant patients for 20 years, says that often individuals know something is wrong with their kidneys but fail to ask for a test to catch CKD early. They tell themselves they just have "active kidneys" or "lazy kidneys" or hide behind some other excuse to avoid the possibility of bad news. In the transplant unit, patients tell Pat "they knew but ignored" hints of ailing kidneys.*

B. Internal Signs

High blood pressure is one of the signs of CKD. However, people usually discover they have kidney disease when a doctor first detects the condition through routine urine and blood tests.

1. Blood Pressure

While high blood pressure, **hypertension**, may lead to kidney disease, it also results from (or is worsened by) kidney disease. In fact, nearly everyone with CKD has hypertension, and strong evidence suggests that high blood pressure is a risk factor for the progression of the disease. The National Kidney Foundation (NKF) identified hypertension as the second leading cause of CKD, just behind diabetes.

Hypertension is both a cause and a consequence of CKD.

Your blood pressure is considered normal if it stays below 120/80 mmHg. Blood pressure consistently higher than 120/80 mmHg, when combined with the results of urine and blood tests, may confirm failing kidneys.

The National Heart, Lung and Blood Institute recommends that those with reduced kidney function maintain blood pressure below 130/80mmHg. We discuss hypertension in more detail in the next chapter.

2. Urinalysis

Healthy kidneys will remove excess fluid and waste products from the blood but leave most protein for use by the body.

> **Even a tiny amount of protein in urine better predicts cardio-vascular disease, diabetes, and CKD than either elevated blood pressure or cholesterol.**

Therefore, protein of any consequence is not normally found in the urine. Impaired kidneys fail to prevent protein from leaking into the urine, creating a condition called **proteinuria** (PRO-tee-NOOR-ee-uh), which means protein in urine. As kidney function worsens, the level of proteinuria increases and can be measured by laboratory tests.

IMPORTANT STUDIES →

In several separate studies of non-diabetic patients with CKD, proteinuria was the strong-est predictor of kidney disease progression.

For a quick check, a doctor can test for protein using a chemically-treated dipstick inserted in a small sample of urine. (You may do this at home, too. Ask your pharmacist for some test strips). The test strip will change color if protein is present in the urine sample. The test strip comes with a scoring chart indicating the presence of protein at +1, +2, +3, +4 levels. A positive reading for protein in the urine, if it shows up twice over a few weeks, suggests some loss of kidney function, perhaps CKD.

> **Proteinuria not only indicates nephron damage but also contributes to the damage.**

A. URINALYSIS

The most routine medical procedure for testing the characteristics of urine is the **urinalysis.** This is the "pee in the cup" test. A lab examines the sample of fresh urine to check for abnormalities in its composition and appearance. A urinalysis will include a report of the urine's:

Appearance. Normal urine will vary from almost colorless to deep yellow, depending on the body's state of hydration. Certain foods, vitamins, and a variety of drugs may cause urine to be pink, brown, green or other colors. Excess white blood cells or pus in the urine may suggest infection in the urinary tract. Blood will tinge the urine pink or brownish and may result from kidney disease, kidney stones, or trauma.

> A CKD patient's blood is too acidic. Patients who take bicarbonate pills to offset the acid may slow kidney decline.
> *Journal of the American Society of Nephrology*
> July, 2009

Odor. Fresh urine is not offensive in smell and is even slightly aromatic. As urine stands, bacteria multiply, making the urine's smell more pungent. Those with diabetes may have fruity or sweet-smelling urine. A rotten odor suggests a urinary tract infection.

pH. Urine is slightly acidic, with a pH range of 4.5 to 8, but usually around 6.0. Diet will markedly influence the pH of urine. For example, a diet high in protein (e.g., meat, eggs, cheese) increases the acidity of urine. A vegetarian diet, in contrast, increases the alkalinity of urine.

> Currently, the guidelines for hypertension from the Seventh Report of the Joint National Committee on Prevention, Evaluation, and Treatment of High Blood Pressure recommend an annual urinalysis to assess proteinuria for all people at increased risk of CKD.

Composition. Urine is 95 percent water and 5 percent solids (i.e., urea, etc.--see chart in Chapter 6). It is abnormal to find protein, glucose, bile, or blood in the urine. Such substances suggest CKD, diabetes, or other disease.

Specific Gravity. This is the relative weight of urine.

Urine normally weighs more than distilled water because it contains solutes. Remember, the glomeruli filter excess chemicals, potassium, and sodium into the urine. These solutes have weight. The urine of someone with CKD may weigh less than normal, because the excess chemicals stay in the blood rather than filter into the urine. Individuals with a kidney infection or kidney stones may have urine with a high specific gravity, because of the concentration of pus cells or other substances in the urine.

A urinalysis also provides the number of milligrams of protein in the urine. Proteinuria greater than 30 milligrams is regarded as abnormal. However, protein excretion rates increase while a patient is in an upright position for standing or walking. Protein excretion rates are also higher in children and adolescents, and they increase with exercise and fever. The potential for "false positives" requires a repeated urine check for protein a few weeks later. Results that consistently show protein indicate kidney disease.

B. URINE MICROALBUMIN TEST

Albumin (al-BYOO-min), the single most abundant protein in the blood, acts like a sponge drawing extra fluid from the body into the bloodstream. The fluid remains in the bloodstream until the kidneys remove it. The albumin molecule itself is relatively small but is too large to filter through normal kidneys into the urine. When the glomeruli are damaged, the small albumin molecules are among the first proteins to enter the urine. Thus, leakage of albumin in the urine is indicative of damaged glomeruli.

If only a tiny amount of albumin is present in the urine, the routine urinalysis may not detect it. In these cases, a urine sample is examined for the microscopic presence of the protein albumin, called microalbuminuria. The presence of albumin at the microscopic level is a very early sign of developing kidney disease.

A test for microalbuminuria is most often performed to detect early kidney damage in those with diabetes. The American Diabetes Association (ADA) recommends that all diabetic patients have an annual screening for micro-albuminuria. The ADA also recommends screening indivi-duals with higher than normal levels of microalbuminuria three times within a 3- to 6-month period. Two elevated tests indicate kidney disease. Individuals without diabetes but otherwise at risk for CKD should be screened annually. Once microalbuminuria is discovered, the ADA recommends further blood and urine testing.

Despite the ADA's recommendations, the NKF found that 60 percent of patients with diabetes and CKD did not receive a urine test for microalbumin during a 12-month period. Similarly, 60 percent of those with CKD and hypertension did not receive the test.

INTERESTING OBSERVATION ➔ Studies show that a urinalysis performed by a nephrologist is more likely to aid in reaching a correct diagnosis than a urinalysis performed by a clinical chemistry lab. Imagine attempting to convince your nephrologist personally to analyze your urine under a microscope!

American Journal of Kidney Disease, 2005

The preferred test for microalbuminuria compares the amount of albumin in the urine with the amount of creatinine (see below). This comparison is used to compensate for variations in the amount of water in the urine, which affects the concentration of albumin. The test result is reported as a ratio of albumin to creatinine, or ACR.

Normally, less than 30 milligrams of albumin per gram of creatinine is found in urine. If the albumin level is 30-300 mg in two separate urine samples, microalbuminuria is present. Albumin greater than 300 mg is proteinuria, and CKD.

3. Creatinine-Based Tests

Creatinine (kree-AT-ih-neen). Remember the word! You will hear it often if you have CKD. Many doctors routinely estimate kidney function by measuring serum creatinine level (SCr). Recall that serum is the liquid part of your blood.

Creatinine is a waste product created from the normal metabolism of a protein called creatinine as muscles burn energy. Creatinine is transported in the blood serum to the kidneys for filtering. Because the muscle mass in the body is relatively constant from day to day, the level of creatinine in the blood normally remains stable. Healthy kidneys maintain that stability by filtering out excess creatinine. When kidneys malfunction, the glomeruli fail to filter creatinine, and it builds up in the blood. Thus, serum creatinine level is used to measure kidney function.

A. BLOOD TEST FOR CREATININE

Routine blood tests will measure how many milligrams of creatinine are in one deciliter of blood serum (mg/dL). This also is called your serum creatinine or SCr. As kidney function decreases, SCr rises.

Creatinine Range in Blood*

	Normal SCr	Loss of Kidney Function	50% Loss of Kidney Function
Men	0.6 to 1.4 mg/dL	1.4 or greater	1.7 or greater
Women	0.6 to 1.2 mg/dL	1.2 or greater	1.4 or greater

The NKF's CKD Guidelines explicitly recommend that clinicians "should not use SCr as the sole means to assess the level of kidney function." The reason for this recommendation? Several factors such as age, muscle mass, and dietary protein intake will impact the amount of creatinine in the blood, causing a variation in the measure of SCr that has nothing to do with kidney function. For example:

- Muscular young/middle-aged adults may have elevated creatinine without a corresponding decrease in kidney function.

- Because of decreased muscle mass, the elderly, infants, and chronically ill individuals may have a misleadingly low SCr, when a better measure of kidney function may show Stage Three CKD.

- A person with a single kidney may have a reading of 1.8 or 1.9, despite no meaningful loss of kidney function.

---

* Laboratories' "normal" ranges vary. The normal range reflected in the chart is common.

Despite the problems with relying on SCr to determine kidney function, it remains a common assessment tool.

B. TIMED CREATININE CLEARANCE

Timed 24-hour urine collections have long been used to measure creatinine clearance for kidney function. The test compares the level of creatinine in the urine with the level in the blood to evaluate how efficiently the kidneys remove creatinine from the blood. The test gauges the rate at which the kidneys clear creatinine from the blood. The rate of creatinine removal is relatively constant, so creatinine levels become a good measurement of kidney filtering function.

Normal Creatinine Clearance Rates

Males (under 40)	97–137 ml/min.
Females (under 40)	88–128 ml/min.

The patient collects urine in a sanitary container for 24 hours and supplies a blood sample. A lab then measures the creatinine concentration in each sample, as well as how much urine the patient collected during the 24 hours. The result, called the clearance rate, reflects how efficiently the kidneys remove creatinine each minute. If the kidneys fail to clear (filter out) enough creatinine, the level in the urine will fall and the level in the blood will rise, indicating decreased kidney function.

Again, the NKF's CKD Guidelines recommend that practitioners not rely solely on the 24-hour urine test to reflect kidney function. A patient's urine collection is notoriously unreliable, either over- or under-collecting the urine. This results in common clearance calculation errors. Also, the creatinine clearance rate naturally decreases with age. Each decade over age 40 corresponds with a decrease in clearance rate of about 6.5 ml/min, and this natural decrease in clearance is not considered kidney disease. Likewise, the creatinine clearance may over-estimate kidney function in those with advanced CKD.

Researchers recently have determined that a single random urine sample is as predictive of creatinine clearance as a 24-hour collection and is substantially less hassle to the patient.

The NKF's CKD Guidelines discourage reliance on random urine samples for monitoring kidney function.

4. Estimate of GFR

A more accurate, but still not perfect, estimate of kidney function is a calculation of your **estimated glomerular filtration rate** (GFR). GFR is generally accepted as the best overall index of kidney function and is one that the NKF encourages clinicians to use. Studies suggest GFR identifies CKD in its early stages better than other creatinine-based tests.

INTERESTING RESEARCH →

In a study, 660 individuals ages 65 and older had normal kidney function when measured by a blood test for creatinine (SCr). Researchers found, though, that up to 39% of those individuals had kidney impairment using estimated GFR instead. Opportunities for slowing the progression of kidney disease in older adults are lost if kidney function is evaluated using SCr alone.

Journal of the American Geriatric Society
June 26, 2007

In a nutshell, GFR is the rate at which all of the nephrons in your kidneys filter a substance from your blood. The more functioning, healthy nephrons you have, the better the per-minute filtration rate and the higher the GFR. The lower the GFR, the poorer the kidney function.

> **If you know your blood creatinine, you can calculate your own GFR at www.K/DOQI.org or www.nephron.com.**

The substance that most labs measure to calculate GFR is creatinine, in addition to the patient's age, weight, and adjustments for gender and race. These factors correlate with muscle mass, which impacts the blood creatinine level. GFR decreases with age, and both African-Americans and men tend to have more muscle mass than other ethnicities or women. The GFR calculation is adjusted to account for these differences, while the 24-hour urine clearance and routine blood tests are not.

Normal kidneys filter out most of the creatinine in the blood at a fixed rate:

- In young adults, GFR hovers around 120-130 ml/min/1.73m^2 and declines with age.

- In women with normal kidneys, GFR is about 105 ml/min/1.73m^2.

- In men, GFR is about 125 ml/min/1.73m^2.

In 2002, the NKF proposed a five-stage classification of CKD based upon GFR[*]. The five stages reflect that CKD is progressive, moving from mild to moderate to severe reductions in GFR. The lower the GFR, the more advanced the CKD. The CKD stages are:

Stage One: GFR 90 or above. An estimated GFR of 90 or above is considered normal. However, some people, even with normal GFR, have other signs of possible kidney damage, such as protein or blood in the urine. Patients remain in Stage One indefinitely or move on to Stage Two.

The level of GFR correlates with the likelihood of developing complications of kidney disease such as cardio-vascular disease, uremia, or anemia.

Stage Two: GFR 60 to 89. Stage Two is kidney damage with a mild decrease in GFR. The glomeruli show damage, and small amounts of blood protein such as albumin leak into the urine, a condition known as microalbuminuria. Normal albumin loss in the urine is less than 5 micrograms per minute, but the rate of albumin loss in Stage Two might increase to 200 micrograms per minute. People with

---

[*] The classification originated from the National Kidney Foundation's Kidney Disease Outcome Quality Initiative (K/DOQI) and is based on the estimation of GFR with an equation developed using data from the Modification of Diet in Renal Disease study. The equation includes SCr, patient's age, gender and ethnicity.

diabetes should have the urine microalbuminuria test to detect protein spillage. With good control over blood pressure and blood glucose levels and with exercise, diabetics could remain in Stage Two without advancing.

Stage Three: GFR 30 to 59*. Stage Three is considered moderate kidney failure. When a patient presents GFR of less than 60 ml/min/1.73m^2 for 3 or more months, the patient is diagnosed with CKD. When CKD has advanced to this stage, signs of bone deterioration, heart and vessel disease, and anemia are common.

Stage Four: GFR 15 to 29. Stage Four constitutes severe CKD. Large amounts of protein leak into the urine and high blood pressure usually exists. Cardiovascular issues commonly develop, as well as anemia and chemical imbalances requiring diet modifications and drug intervention. During Stage Four, the patient must consider options such as dialysis or kidney transplantation.

Stage Five: GFR less than 15. Stage Five is considered end-stage renal disease (ESRD), and the kidneys do not work well enough to keep the patient alive without dialysis or a transplant.

You will want to memorize these five stages of CKD. After each blood test, find out your current estimated GFR. The NKF's most recent definition for CKD is either a GFR of less than 60 (Stage III) or the presence of protein in the urine for at least three months.

GFR declines normally with age, with older individuals showing decreased kidney function. Such decrease is not kidney disease, but the naturally aging kidneys become more

---

* The Kidney Disease: Improving Global Outcomes (KDIGO) data consortium, at the National Kidney Foundation's 2010 Spring Clinical Meetings, proposed that Stage Three be subdivided into two stages (GFR 30-44 and GFR 45-59) because of noticeable differences in impact of CKD in those substages.

susceptible to glomerular injury from hypertension, diabetes, common drug use, and numerous other health conditions that more commonly develop in the elderly (revisit Chapter 7).

Although the NKF recommends estimating GFR with creatinine, it is not a perfect measure of kidney function. Blacks often have higher GFR than whites at the same level of serum creatinine because blacks generally have higher average muscle mass and creatinine generation. Men have higher GFR than women at the same level of serum creatinine because men usually have higher average muscle mass, which results

Average Decline with Age

Age	GFR
20-29	116
30-39	107
40-49	99
50-59	93
60-69	85
70+	75

in an increased creatinine generation rate. In the very obese, the malnourished, or people with liver disease, creatinine measurements will not properly reflect kidney function. The GFR calculation cannot take into account and correct for all the variables that affect SCr levels.

Because of the variables that impact serum creatinine, a substance known as cystatin C is increasing in popularity as an alternative to creatinine to monitor kidney dysfunction and determine GFR. Cystatin C is a small protein molecule produced by all cells in the body at a constant rate. It is removed from the blood in the glomeruli of the kidney, so its presence in the blood stays constant if the kidneys work efficiently, which makes it an ideal marker for kidney function. As the kidneys deteriorate, the level of cystatin C in the blood climbs. Unlike creatinine, cystatin C is not influenced by age, weight, gender, or race.

Recent studies suggest that elevated cystatin C also indicates an increased risk of heart disease and stroke.

5. Blood in the Urine

While a consistent finding of proteinuria indicates kidney disease, the presence of blood in the urine also may be a sign. The abnormal presence of red blood cells (RBC) in urine is called **hematuria** (hee-muh-TOOR-ee-uh).

Hematuria at low levels requires a microscopic exam to detect. At higher levels, the urine may appear red or smoky-brown.

In healthy individuals, RBCs occasionally may appear in the urine after vigorous exercise, so-called joggers' nephritis. Occasional appearances of RBCs do not indicate kidney disease. Also, hematuria may be unrelated to the kidneys; but, the RBCs may indicate a urinary tract infection, kidney stones, urinary tract cancer, or may even result from the consumption of large amounts of vitamin C.

Several kidney diseases do cause hematuria, including several forms of glomerulonephritis, polycystic kidney disease, and Alport's syndrome. Urine tests routinely include a check for the presence of RBCs.

6. Other Tests

If your nephrologist is not sure what is causing your kidney disease, he/she may order other tests, such as:

A. BLOOD UREA NITROGEN (BUN)

In addition to measuring the level of creatinine in your blood, a measurement of the level of urea in the blood can reveal kidney dysfunction. You will recall from Chapter 7 that urea is a toxic byproduct from your cells' metabolism of protein. The cells discard urea into the blood; the kidneys remove the urea from the blood in the filtering process; and, urea ends up in the urine. In people with malfunctioning kidneys, abnormal amounts of urea stay in the blood, rather than being filtered into the urine.

Normal blood contains 7 to 20 milligrams of urea per deciliter. If a blood test reveals a urea or BUN level greater than 20 mg., the kidneys may not be filtering properly.

RECENT STUDY ➜ A recent study suggests that elevated levels of urea in people with CKD are more toxic than originally thought and can lead to insulin resistance.

Journal of Clinical Investigation, 2010

B. IMAGING TESTS

The following renal imaging tests are used to obtain a picture of your kidneys and can reveal tumors, kidney stones, or other obstructions of the urinary system or vessels leading to and from the kidneys. The tests also are used to determine kidney size. For example, small kidneys may indicate damaged kidneys.

1. Ordinary X-ray

An X-ray or radiograph of the abdomen to evaluate kidney size and shape was regularly used in the past but is less common today, generally replaced by the CT scan. X-ray films are still valuable to follow a kidney stone through the urinary system or to detect a tumor. The advantage of an X-ray is the considerably lower radiation dose compared with a CT scan.

2. IVP

The **intravenous pyelogram (IVP)** is an X-ray accompanied by a contrast dye. In an IVP, contrast dye is injected in the patient's arm vein, and the radiologist takes a series of X-rays as the dye circulates in the blood, through the kidneys, and into the ureters. The kidney structures are visible as the dye moves through, providing clearer images of the kidney's anatomy and any defects.

3. Ultrasound

Ultrasound is the preferred method for screening kidney abnormalities. It is inexpensive and does not emit radiation. During the ultrasound test, the patient lies on a table in a darkened room. The ultrasound technician conducting the test spreads a clear conducting gel on the skin over the area of the kidneys. This gel helps transmit the sound waves used in the test. The technician then glides a handheld probe (transducer) that sends the harmless sound waves over the area of the kidneys, which bounce back and produce a picture on a monitor.

The ultrasound does not determine renal function but will reveal obstructions, tumors, and cysts that damage kidneys. The ultrasound provides accurate measurement of overall kidney size and thickness. It can also be used to evaluate blood flow in the kidney vessels.

4. CT Scan

The CT (computed tomography) scan uses X-rays to produce pictures of the urinary tract. The patient lies on a table that moves into the center of a CT scanner. The scanner's X-ray beam rotates around the patient. The X-rays can offer a three-dimensional view of the kidneys.

A downside of CT scans is the high level of radiation to which the patient is exposed. An abdominal CT scan has a radiation dose up to 800 times greater than that of a chest X-ray.

> **To calculate the radiation dose from any imaging procedure, see X-rayrisk.com**

CT-based imaging is routinely used to evaluate a potential living donor's renal anatomy. The CT generates images that allow the surgeon to assess the quality of the kidneys and connecting blood vessels.

RECENT RESEARCH → Researchers at the Mayo Clinic examined nearly 2000 potential kidney donors who underwent a CT scan for kidney donation purposes. Abnormalities (most not harmful) were found in 1 out of 4 adults. Kidney stones were present in 1 out of 10 adults.

Clinical Journal of the American Society of Nephrology, 2010

CT's are performed with or without a contrasting dye. CT without contrast is often used to detect kidney stones, even tiny ones. If the CT scan is a contrast scan, an iodine-based contrast dye is given intravenously to enhance the quality of the scan. Contrast agents can damage kidneys, particularly in those already vulnerable because of CKD, age, or diabetes. The American College of Radiology Guidelines require caution when using contrast agents in individuals with decreased kidney function.

5. MRI Scan

The MRI (magnetic resonance imaging) scan uses powerful magnets and radio waves. This lack of radiation is an important advantage. The patient is placed in a scanner with a strong magnetic field to create images based on molecular composition of the kidneys. Often the MRI procedure includes contrast dye. The MRI provides better detail than the ultrasound or CT scan, and one MRI exam can produce dozens of images. An MRI process can take an hour or longer, and people who do not like enclosed spaces may find the process difficult.

C. KIDNEY BIOPSY

A biopsy is a test in which a surgeon removes small pieces of kidney tissue to examine under a microscope. A biopsy is indicated only when the cause of the kidney disease cannot be determined by less invasive procedures, and the patient's symptoms suggest the biopsy will result in a diagnosis that has a treatment.

An ultrasound or CT scan locates the kidney as the lightly-sedated patient lies face-down on a table. The surgeon marks the area above the kidney and injects the patient with a local painkiller. The surgeon then inserts a spring-loaded needle through a small incision in the back to remove two or three tiny portions of one kidney. A microscopic examination of the removed tissue sometimes helps to identify the type of kidney disease or the degree of kidney loss.

D. PHYSICAL EXAM

A physical examination by your nephrologist is not used to diagnose CKD. However, certain outward symptoms, if present, can support a diagnosis, particularly if you show signs of **edema** (eh-DEE-muh). Edema is the accumulation of excess fluid in body tissues. This excess accumulation often results in swelling of the face, fingers, ankles, or abdomen, but concurrently impacts internal organs where its effects are invisible. Edema is common in individuals with CKD and occurs when water filters from the blood into tissue faster than it is reabsorbed. Both high blood pressure in people with impaired kidney function and the loss of albumin lead to the edema.

Edema has multiple consequences. When tissues are congested with excess fluid, waste removal and oxygen delivery are impaired, and the tissues may die. Edema in lung tissue, pulmonary edema, presents a threat of suffocation as fluid replaces air in the lungs. Cerebral edema produces headaches, nausea, and even seizures and coma.

Edema, when combined with blood and urine test results, may reveal **nephrotic syndrome** (NS). NS is a set of symptoms commonly associated with several kidney diseases. Your nephrologist may note the cluster of symptoms of NS after reviewing your blood and urine tests and making a physical examination. The symptoms of NS are:

- Severely high levels (more than 3500 mg) of protein in the urine (proteinuria);

- Low levels of protein in the blood (hypoalbuminemia);

- Swelling around the eyes or in the feet or hands (edema);

- High cholesterol (hyperlipidemia); and

- Fat bodies in the urine (lipiduria).

While NS can result from other health issues, many with CKD will exhibit NS, and its symptoms and complications are serious. Besides indicating CKD, NS may lead to:

- Malnutrition from insufficient retention of protein.

- Fluid overload.

- Frequent bacterial infections.

- Heart and vessel disease and also clots.

A patient with NS may also have a swollen abdomen, unintentional weight gain from water retention, and poor appetite.

C. Early Detection Important

One study found that only 12% of men and 6% of women with CKD knew it.

While a cure for CKD is not available, early detection of failing kidneys combined with available treatment can slow further kidney deterioration in many patients. The American Society of Nephrology reports that CKD currently affects nearly 30 million Americans--or 13 percent of all U.S. adults--and is on the rise, due in part to the surge in high blood pressure and diabetes.

The peril of CKD is its silent progression through its early stages when it is most treatable. In many patients with developing CKD, the disease is detected too late to prevent the often-deadly end stage. The damaging impact of CKD is not restricted to ESRD, but includes the complications of decreased kidney function in Stages Three and Four, where the patient may suffer hypertension, anemia, bone disorders, nerve damage, and cardiovascular disease, all related to the progressing CKD.

For most people, advancing CKD and ESRD are preventable if the kidney disease is addressed in its earliest stages. The NKF's 2002 position statement recommends two simple tests to detect CKD in patients: a urine test for proteinuria and a blood test for estimated GFR. These tests should be included in a normal annual exam, but often are not.

A panel of experts commissioned by the U.S. Centers for Disease Control and Prevention (CDC) designed a public health strategy released in 2009 to encourage clinicians to target at-risk individuals for testing and treatment to reduce the incidence of CKD and ESRD. The strategies include:

- Awareness of the risks of CKD (see Quiz 1 in this survival guide, as well as Chapters 7 and 9 for the risks)

- Routine testing of urine for proteinuria and blood to estimate GFR (this Chapter 8)

- Blood pressure control and treatment of hypertension with ACE inhibitors or ARBs (see Chapters 9 and 14)

- Blood sugar control in people with diabetes (see Chapters 9 and 14)

> **Rates of CKD have increased by more than 20% over the last decade.**
> *National Kidney Foundation*
> **January, 2009**

Researchers actively seek mechanisms that will help identify CKD earlier, especially in patients most likely to advance to ESRD. For example:

RESEARCH ➜ Researchers in Israel have isolated 5 compounds in the exhaled breath that signal CKD. They are developing sensors to diagnose and monitor CKD, in hopes of earlier detection to slow progression   *ACS Nano,* 2009

RESEARCH ➜ Researchers identified a tiny protein (NGAL) in the blood and urine of CKD patients and found that NGAL level is increased in patients whose CKD progresses significantly. This protein might be used to identify at-risk patients earlier to slow the progression of their CKD.

Current Diabetes Reports, February, 2010

In summary, earlier detection of CKD allows for evaluation and treatment. For individuals who wait too long, CKD becomes untreatable.

9.

COMMON CAUSES OF
CHRONIC KIDNEY DISEASE

If you took Quiz One in KidneyStep 1 of this Guide, you are familiar with the prominent risk factors for chronic kidney disease (CKD). Each of those Quiz One questions presents a factor that increases the odds of kidney disease. The two most common risk factors for, and causes of, CKD are diabetes and hypertension.

A. Diabetes

The American Diabetes Association (ADA) reports that nearly 26 million Americans (over 11% of the adult population) have diabetes, and 79 million have prediabetes, a precursor to the disease. Over one-third of diabetics will develop CKD. In fact, **diabetic nephropathy** (neff-RAH-puh-thee), kidney disease caused by diabetes, is the single most common cause of both CKD and end-stage renal disease (ESRD) in U.S. adults. Nearly one-half of patients starting dialysis each year have diabetes and most of these, about 90 percent, have type 2 diabetes. The death rate of patients with diabetic nephropathy is high when compared to the general population, with cardiovascular disease killing more than half.

> **The Centers for Disease Control and Prevention estimates that 1 in 3 Americans will develop diabetes, and 40% of diabetics develop CKD.**

The current ADA statistics illustrate that diabetes is prevalent, getting worse, and has perilous implications:

> **Having a family member with diabetes raises your diabetes risk by up to 30%.**

❖ Over 1/4 of U.S. adults over age 65 has diabetes.

❖ Each year brings 1.9 million new cases of diabetes.

❖ An estimated 1/3 of people who have diabetes do not know it.

❖ African-Americans and Native Americans are up to 4 times more likely than whites to reach ESRD with diabetes.

❖ Adults with diabetes have a heart disease rate 2 to 4 times higher than those without diabetes.

❖ Three-fourths of diabetic adults also have hypertension.

Despite increased knowledge and better medical treatments, the rate of diabetes continues to grow and is expected to double over the next 25 years.

1. What is Diabetes?

The two most common forms of diabetes are diabetes insipidus, which is a disorder of the pituitary gland, and **diabetes mellitus,** which stems from a pancreatic disorder. Diabetes mellitus is the most common form. When you see the word "diabetes" standing alone, it refers to diabetes mellitus and that is how we use it here.

A. TYPE 1 AND TYPE 2

In diabetes, the pancreas either fails to make enough **insulin** to control the amount of glucose (sugar) in the blood, or the body's cells ignore the insulin. Insulin is the hormone that transports glucose from the blood into the cells of the body, where it becomes an energy source. The amount of glucose in the blood increases after a meal. This increase in glucose is the signal to the pancreas to release insulin. Insulin also helps the cells synthesize protein and store fats. In people with diabetes, the glucose stays in the blood instead of entering the body's cells. This disturbs the ability of cells to metabolize and use sugars, protein, and fats, starving the cells.

Diabetes mellitus comes in two types:

Type 1 – Type 1 diabetes is an autoimmune disease that destroys the insulin-producing beta cells in the pancreas. Only about 5 to 10 percent of diabetics have type 1. Nearly 30 percent of those will develop CKD, generally after 20 years with diabetes. Type 1 diabetes, once called juvenile-onset diabetes, usually begins earlier in life, but can occur at any age. The person must take insulin by injection or pump and must also eat carefully planned meals to control glucose levels. Unlike type 2 diabetes, type 1 is neither caused nor reversed by diet and exercise. The only cure for type 1 is a pancreas transplant.

> **Of 1132 patients hospitalized over 4 months in one city, 34% had undiagnosed diabetes.**
> *Journal of Clinical Endocrinology and Metabolism*
> **2010**

Type 2 – Type 2 diabetes accounts for 90 to 95 percent of all diabetes cases. In type 2 diabetes, the pancreas makes insulin, but the cells of the body cannot respond correctly to it, a condition termed **insulin resistance**. The insulin resistance requires the pancreas to make extra insulin just to keep blood glucose levels normal. However, this excess glucose also injures other organs and muscles, including the heart, blood vessels, brain, and nerves.

The overweight are more likely to have type 2 diabetes, because body fat interferes with insulin use. However, it is not always the "inch you can pinch" that is the problem; rather, it is the fat wrapped around the internal organs. Researchers believe this visceral fat is more likely to leak fatty acids that damage the insulin-producing cells of the pancreas, worsening the insulin distress. About 15 percent of individuals with type 2 diabetes appear slim, but they may have higher concentrations of visceral fat.

Interview: Dr. Bonnie L. Blazer-Yost.

"Recent studies show that in addition to glucose, insulin itself can have detrimental effects. In most cases of prediabetes or metabolic syndrome, the body's cells have become insulin resistant, and it takes more insulin to cause a normal amount of glucose uptake into cells. Since the signal for insulin release is the blood glucose, the extra glucose causes an increase in insulin release. Now as far as glucose uptake is concerned, all is well. The increased insulin has caused normal glucose uptake. However, the excess insulin now over-regulates processes that are not insulin resistant--such as protein synthesis, growth of cells lining the blood vessels, and lipid storage.

What we are particularly interested in is that insulin causes sodium retention by the kidneys. Sodium retention makes sense in a healthy person because our ancestors lived in a salt-poor environment, and insulin is a great hormone for extracting all nutrients from a meal. However, in a person releasing excess insulin, the kidneys retain too much sodium. The resulting increased sodium in the blood causes an increase in water in the blood by simple osmosis. The increased blood volume, in turn, increases blood pressure. A lot of my research has been exploring what sodium transporters are influenced by insulin."

[Dr. Blazer-Yost is a research professor at Purdue University in Indianapolis, where she focuses her research on issues resulting in kidney damage.]

A. PREDIABETES

Many people destined to develop type 2 diabetes exist for years in a prediabetic state, where their blood glucose and insulin levels are higher than normal but not yet high enough for the type 2 diagnosis. As Dr. Blazer-Yost emphasized in her

> An estimated
> 79 million
> U.S. adults
> currently suffer
> prediabetes.

interview (above), damage caused by the increased insulin already is occurring, and blood pressure may be rising.

The CDC now estimates that 35 percent of Americans under age 65 have prediabetes. Nearly two out of three people over age 65 have pre- or full diabetes, most likely stemming from obesity and inactivity.

We discuss prediabetes in more detail in Chapter 14.

RECENT RESEARCH → Researchers funded by the CDC analyzed 8,200 American adults for prediabetes, diabetes, and CKD. They found 42% of subjects with undiagnosed diabetes had CKD, in addition to 18% of individuals with prediabetes.

Clinical Journal of the American Society of Nephrology
March, 2010

C. DAMAGE TO KIDNEYS

Diabetes damages the kidneys in a couple of ways:

1. The kidneys of someone with diabetes initially become enlarged and appear to filter blood exceptionally well. This **hyperfiltration** is caused when the glomeruli within the kidneys become overloaded with the large amount of water drawn into the blood by the excess glucose. The resulting glomeruli overload increases the glomerular filtration rate (GFR) above normal, straining the glomeruli's ability to filter and raising blood pressure.

> **In diabetes, the urine is sweet. Before the development of tests for diabetes, doctors would taste the patient's urine for sweetness.**

2. The excess glucose in the blood also causes the membrane surrounding the glomeruli to thicken and expand, taking up the space occupied by the glomeruli capillaries. Those scarred and inflamed capillaries cannot filter the blood as they should.

> **The USRDS reports that 1 in 2 adults with CKD also has diabetes.**

The combined damage to the glomeruli and the resulting high blood pressure eventually lead to diabetic nephropathy. The excess glucose also can damage the nerves of the bladder. The nerves then fail to carry the message to the brain that the bladder is full. Excess pressure from a full bladder can cause urine to back up into the kidneys, further destroying nephrons.

The normal blood level of glucose is less than or equal to 80 to 120 milligrams per 100 milliliters of blood. Without insulin, blood levels of glucose can rise to 600 milligrams per 100 milliliters of blood, for example. At such levels, glucose spills into the urine, because the tubule cells of the nephrons cannot reabsorb it fast enough. Without insulin, body cells cannot use the glucose to transport it into the cells, and the cells metabolize fats and protein for energy. As a result, weight may decline and lack of protein leads to a diminished ability to fight infections.

2. Stages of Diabetic Nephropathy

The course of kidney disease as it develops in someone with diabetic nephropathy is divided into stages. The 5 stages are based on GFR, albumin in the urine, and blood pressure. While the stages of diabetic nephropathy were established for type 1 diabetes, studies also apply them to type 2. These stages are a guide only and are not always accurate of true kidney disease progression in diabetics.

CKD Stage	Years with Diabetes	Symptoms
I	0	GFR above normal level Blood pressure normal
II	5–15	Microalbuminuria Blood pressure rising
III	10–20	Proteinuria Blood pressure elevated
IV	15–25	Proteinuria Hypertension GFR decreased High risk of heart disease
V	20–30	ESRD

A person with type 2 diabetes may halt the progression of kidney disease at each stage with strict glucose control, a healthful diet, and regular exercise (see KidneySteps 4 and 5).

Because of increased risk of cardiovascular disease in diabetics, many die before reaching ESRD. A patient with diabetes who has microalbuminuria (see Chapter 8) and proteinuria has a 2- to 4-times increased risk for cardiovascular disease. Even in dialysis, the cardiac death rate of diabetic patients is 50 percent higher than in non-diabetics.

The important factors in determining the risk of reaching ESRD for anyone with diabetes are:

- **Glycemic control--**
  Studies show that blood sugar control reduces the risk of CKD.

- **Blood pressure--**
  Blood pressure control is associated with reduced microalbuminuria.

> **The ADA reports that glycemic control is achieved in only 12.3% of diabetics.**

- **Genetic factors--**
  Patients with diabetes also can be genetically disposed to CKD and hypertension, which makes CKD more likely.

- **Lipid levels--**
  High blood lipid levels increase the risk of cardiovascular disease, which is already abnormally high in diabetics.

- **Vitamin D intake--**
  Vitamin D is receiving much research interest. In one study, vitamin D replacement reduced proteinuria in about half of diabetic patients with Stage III or IV of CKD.

During the prediabetic state and the progression to type 2 diabetes, damage to the kidneys occurs. Prediabetes can nearly always be prevented from progressing to diabetes if the condition is identified and treated with a healthful diet, regular exercise, and medication, if necessary. Even type 2 diabetes can be halted with proper and consistent measures. We will address both prevention and control of diabetes in KidneyStep 3.

B. High Blood Pressure

According to the American Heart Association (AHA), most people over age 50 in the U.S. suffer from high blood pressure, also called **hypertension**. You must measure your blood pressure to know if it is high. Nearly everyone with kidney disease has hypertension, and hypertension is the second leading cause of kidney disease, accounting for 25 percent of all CKD cases. Even otherwise healthy people with high blood pressure who excrete a slight excess of protein in their urine have an increased risk of developing kidney and heart complications:

RECENT RESEARCH → Over 12 years (1993-1997), researchers followed 917 hypertensive, non-diabetic patients. The researchers found that patients with microalbuminuria at the start of the study were 7.6 times more likely to develop CKD and 2.1 times more likely to develop cardiovascular complications as individuals without microalbuminuria. They also had a 3.2 times higher risk of developing both kidney and cardiovascular conditions.

Clinical Journal of the American Society of Nephrology, 2010

While controlling high blood pressure may not save you from kidney failure, it may delay progression of the kidney destruction. Also, blood pressure control will lessen the likelihood of death from heart failure or stroke, common threats in people with kidney disease and with diabetes. In fact, if you have CKD, you are more likely to die early from accompanying cardiovascular disease than from the CKD.

1. Mini-Quiz for Risk of Hypertension

To learn whether you are at risk for high blood pressure, take the following mini-quiz:

- Are you overweight?

- Are you male or a post-menopausal female?

- Do you eat out often, or eat prepackaged foods?

- Do you have a family history of cardiovascular disease?

- Do you smoke?

- Do you have high cholesterol?

- Do you have more than 1 or 2 drinks of alcohol daily?

- Are you African-American?

- Is your life stressful?

- Do you have diabetes?

- Do you have loss of kidney function?

> **African-Americans develop high blood pressure earlier and twice as often as whites. Over 40% of African-Americans over age 20 have high blood pressure compared to 10-15% of whites, and they reach ESRD 6 times more often.**

If you answered "Yes" to any of these questions, you are at an increased risk for high blood pressure. High blood pressure has a variety of associations, including race, age, diet, family history, health status, etc. While all the causes of high blood pressure are not known, scientists do know that CKD and high blood pressure are intertwined, with one leading to the other.

2. When Blood Pressure is High

Blood pressure is the force of blood pushing against the artery walls as the blood moves from your heart to all of your organs. When the left ventricle, the pumping chamber of the heart, contracts, blood pressure temporarily increases–**systolic pressure**. When the left ventricle relaxes between beats, blood pressure temporarily decreases–**diastolic pressure.**

High blood pressure results when the force of blood pumping against your artery walls is too high. Extra fluid in the blood vessels increases the blood pressure, as do clogged or rigid blood vessels. Hypertension is defined as systolic pressure readings of 140 (or higher) **or** diastolic pressure of 90 or higher. Either or both numbers may be too high.

Occasional high readings in blood pressure do not necessarily mean hypertension, as your blood pressure fluctuates naturally throughout the day and depending upon stress and activity. It generally is highest in the morning and lowest at night, during sleep.

Normal Blood Pressure	
Less than:	
120	←Systolic pressure (when the heart beats)
80	←Diastolic pressure (between heartbeats)

However, if blood pressure remains elevated, it can damage your heart, vessels, and kidneys.

In 2003, a coalition of the AHA and 45 other organizations issued revised blood pressure guidelines that redefined "normal" blood pressure to be **less** than 120/80 mmHg. Here are the blood pressure guidelines:

Category	Systolic (mmHg)	Diastolic (mmHg)
Normal	Less than 120 AND	Less than 80
Pre-hypertension	120-139 OR	80-89
High/Stage 1	140-159 OR	90-99
High/Stage 2	160 or higher OR	100 or higher

Falling into any category other than "Normal" is a signal to cut down on salt, exercise more, and check kidney function. If you have CKD, you should aggressively strive to lower your blood pressure. Following Kidney Steps 4 and 5 can help.

Every year, high blood pressure results in more than 30,000 new cases of end-stage renal failure in the United States.

3. The Impact of Hypertension

High blood pressure can be a silent killer, as you generally feel no symptoms. But left undetected or untreated, high blood pressure will damage the overworked heart and blood vessels, including blood vessels in the kidneys, brain, eyes, and other organs. It is a leading cause of heart attacks, strokes, and CKD.

High blood pressure is the most common association with kidney disease and the second most common cause of CKD. According to the USRDS, "hypertension control is achieved in only 10 percent of patients with early stage CKD." With such poor control of high blood pressure, it is not surprising that it also is a leading cause of kidney failure and end-stage renal disease.

> **The AHA reports that medication alone is inadequate for successful treatment of high blood pressure. Finding the right medication, plus lifestyle changes (exercise, weight loss, salt restriction) are necessary.**

Persistent high blood pressure that is untreated or inadequately treated, often results in CKD that leads to ESRD, if the person does not die first from heart failure or stroke. Because of the close and severe relationship between high blood pressure and CKD, the National Heart Lung and Blood Institute recommends that people with CKD use whatever therapy is necessary, including lifestyle changes and medications, to keep blood pressure below 130/80.

C. Glomerular Diseases

As the third leading cause of CKD, glomerular diseases are associated with slow, progressive loss of kidney function resulting from injury to the glomeruli. This slow, progressive kidney loss often is termed **chronic glomerulonephritis**. Chronic glomerular diseases fall into two major categories:

- **glomerulonephritis**, which describes inflammation of the glomeruli in the kidneys; and,

85

- **glomerulosclerosis**, which describes scarring or hardening of the glomeruli. The glomeruli are prompted by growth factors in the blood or in the glomeruli themselves to produce scar material.

All glomerular diseases impact the kidneys similarly; they are characterized by inflammation, scarring, and eventual destruction of the glomeruli, the tiny filtering capillaries and tubules in the nephrons of the kidneys (revisit Chapter 6). This damage impairs the kidneys' ability to retain protein and red blood cells, which then show up in the urine. Damage also impairs the kidneys' ability to eliminate blood waste products and excess fluid.

> **Nearly all causes of CKD harm the glomeruli, even when not classified as glomerular disease.**

Some glomerular diseases rapidly progress to end stage without treatment, while others follow a slower course or may even remit spontaneously. Typical signs of several glomerular diseases include:

- significant protein in the urine (**proteinuria**) caused by leaking of the glomeruli

- blood in the urine (**hematuria**) caused by leaking of the glomeruli

- hypertension caused by water retention and renin disruption

> **Not counting diabetic nephropathy, glomerular diseases comprise 14% of CKD cases.**
> USRDS 2010 Annual Report

- swelling of hands, leg, etc. (**edema**) caused by water and salt retention

- high level of urea/nitrogen in blood (**azotemia**)

- gradual loss of kidney function

As you will recall from Chapter 8, these symptoms comprise the nephrotic syndrome, the set of symptoms associated with CKD. As a patient's glomerular injury increases, nephrotic syndrome symptoms intensify.

The most common glomerular disease is diabetic nephropathy, kidney disease resulting from diabetes and causing scarring of the glomeruli. This scarring of the kidneys occurs from the elevated blood glucose and the resulting increased blood surge through the kidneys. Diabetes was discussed earlier in this chapter. Other common glomerular diseases include:

1. Membranous Glomerular Nephropathy

Membranous glomerular nephropathy (MGN) is a common cause of kidney disease, and the most common cause associated with nephrotic syndrome in adults. Up to 70 percent of patients will have nephrotic syndrome symptoms of high levels of protein and blood in the urine, high cholesterol, and edema. Up to 30 percent of patients also develop dangerous clots in the renal veins.

The cause of MGN is unknown, or **idiopathic**, in 70 to 80 percent of patients. In the remaining patients, MGN is a secondary disease to:

- cancer
- infections (*e.g.*, hepatitis B and C, malaria, syphilis, leprosy)
- drugs (*e.g.*, penicillin, gold)
- lupus, thyroiditis
- sickle cell anemia

Malignancy is found in up to 20% of people over age 60 with MGN.

The primary disease, which could have occurred years earlier, elicits an autoimmune response that results in a thickening and destruction of the glomeruli when self-attacking antibodies deposit in the glomeruli.

In about 50 percent of patients, MGN will go into spontaneous remission. However, up to half of those patients eventually relapse. While most patients have less damage to the kidneys, nearly 30 percent of MGN patients advance to ESRD. Increased proteinuria indicates an increased risk of progression to ESRD.

Unless the MGN patient has a low risk of ESRD measured by the level of proteinuria, immunosuppressants are used to treat MGN, which can slow kidney damage. Also, ACE inhibitors and ARBs are given to reduce blood pressure and proteinuria.

2. Focal and Segmental Glomerulosclerosis

Focal and segmental glomerulosclerosis (FSGS) is a pattern of destruction in the nephrons, appearing as scarring of the glomeruli in scattered regions of the kidneys. Nephrotic syndrome is characteristic of FSGS. In fact, FSGS accounts for over half of the cases of nephrotic syndrome in adults and up to 28 percent in children. Nearly 50 percent of the adults and children with FSGS have hypertension and blood in the urine. Virtually all have proteinuria.

In many cases, FSGS is idiopathic, without a known cause. Often though it is secondary to other disorders or causes, such as:

- viral – parvovirus B19

- drug-related – heroin, lithium

- genetic – mutation-based

- other – obesity related, sickle cell anemia, lymphoma

Untreated FSGS frequently progresses to ESRD within 5 to 20 years. Progression is faster in African-Americans. If untreated and accompanied by nephrotic syndrome, only about one-third of those with FSGS have kidney survival at 10 years.

RECENT RESEARCH → In a small study of 10 bodybuilders who had long-term use of steroids, 9 developed FSGS. When the bodybuilders discontinued the steroid use, the proteinuria improved, except in one who suffered ESRD and required dialysis.
Journal of the American Society of Nephrology, 2010

Treatment for FSGS generally includes immuno-suppressants, but this treatment is controversial, and studies of effectiveness are under way. At least one-half of FSGS patients are unresponsive to such treatment and continue to progress to ESRD. Scientists are also studying the use of antifibrotic agents in delaying ESRD.

3. Autoimmune Related Glomerular Diseases

The body's immune system creates protein-like substances called antibodies and immunoglobulins that protect the body against invading organisms. In an autoimmune disease, the body's immune system also creates autoantibodies that attack specific organs in the body, depending on the disease. Certain of these self-destructing antibodies can deposit in the glomeruli of the kidneys, causing inflammation and scarring and damaging the filtering ability of the glomeruli. Immunosuppressants that suppress the ability of the body to form antibodies may slow the damage to the kidneys.

Examples of autoimmune diseases particularly impacting the kidneys include:

A. IgA NEPHROPATHY (IgAN)

IgAN is a form of glomerular disease that results when immunoglobulin A (IgA), an antibody created by the immune system, forms deposits in the glomeruli of the kidneys, creating inflammation, scarring, and eventual damage. These deposits are identified through a biopsy. Originally coined "Berger's disease," the condition has been renamed IgAN.

> **In Asia, IgAN accounts for 40% of glomerulonephritis cases.**

IgAN ranges from mild to severe glomerulonephritis. The cause is unclear. Some researchers compare IgAN to an infection and others to a food allergy. Most scientists agree it involves a faulty IgA immune response to different antigens. IgAN runs in some families and is the most common form of glomerulonephritis in some countries. IgAN affects males more often than females and is found in all age groups.

> **Some studies suggest omega-3 fatty acid supplements may slow CKD in those with IgAN.**

Blood in the urine is a common symptom of IgAN, often present following an upper respiratory tract infection. However, the disease generally remains silent and undetected until significant damage to the kidneys causes other, detectable symptoms or complications, such as high blood pressure and proteinuria.

About 30 percent of adults diagnosed with IgAN progress to ESRD. Currently, no cure or treatment for IgAN exists. Controlling blood pressure and reducing proteinuria with ACE inhibitors or ARBs seems to be the prevalent treatment. For severe cases, the patient receives immunosuppressants.

B. SYSTEMIC LUPUS ERYTHEMATOSUS (SLE)

SLE is a complex autoimmune disease that affects many parts of the body, including the kidneys, where it causes **lupus nephritis**. About 90 percent of SLE patients are women, and many are young. As in other autoimmune kidney diseases, antibodies form and deposit in the glomeruli, causing inflammation. The inflammation causes scarring that prevents the glomeruli from filtering properly.

Why a person develops this autoimmune response in SLE is not completely understood, but there appears to be a genetic association. Also, environmental factors such as sunlight, drugs, or infections may provoke the release of the damaging antibodies.

RECENT RESEARCH → A recent study of smokers with SLE links permanent skin damage, hair loss, and rashes with the smoking.
Journal of Rheumatology, November, 2009

Patients with lupus nephritis will exhibit a variety of symptoms, most commonly inflammation of the skin and joints and in the kidneys. A urinalysis determines the presence of protein, blood, and other sediments. A biopsy of the kidney helps identify the type and severity of SLE. The International Society of Nephrology/Renal Pathology Society has developed a recently updated classification system for identifying the characteristics and severity of SLE. You may link to it at KidneySteps.com.

Lupus nephritis regularly progresses to ESRD. Also, kidney transplant patients with SLE may reject the transplanted kidney because of the continuing SLE disease. No cure exists for SLE. Treatment includes drugs to suppress the faulty immune system and steroids to ease inflammation, which slows the progression of kidney destruction. A rheumatologist is typically involved in treatment to address associated joint inflammation.

C. GOODPASTURE'S SYNDROME OR ANTI-GBM DISEASE

Goodpasture's syndrome is named for the scientist who first discovered the condition in 1919. Today, the term describes a condition of rapidly progressing glomerular nephritis, pulmonary hemorrhage (bleeding in the lungs), and self-destroying antibodies. In this auto-immune disease, the body creates an autoantibody, anti-GBM, that targets the kidneys and lungs. Because of this autoantibody, some use the term anti-GBM disease rather than Goodpasture's syndrome.

Hemorrhaging in the lungs occurs in about two-thirds of patients and is slightly more common in young men. Patients often complain of breathlessness and cough.

> ***Patient Interview:*** *Iris is a six-year dialysis patient with anti-GBM disease. She is on oxygen and notes that her daily tank use is increasing. Over the last four months, her left lung has collapsed three times, requiring hospitalization.*

Goodpasture's disease may have a genetic basis and is seen in siblings. Several cases have resulted from exposure to industrial pollutants, cigarette smoke, inhaled toxins, or infection. In all cases, it is the autoimmunity that results in the kidney damage.

Often, Goodpasture's results in acute kidney injury. If the acute kidney injury is not treated, death results. If the patient survives, kidney function remains damaged.

Goodpasture's disease accounts for about seven percent of patients with ESRD. It is less common in people of African or Asian origin than in whites. While no cure for the disease exists, immunosuppressants slow kidney damage. If the patient receives a kidney transplant and still possesses the anti-GBM, it may damage the transplanted kidney.

91

4. Infection-Related Glomerular Diseases

Glomerular disease can quickly develop after an infection elsewhere in the body. In fact, infection is a common cause of glomerulonephritis (GN). Examples include:

A. STREP, STAPH, OR OTHER INFECTION

A staphylococcal or streptococcal infection (strep throat, for example) or some other bacterial infection, particularly in children, can lead to damage of the glomeruli. The presence of the bacteria stimulates the body to make antibodies to fight the infection. An overproduction of antibodies results, and the antibodies in the circulating blood enter the kidneys and deposit in the glomeruli during filtering, causing damage and GN. Sometimes the damage is permanent.

B. BACTERIAL ENDOCARDITIS

Bacterial endocarditis is an infection of heart tissue, which can result in damage to the glomeruli of the kidneys, from the overproduction of antibodies that enter the kidneys in the blood.

C. HIV

The HIV virus leads to AIDS and frequently impacts the kidneys. Up to 10 percent of HIV patients will experience CKD. Many of the complications impacting the kidneys are treatable with early detection. If the kidneys fail, the HIV patient has the same treatment options as an HIV-negative patient--dialysis and transplant. Patients with the HIV infection suffer a variety of kidney disorders, including acute kidney injury and injury caused by the drugs used to treat the HIV infection.

D. HEPATITIS B AND C

Hepatitis infection can result in GN. In the U.S., hepatitis B-induced GN is seen in drug addicts, in individuals receiving tainted blood transfusions, or in those otherwise exposed to the virus. Nephrotic syndrome is common. Again, the immune system creates antibodies to fight the hepatitis virus, and those antibodies deposit in the glomeruli, damaging them.

D. Inherited Kidney Diseases

Individuals can inherit kidney disorders that may result in CKD. First degree relatives of family members with ESRD are at an especially high risk for CKD. Examples of inherited kidney diseases are:

1. Polycystic Kidney Disease (PKD)

PKD is the most common of the inherited kidney disorders, affecting all ethnic groups equally. Nearly all cases of PKD are "autosomal dominant," resulting from a gene inherited from a parent. In PKD, the kidneys form multiple cysts (blister-like sacs containing fluid) that enlarge the kidneys and interfere with function. Cysts typically develop in other systems of the body, most commonly in the bile ducts of the liver, but occasionally in the heart, pancreas, thyroid, or brain.

On average, half of the children inheriting the PKD gene will develop the cyst-forming disease. The half developing PKD will develop CKD by age 50. By around age 20, an ultrasound examination of the kidneys can detect PKD. The ultrasound reveals the multiple cysts and enlargement of the kidneys, sometimes over 3 times the normal size. The cysts themselves may consume 95 percent of the enlarged kidney volume.

> **Increases in kidney volume over a 6-month period in young PKD patients best predicts kidney function decline.**
> *Kidney International,* **2009**

RECENT RESEARCH → Researchers believe the drug rapamycin (also called sirolimus) may slow the progression of PKD. Rapamycin is an immunosuppressant often used with transplant recipients. Mice given the drug showed a 50% reduction in cyst growth and appeared to reverse existing kidney deterioration. Studies are underway to determine if the drug is safe for PKD patients.

Journal of the American Society of Nephrology,
January, 2010

PKD causes chronic high blood pressure, kidney infections, shortness of breath, fatigue and decreased appetite. Back pain is common, resulting from the enlarged kidneys and, perhaps, liver. The cysts can become infected or leak. Blood in the urine and kidney stones are common in PKD patients.

People with PKD may maintain normal kidney function for decades, despite cysts and kidney enlargement. PKD is the fourth leading cause of CKD and causes 10 percent of all ESRD, usually between the ages of 40 and 60. Kidney transplant recipients with ESRD resulting from PKD survive longer than patients receiving transplants for other causes.

Scientists have discovered the specific chromosomes and individual genes responsible for PKD, and gene mutation screening for PKD is available.

RECENT RESEARCH
➔
PKD is linked to the malfunction of certain proteins (polycystine proteins 1 and 2) coded by faulty genes.
Journal of the American Society of Nephrology,
2010

Scientists have learned how the faulty genes interfere with proper operation of the impacted organs. This knowledge may lead to an eventual cure for PKD.   Current treatment is limited to antihypertensive drugs, and no established treatment exists to retard the progression of PKD. However, researchers are testing several promising drug options.

2. Alport's Syndrome

Alport's syndrome, another hereditary disease, is the disease that led to ESRD in your author. The genetic mishap causes a defect in the collagen that normally helps to form the basement cell membranes of many organs in the body, including the kidneys, ears, and eyes. Some unfortunate individuals with Alport's syndrome not only have CKD, but also become deaf and blind.

Women transmit the mutated gene that causes the disease but sometimes will not show severe symptoms of CKD themselves. Males who inherit the disease evidence CKD in childhood and may reach end-stage between adolescence and age 40. Females may not reach end stage, and if they do, it is usually after age 50.

Signs of CKD in people with Alport's include blood in the urine (often only microscopic amounts), proteinuria, and hypertension. Individuals suspecting the inherited disease can have a skin biopsy to identify the existence of the genetically deficient collagen (protein), as did your author.

No cure for Alport's exists. Treatment simply involves blood pressure control, but no study has demonstrated that even this delays ESRD. In other words, the disease progresses as the genetic timetable determines.

RECENT RESEARCH → A new study using mice with a genetic defect similar to Alport's shows a slowing of the CKD with stem cell treatments. Stem cells from the bone marrow of healthy mice were transplanted into the mice with Alport's. The recipient mice showed significant improvement of kidney function.

Journal of the American Society of Nephrology,
2009

3. Sickle Cell Anemia

Sickle cell anemia is an inherited disease in which red blood cells become hard and sticky and have an abnormal C or "sickle" shape rather than the normal round, disc shape. The disease occurs most frequently in African-Americans, Hispanics, Asians, and those of Middle Eastern descent. In the U.S., about 8 percent of African-Americans inherit the sickle cell genetic trait, and one in 500 is born with actual sickle cell anemia.

People with the sickle cell gene are less likely to be infected with malaria, which explains why the lethal gene continues to exist.

The abnormal red blood cell shape is caused by a faulty hemoglobin molecule. The C-shaped red blood cells cannot carry normal amounts of oxygen, and the cells die earlier, often causing anemia. These misformed blood cells clog smaller vessels rather than slipping through easily as round blood cells do. The tiny capillaries comprising the glomeruli in the kidneys are particularly vulnerable to clogging, resulting in their destruction.

High blood pressure is uncommon in sickle cell patients, but proteinuria is likely. Use of angiotensin-converting enzyme (ACE) inhibitors is the treatment of choice to reduce the protein in the urine. Individuals with sickle cell anemia may not tolerate dialysis as well as others with ESRD, and rejection of a transplanted kidney is somewhat higher than average.

E. Drugs / Poisons

Individuals can gradually destroy the glomeruli in their kidneys by taking certain over-the-counter or prescription medications for extended time periods. Drugs used for diagnostic purposes, such as contrast dyes used in imaging tests, can also harm the kidneys. The kidneys are a major excretion route for a variety of drugs. The drugs become concentrated in the kidneys as blood flows through these small organs. This concentration can be toxic to the glomeruli and tubules.

> **76% of the U.S. population age 17 and older (143 million adults) reported using NSAIDs or acetaminophen in a 1-month period.**

Kidney-threatening drugs include:[*]

- **Nonsteroidal anti-inflammatory drugs (NSAIDs).** NSAIDS include aspirin, ibu-profen, Actron, Advil, Aleve, Alka-Seltzer, aspirin, Bayer, Excedrin, Nuprin, Medipren, Ibuprofen, Motrin-IB, and Pediacare Fever, among other over-the-counter drugs.

> **As it announced January 2011, the FDA will require drug manufacturers to reduce the amount of acetaminophen in pain relievers to no more than 325 mg., down from 500 mg.**

- **Acetaminophen.** A common over-the-counter drug found in the following products:

    Tylenol, Anacin, Backaid Maximum Strength Back Relief, Benadryl Allergy and Sinus Headache Caplets, Contac Day & Night Cold/Flu Caplets, DayQuil Cold & Flu, Excedrin (all products), Midol Menstrual

---

[*] Capitalized products have registered trademarked brand names.

Complete, Nyquil Cold & Flu Relief, Pamprin Multi-Symptom, Theraflu Packets Severe Cold & Cough, Triaminic Cough and Fever

- **Laxatives.** Overuse can cause chronic potassium deficiency, which damages kidneys.

- **Lithium.** Used for bipolar disorder.

- **Heroin.** This illegal drug can lead to rapid loss of kidney function.

- **Diagnostic and Prescription Drugs.** Radiocontrast dyes, ACE inhibitors, ARBs, some immunosuppressants, penicillin.

Older people are particularly vulnerable to harm from drugs. Kidney function naturally declines with age, impairing the kidneys' ability to eliminate accumulated drugs. Accordingly, the elderly often need lower doses of many drugs compared to the dose tolerance of younger people, and they are two to seven times more likely to experience side effects. Approximately one-third of hospital admissions for older adults is associated with a problem with medication use. Age-related decline of kidney function increases the chance that long-term use of common pain relievers like NSAIDs and acetaminophens will damage the kidneys.

> *Patient Story*: *Arlene donated a kidney to her sister 25 years ago. In recent years, Arlene suffered from arthritis and regularly took aspirin, ibuprofen and related pain relievers. Extended use of the pain medications damaged her remaining kidney. On a Friday, Arlene qualified to receive a kidney transplant. The successful surgery occurred the following Monday. Because she was a prior kidney donor, Arlene received priority on the transplant waiting list.*

If you already have kidney damage, diabetes, or hypertension, use of these drugs--even briefly--is harmful to the kidneys. Only take such drugs after consulting with your nephrologist.

10.

Dialysis

Dialysis is one of two available treatment methods used when chronic kidney disease (CKD) has reached end stage. The second method is kidney transplantation, which is the superior treatment. When the kidneys stop functioning, a buildup of fluids and chemicals in the blood reaches deadly levels. Dialysis is the less-than-perfect medical solution for removing those toxins in most patients with Stage V, or end-stage renal disease (ESRD). Over 90 percent of U.S. patients with ESRD are on dialysis, which generally is initiated when the patient's GFR is below 10 mL per minute.

Dialysis has two forms:

❖ **Hemodialysis**

❖ **Peritoneal Dialysis (PD)**

A. Hemodialysis

The USRDS reports that the dialysis population increased 35% between 2000 and 2008.

During hemodialysis, the patient's blood is slowly removed from the body and is pumped through a dialysis machine containing a special filter called a **dialyzer,** or "artificial kidney." The dialyzer filters waste products and extra water. The filtered blood is sent back to the body. Here is an outline of the hemodialysis process:

1. The Hemodialysis Process

❖ Before beginning hemodialysis, the patient goes through a painless ultrasound evaluation of the blood vessels in the arms. This evaluation, called **vein mapping,** assists in determining the best arm vessels to use as a vascular access point during hemodialysis treatments. Three access types exist:

o **Arteriovenous (AV) Fistula** – An AV fistula is the
recommended access type because it is less likely
to cause infections, form
clots, or require hospitalization; and, it lasts longer than other access
types. An artery and
vein, usually the radial
artery and the cephalic
vein in the arm, are
joined to make a larger
blood vessel. This

> **A fistula is an
> opening or con-
> nection between
> 2 parts of the
> body that usually
> are separate.**

unnatural joining of the two vessels is the fistula.

The National Kidney Foundation's (NKF) K/DOQI
Guidelines* recommend the AV fistula be placed
at least 3 to 6 weeks, and ideally 3 to 4 months,
prior to dialysis.

o **AV Graft** – Sometimes a piece of artificial tubing (a
graft) is used to connect the artery and vein if
these vessels are too small for a satisfactory
fistula. Natural AV
fistula connections are
preferred over grafts
because they last
longer and are less
susceptible to clotting
and infection. The
USRDS reports that
about 80 percent of AV
fistulas last 3 years, while

> **According to
> the USRDS,
> only about 14% of
> patients begin
> dialysis with a
> fistula. The rest
> have a catheter.**

less than 50 percent of grafts last that long.

One of the Healthy People (HP)** 2010 goals calls
for an increase to 50 percent of patients that

---

* The National Kidney Foundation publishes Kidney Dialysis Outcomes Quality
   Initiative (K/DOQI) dialysis guidelines as recommendations to practitioners
   regarding dialysis quality care.
** Healthy People began in 1979 and is a national program supported by the
   federal government, that identifies the most significant and preventable health
   threats and establishes national goals to reduce the threats. Many of the goals
   are aimed at healthcare professionals and call for improved recognition of risk
   factors for diseases such as diabetes, CKD, and cardiovascular disease and

begin dialysis with the preferred AV fistula. The 2010 USRDS Annual Report indicated that only 14 percent of patients started dialysis with a mature AV fistula.

o **Venous Catheter (CVC)** – If the fistula is not ready for use when dialysis must begin, a CVC is inserted into a large vein in the neck (commonly, the jugular or subclavian vein) for access to the blood. A CVC is the least desirable access method for long-term use because of increased infection risk, clotting damage to the vein, and death. The infection rate from a CVC is about 4 times higher than with an AV fistula. Studies indicate that patients without a nephrologist are more likely to start dialysis with a CVC, often because the patient delayed in obtaining an AV fistula and dialysis has become an emergency.

❖ Following vein mapping, a surgeon connects the chosen artery and vein to form a fistula. Over the next few months, the increased blood flow through the fistula causes the joined vessels to grow larger and stronger so they are usable for repeated needle

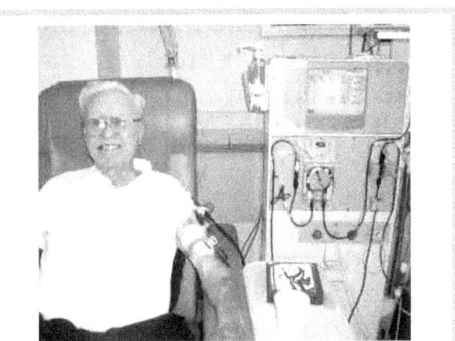

The hookup is illustrated by Bob, an Indiana dialysis patient.

insertions and provide an increased blood flow during the dialysis treatments.

❖ Dialysis usually occurs three times per week for 3 to 5 hours per time. The patient sits beside a hemodialysis machine, and a needle is inserted into the fistula to remove the patient's blood and filter it through the dialyzer. A second needle is also inserted into the fistula for return of the filtered blood to the body.

---

more aggressive and appropriate care of such patients. The goals are adjusted each decade.

❖ The patient's blood travels through semipermeable cellophane membranes that are surrounded by a warm water bath of dialysis fluid in the dialyzer. The semi-permeable membranes have tiny holes and work much like a coffee filter. The holes are too small to let blood cells, protein, and certain other important chemicals leave the blood and move into the dialysis fluid (the dialysate). However, excess water, urea, potassium, and other substances that are more concentrated in the blood than in the dialysate leave the blood through the semi-permeable membranes and move into the fluid, which is later discarded. Chemicals needed by the patient can be administered by adding them to the fluid so they diffuse through the membranes into the blood.

❖ Dialysis removes blood waste by diffusion. Diffusion is the natural movement of molecules from an area of higher concentration to one of lower concentration. A dialysis patient, for example, will have a high urea level in the blood. The dialysate in the dialyzer will not have urea molecules. As the blood flows through the dialyzer, urea molecules naturally will diffuse out of the blood and into the fluid. Conversely, bicarbonate needed by the body and contained in the dialysate will diffuse from the dialysate into the blood.

RECENT RESEARCH ➔ Scientists are developing a wearable artificial kidney (WAK) for continuous, 24-hour dialysis. The WAK weighs about 10 pounds and is powered by two 9V batteries. The continuous dialysis more closely approximates normal kidney function.

Clinical Journal of the American Society of Nephrology, August, 2009

2. The Hemodialysis Location

Hemodialysis is most commonly performed in a dialysis center but may also be performed at home.

A. IN-CENTER DIALYSIS

Most dialysis patients travel to a dialysis center for their treatments. Medicare will pay for three in-center dialysis treatments per week if the patient does not have employer-sponsored insurance. Medicare has no age restriction for payment.

The in-center dialysis treatment normally lasts 3 to 5 hours. After dialysis, the patient spends additional time waiting for excess bleeding to stop and blood pressure to normalize. Schedules at the dialysis center generally are tight, and if a patient arrives late, treatment may be cut short. This means toxins remain in the blood, and the patient will feel poorly sooner.

The 2010 USRDS Report reports that about half of dialysis patients are over age 65; 45% are African-American; and men outnumber women.

The hemodialysis patient must follow a strict diet and limit fluids to avoid weight gain, heart failure, and increased blood pressure. The patient usually takes several drugs to control blood pressure, anemia, high phosphorus levels, high acid levels, clotting, and a host of other complications.

> *Patient Interview:* *Miles, a school psychologist, began dialysis 5 months before the interview. His kidney failure resulted from diabetes and high blood pressure. Miles reports that he was "pushed over the edge and onto dialysis" after he was hospitalized for the hypertension. Miles has closely monitored his fluid intake and weight since beginning dialysis. "If my weight increases or I take in too much fluid, I feel wrung out like a sock following my dialysis treatment. I look forward to beginning longer, nocturnal dialysis next week so that I feel better between treatments."*

Chain-owned dialysis units treat nearly 66 percent of hemodialysis patients. Recently, attention has focused on the quality of care in the U.S. in such units as compared to that in other countries. According to the director of the Kidney Research Institute, the U.S. has one of the highest dialysis-care mortality rates in the world.

RECENT RESEARCH

➔

In a recent study, researchers looked at hospitalization and mortality rates in patients in for-profit compared to not-for-profit dialysis facilities. Both hospitalization and mortality rates were significantly higher in the for-profit centers. The researchers concluded that Medicare's current payment system may be insufficient to achieve optimal patient care.

Health Services Research, 2010

B. HOME DIALYSIS

Some patients are using dialysis machines at home with better health results. The patient may dialyze 5 or 6 days per week or have a long, slow treatment during sleep, either every night or every other night, depending on medical requirements. Night treatments last 6 to 8 hours, and these slower treatments are easier on the heart. Having longer treatments more frequently helps to avoid the build-up of toxins that occurs when treatments are only 3 days per week for fewer hours.

Research indicates that frequent or 8-hour overnight hemodialysis reduces the risk of death by 80 percent when compared to conventional dialysis. In a 2009 study, lengthy dialysis led to better

Nearly 40% of new Illinois dialysis patients use home hemodialysis.

blood pressure control, both during and after dialysis. Two-thirds of patients were able to lower their blood pressure medication dosages and had reduced levels of phosphates. Frequent home treatments allowed better control over blood fluids, phosphorus levels, anemia, and blood pressure. The patients felt more energetic and suffered fewer headaches, nausea, and other physical symptoms. Patients with frequent home dialysis have fewer diet and liquid restrictions, reverse some heart damage, and live longer.

RECENT RESEARCH
→

Researchers concluded that patients receiving long, frequent nocturnal dialysis treatments may survive as long as patients who receive a transplanted kidney from a deceased donor. Over a 12-year period, 14.7 percent of those receiving night dialysis died, and 14.3 percent of transplant recipients of deceased donor kidneys died.

Nephrology Dialysis Transplantations
September, 2009

Home hemodialysis has the same risks as in-center dialysis, including the possibility of excess blood loss or an air embolism. The training that patients and their at-home helpers receive teaches them how to respond to such events.

Patient Interview: *Arthur, a well-built 42-year-old, has dialysis at home 6 days per week for 4 hours at a time, using NxStage®, a smaller, portable dialysis machine. He enjoys choosing his dialysis schedule and feels better than he did when he had 3-days-per-week, in-center dialysis. "I work as a guidance counselor, which allows me to keep my employment health insurance to pay for six days of treatments and the supplies," he says. Arthur was in the hospital dialysis unit on his dialysis machine when we interviewed him. "My wife is my at-home helper, and we had a tiff. They let me come here once in a while to give her a break." Arthur has waited for a transplant for 6 years. "I occasionally have health issues that cause me to become inactive on the waiting list until the problem is resolved."*

Despite the substantial advantages of home hemodialysis, only 3,800 patients in 2008 received home dialysis. Some of those were nursing home patients still receiving the inferior but common 3-times-per-week treatments. When it comes to dialysis, more is better and more closely approximates natural kidney function. Most dialysis patients, though, rely solely on Medicare to cover dialysis expenses; and, it only pays for the customary 3 treatments per week.

3. Complications of Hemodialysis

Having blood cleaned only 3 times per week for only 3 to 5 hours leaves long periods when no fluids and toxins are removed, which results in buildup in the body. Then, during hemodialysis, this buildup is removed much more rapidly than is natural, resulting in a sudden change in the fluid and electrolyte contents of the blood. This swift change in body chemistry is not one the body is prepared to endure and induces many of the following complications:

- Cardiac arrhythmias

- Muscle cramping, headaches, nausea and vomiting

- Altered mental states, seizures, coma, death

- Hypotension, low blood pressure.

The most common post-hemodialysis symptom is a "washed-out" feeling, called **asthenia** (az-THEE-nee-yuh), also resulting from the rapid changes in fluids and blood chemistry. Some patients suffer from asthenia only a few hours following dialysis, and others experience it consistently.

> ***Patient Interview:*** *Carol is a lovely woman with multiple health problems, including uncontrolled high blood pressure that she believes caused her kidney failure. Carol takes 5 different classes of hypertension drugs, and still has high blood pressure. Carol chooses in-center dialysis over home dialysis "to separate my family life from this," she says. "I do pretty well with the 3-hour dialysis sessions, but about two-thirds of the way through a treatment, I get a horrid headache and my heart pounds. I am completely wiped out for the rest of the day."*

Access problems are common for dialysis patients, often resulting in hospitalization. The access point becomes infected, blocked from clotting, or offers poor circulation. Many patients also have episodes where the access needle is dislodged or the patient receives a heparin overdose, leading to blood loss. Contamination of the dialyzer or the dialysate fluids can cause fever and infections, including hepatitis.

Dialyzer reuse is common in the U.S., which increases the odds of infections.

About 92 percent of kidney patients reaching ESRD choose hemodialysis. The total number of patients reaching ESRD grows every year. The 2010 USRDS Report showed over 548,000 ESRD patients. Of those, over 382,000 remained on dialysis and about 165,000 had a functioning transplant. Over 88,600 ESRD patients had died during the survey year.

B. Peritoneal Dialysis

The abdominal cavity is lined with a natural filtering tissue called the peritoneal membrane, or **peritoneum** (pair-uh-tuh-NEE-um). The peritoneum lets in the liquid part of the blood but prevents large molecules in the blood (such as protein and blood cells) from passing through to the abdomen. Peritoneal dialysis (PD) takes advantage of this natural filtering ability of the peritoneum.

1. The PD Process

❖ For peritoneal dialysis, a surgeon places a permanent catheter (access hole and tube several inches long) into the patient's abdominal wall. The section of the tube in the abdomen has tiny holes over it so fluid can drain out of the tube and throughout the abdomen. A small portion of the tube protrudes outside the abdomen and has an adaptor on it to connect to the bags of solution that drain into the abdomen.

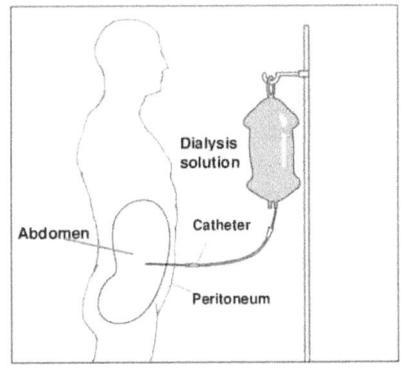

Diagram used with permission of NIDDK.

❖ The patient places a bag of solution called dialysate into the abdomen through the catheter. This process takes about 15 minutes. Dialysate bags are a concentrated mixture of salt and sugar (dextrose) dissolved in liquid. The body waste products and water in the abdomen naturally move or diffuse into the solution.

❖ The dialysate washes through the abdomen, absorbing the waste products and extra water that filter into the abdomen through the peritoneum from the blood. The dialysate remains in the abdomen for several hours (the "dwell time") to absorb all the waste collected from the blood.

> **Because the dialysate contains glucose, most diabetic patients on PD require insulin.**

❖ After the dwell time, the patient drains the dialysate (along with the waste and extra water) out of the abdomen, through the catheter, and into an empty bag. This takes about 20 to 30 minutes.

❖ The patient then places a fresh bag of dialysate into the abdomen for several more hours.

❖ Each cycle of putting in and then removing the dialysate is an "exchange." Several exchanges are required each day.

2. Forms of PD

Peritoneal dialysis comes in three forms:

❖ **Continuous Ambulatory Peritoneal Dialysis (CAPD).** CAPD is the most common form of PD. It requires three to five exchanges every 24 hours. No machine is involved. The patient hangs a bag of dialysate higher than the abdomen; gravity then causes the dialysate to enter the abdomen. The fluid sits in the abdomen for a few hours as the patient proceeds with normal tasks. Later, the patient allows the dialysate (which is then full of wastes) to flow out of the abdomen, through the catheter, and into a bag positioned lower than the abdomen. The patient then fills the abdomen with a clean bag of dialysate to begin the next exchange. Each emptying and filling takes about 30-40 minutes.

❖ **Continuous Cycle-Assisted Peritoneal Dialysis (CCPD).** With CCPD, the patient uses a machine (cycler machine) to make 3 to 5 exchanges during the night as the patient sleeps. In the morning, the patient begins a longer exchange that lasts all day.

Pros and Cons of Peritoneal Dialysis

Pros	Cons
• The patient can time exchanges to schedule outside events. • The patient can perform the exchanges alone and at home, work or elsewhere, rather than at a dialysis center. • The patient can travel, but must ship or take supplies. • The patient may exercise. • Diet is less restricted than with hemodialysis but still is planned. • The patient feels better than many on in-center hemodialysis.	• Training is required. • Peritonitis (infection of the peritoneal cavity) is common, serious, and requires antibiotics. • PD is performed all 7 days/week and is less efficient in removing wastes than hemodialysis. • The dialysate bags and equipment require storage space. • The cycler machine requires help from a partner. • Weight gain is likely if dialysate contains sugar (dextrose).

❖ **Nocturnal Intermittent Peritoneal Dialysis**.
The patient uses the cycler machine to make only night-time exchanges, with no exchange during the day. This type of dialysis is not as efficient unless the patient has some remaining kidney function.

3. Complications of PD

According to the USRDS 2010 Annual Data Report, 6 percent of patients beginning dialysis select peritoneal dialysis. Of the total U.S. population on dialysis, only 1 out of 20 chooses PD. In contrast, PD is widely used in other countries. For example, 66 percent of patients prefer PD in Mexico and 80 percent in Hong Kong.

Some people do not do well with PD because:

• Their peritoneum does not allow efficient exchanges;

• They have inflammatory bowel disease;

• They cannot self-care adequately; and

- Prior abdominal surgery left scarring, thus interfering with the PD process.

Patient Interview: Bob, a former B-24 bomber pilot, has received hemodialysis treatments for 3 years. Bob told us his diabetes and hypertension caused a decrease in kidney function, but when he was hospitalized for heart by-pass surgery, he "received a dye during tests that put me on dialysis." Bob tried PD but "it kept getting clogged." Like many other dialysis patients, Bob prefers in-center hemodialysis. "I lose 3 days of each week of my life, but I like the comfort of the facility and the supervision of the staff."

The major complication of PD is peritonitis, infection of the peritoneum. It accounts for 15 percent to 35 percent of hospital admissions for PD patients. Bacteria enter the catheter during exchanges. If peritonitis exists, the patient usually observes cloudy fluid after an exchange. Abdominal pain is present in up to 95 percent of cases, and chills and fever are evident about 25 percent of the time. Because of aggressive antibiotic treatment, death from peritonitis is rare (one percent to three percent of reported cases).

> **Dialysis patients take an average of 19 pills each day, with a quarter taking more than 25 pills.**
> *Clinical Journal of American Society of Nephrology, May 2009*

Life with PD may be slightly better than with hemodialysis, not only because of the greater freedom PD offers, but also because the PD patients experience less anemia and vitamin D deficiency and have fewer hospitalizations. The PD population, however, has a higher risk of certain cardiovascular events. According to the USRDS, PD patients are 10 percent more likely to suffer cardiac arrest, and they have a 19 percent higher risk of acute myocardial infarction. At the same time, they are 20 percent less likely than those on hemodialysis to develop congestive heart failure.

C. How Much Dialysis is Enough?

Whether the patient chooses hemodialysis or peritoneal dialysis, lab tests determine the proper dialysis amount. Time spent on hemodialysis or peritoneal dialysis will depend on:

- How much kidney function the patient still has: the more function, the less dialysis needed.

- The patient's size: large people need more dialysis.

- How much waste collected in the blood: the more waste, the longer the dialysis.

- The patient's general health and subjective reports of symptoms: if the patient has poor appetite, nausea, or general weakness, the patient may need more dialysis.

The major goal of dialysis is to remove excess fluid that accumulates between treatments and to normalize plasma levels of electrolytes such as potassium and bicarbonate. The removal of urea, the most significant nitrogen-based waste product in the body, is used to quantify the dose of hemodialysis.

About once a month, a blood test is used to determine if the dialysis treatment is removing enough urea from the blood. This test is called the Kt/V urea. For hemodialysis patients, the Kt/V number should be at least 1.25. For PD patients, the number should remain above 1.7.

Think about it:
The average dialysis patient receives 12 to 15 hours of hemodialysis each week. The functioning kidneys of most people clean blood 168 hours per week.

K = hemodialyzer urea clearance (in millimeters per minute)

t = the numbers of minutes of dialysis

V= the volume of urea in the body in millimeters

The NKF's K/DOQI dialysis guidelines recommend that urea Kt/V be maintained at 1.2 or higher for all patients. In a large U.S. multicenter study in 2003, called the Hemodialysis or HEMO study, researchers compared a Kt/V of 1.25 and a higher Kt/V of 1.65. The higher Kt/V was associated with a decreased mortality in women. This and many other similar findings suggest that more dialysis is better than less.

Patients treated with dialysis often remain unwell. Even in patients adequately treated with dialysis, progressive cardiovascular disease, nerve damage, and bone disease are common. Fatigue is universal, despite management of anemia. All of this is not surprising given that the most efficient hemodialysis regimens provide less than 15 percent of the small solute removal of two functioning kidneys.

D. Dialysis - Survival Facts

The NKF states in the Background Section of its K/DOQI Guidelines:

> Despite advances in dialysis, the annual mortality rate of dialysis patients is in excess of 20 percent. Expected remaining lifetimes of patients treated by dialysis were far shorter than the age-matched general population, varying (depending on gender and race) from 7.1 to 11.5 years for patients ages 40 to 44 years, and from 2.7 to 3.9 years for patients ages 60 to 64 years.

Medicare regulations require medical providers to provide information about dialysis and transplant options to all patients starting dialysis, regardless of insurance status. The USRDS compiles the associated data regarding such patients. The USRDS' 2010 Annual Data Report reveals the following outcome information for dialysis patients:

- The average dialysis patient is hospitalized between two and four times during the first year of dialysis for infections, catheter or fistula clotting, or excessive bleeding, among other issues.

- The first few months of dialysis are the deadliest for patients; over 15 percent die.

- Infections cause nearly 20 percent of deaths in the first dialysis year.

- Dialysis patients have three times the risk of stroke during the first two months of dialysis, and 60 percent of those suffering a stroke will die.

Continued survival with dialysis is tentative. Death from any cause is 3.5 times greater for patients on dialysis than for people without kidney failure. The annual mortality rate of dialysis patients is approximately 23 percent, compared with less than 0.01 percent in the general U.S. population. In the first two years of dialysis, PD patients have a slight survival advantage over those on hemodialysis. The 5-year survival rate is about equal; less than 40 percent of dialysis patients survive.

> **Almost a quarter of dialysis patients die each year, primarily from cardiovascular disease.**

Despite these poor outcome statistics, dialysis patients who are able to avoid cardiovascular disease and other co-morbidities can have good survival results. For example, dialysis patients with other problems (uncontrolled diabetes or cardiovascular disease, etc.) have a 2-year survival rate of only 40 percent. Dialysis patients who carefully control and avoid such coexisting health problems have a 2-year survival rate of 95 percent.

> ***Patient Interview:*** *Bob, the former B-24 bomber pilot mentioned earlier in this chapter, says that he had great difficulty deciding whether or not to accept dialysis. "My daughter begged me to try it for just one year. I promised I would, and here I am 3 years later. My doctor says I'm a walking miracle. My vessels are bad and so is my heart. My doctor says I have heart failure."*

Dialysis patients like Bob generally have multiple health issues. The common comorbidities for dialysis patients and for others with progressing CKD include the following:

1. Cardiovascular Disease

Cardiovascular disease is epidemic in dialysis patients and is the primary cause of death. Cardiovascular disease accounts for 50 percent of deaths of dialysis patients, a rate that is 10 to 20 times greater than in the general population.

Patients with CKD often develop left ventricular hypertrophy (LVH), a heart abnormality in which the left chamber of the heart enlarges. The less kidney function the patient has, the greater

> **A high fatigue rating is a predictor for cardiovascular outcomes in hemodialysis patients.**
> *American Journal of Kidney Disease*, 2010

the chance of LVH. Up to 80 percent of patients starting dialysis have LVH, and the prevalence of associated coronary artery disease may reach 40 percent.

2. Metabolic Syndrome

A study of dialysis patients found nearly 70 percent had metabolic syndrome at initial dialysis. Metabolic syndrome is a set of symptoms that is a predictor for cardiovascular disease. This further illuminates the relationship between heart and kidney disease. Metabolic syndrome applies to anyone with three of the following five symptoms:

- Abdominal obesity;
- Elevated triglyceride levels;
- Low HDL levels;
- High blood pressure; and
- High glucose levels.

According to one study, female dialysis patients had a higher incidence of metabolic syndrome, but male patients with metabolic syndrome were more vulnerable to cardiovascular disease.

3. Anemia

Anemia is common in many patients with CKD, including nearly all who reach ESRD. The administration of erythropoietin (EPO) has helped enormously (revisit Chapter 6 about anemia and EPO). Fatigue, depression, cognitive impairment, and heart abnormalities improve with anemia treatment. The NKF's K/DOQI anemia guidelines guide clinicians on successful anemia treatment. You may link to these guidelines at KidneySteps.com.

4. Renal Osteodystrophy/PTH

Patients who approach end stage and are on dialysis typically develop hyperparathyroidism and bone disease. Deteriorating kidneys fail to produce sufficient calcitriol, the active form of vitamin D. Inadequate calcitriol is expressed as a vitamin D deficiency (see Chapter 6). This deficiency leads to inadequate calcium stores.

In response, the parathyroid glands in your neck kick into overdrive to produce the parathyroid hormone (PTH). PTH is the most important regulator of calcium metabolism. It enters the blood, stimulating the kidneys to increase production of calcitriol. PTH also stimulates bones to release calcium into the blood, weakening the bones but insuring that cells have adequate calcium to perform their functions.

> **Investigators recently found that 79% of dialysis patients were vitamin D deficient.**
> *Clinical Journal of the American Society of Nephrology*
> **February, 2010**

When kidney function is decreased, or non-existent, the kidneys are unable to respond to PTH. As a result, the parathyroid makes more PTH, and the non-functioning kidneys still fail to make sufficient vitamin D; however, the bones continue to respond by releasing calcium. The excess calcium from the bones enters the bloodstream and deposits in the heart, vessels, and other places where it doesn't belong. The ultimate result is an overactive parathyroid gland, faulty bone formation, bone pain, bone fractures, and cardiovascular disease. Many dialysis patients become wheelchair-bound as a result of their frail skeletal system.

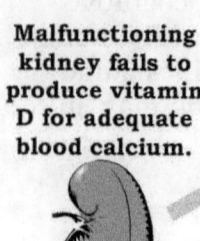

Malfunctioning kidney fails to produce vitamin D for adequate blood calcium.

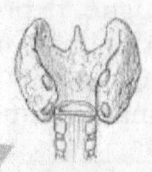

In response, parathyroid gland overworks to make PTH (hyperparathyroidism).

Excess PTH causes too much calcium to leave bones.

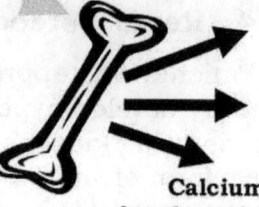

Calcium is released; bones weaken.

Excess calcium builds up in heart and vessels, damaging them.

Higher blood levels of calcium, and both high and low levels of PTH, are associated with poor vascular health and mortality. In a 2008 study, dialysis patients who took a phosphate binder to reduce phosphorus levels in the blood appeared to reduce their risk of death up to 30 percent in the first 90 days of treatment.

E. Paying for ESRD

Medicare. In 1972, Congress passed legislation making people of any age with ESRD eligible for Medicare, a program ordinarily only available to those age 65 or older. Medicare covers up to 80 percent of dialysis and transplantation costs if the person does not have health insurance. To qualify for Medicare, the person must require regular dialysis or have had a kidney transplant

> I completed the Medicare Part A and B applications in the hospital the day following transplant surgery. However, I had employer-sponsored health insurance that covered all the costs.

and must have paid social security through previous employment (or be the child or spouse of someone who has).

Health Insurance. Those who can remain employed despite ESRD often have employer-provided insurance that will pay the entire cost of treatment (or the 20 percent not paid by Medicare).

Medicaid. Medicaid is a need-based joint federal and state program available for those who have minimal income and assets. Guidelines for the program vary by state. Medicaid pays the 20 percent that Medicare does not pay for dialysis.

SHIP. The State Health Insurance Program (SHIP) provides free counseling and assistance to Medicare recipients regarding insurance matters. SHIP can assist in finding ways to cover the 20 percent of costs not covered by Medicare. Find your state program at www.shipusa.com.

VA Benefits. Veterans can contact their local VA office for help paying for treatment. Military retirees can contact the U.S. Department of Defense.

SSDI. Many on dialysis qualify as disabled and can seek Social Security Disability Income to help with daily living costs.

PAPs. Most drug companies who participate in Partnership Assistant Programs (PAPs) give discounts to patients who show they cannot afford the prescribed drug costs, which can be the case for those on dialysis or with a transplanted kidney. Medicare Part B pays for EPO to treat anemia for those on dialysis or with a kidney transplant. Medicare also pays 80 percent of immunosuppressants, which can cost $1,500 per month for kidney transplant recipients, but only for 3 years after transplantation (unless the person has reached age 65 and is otherwise eligible for Medicare).

11.

Deceased Donors and Waiting List

For those needing a transplant, a kidney can come from a recently deceased donor, a living relative, a friend, or a stranger. Living donation is discussed in detail in Chapter 12. This chapter focuses on the national transplant waiting list for a deceased donor's kidney.

I (author with CKD) was in late Stage IV, approaching end stage. My nephrologist repeatedly encouraged me to locate a living person who would donate a kidney to me. That would allow surgery to proceed immediately and preemptively, before dialysis and before my health deteriorated from the continuing waste buildup in my body. However, many of my blood relatives also inherited Alport's syndrome, eliminating them as potential donors. I could not bring myself to seek the kidney of a friend or acquaintance, so I began the process to qualify for the national transplant waiting list to receive a deceased donor kidney.

A. Transplant Waiting List

1. UNOS / OPTN / OPO

Surgeons in the U.S. have transplanted kidneys since 1950, but it wasn't until 1984 that Congress passed the *National Organ Transplant Act* (NOTA) to control the distribution of organs from deceased donors. NOTA was necessitated by the development of effective immuno-suppressant drugs that had opened organ transplantation to a greater number of people, all needing the limited supply of donated organs. NOTA also was prompted by a fear of the sale of organs to the advantage of the wealthy (particularly the foreign wealthy who would come to the U.S. seeking organs because of our advancements in transplantation) and to the disadvantage of terminally ill U.S. citizens in need of a transplant. There are only so many deceased-donor organs to go around.

NOTA required the creation of a national *Organ Procurement and Transplant Network* (OPTN) as the exclusive means to facilitate matching and placement of organs from deceased donors. The Department of Health and Human Services awarded a contract to the *United Network of Organ Sharing* (UNOS), a non-profit company, to operate the OPTN and to keep data regarding all organ donors and recipients.

In 1987, UNOS implemented nationwide policies on organ allocation, fair access to organs without regard to race or wealth, and safety in organ procurement. It also adopted a waiting list format and point system to determine the order in which recipients are matched with donor organs.

The national transplant waiting list is a computer list of individuals waiting to receive organs from deceased donors. A patient on the list might be waiting for a kidney, pancreas, heart, liver, lung, or small intestine. UNOS, at its Organ Center in Richmond, Virginia, maintains the computerized network 24 hours a day, every day of the year, to provide instantaneous information to all linking transplant centers, histocompatibility laboratories, and *Organ Procurement Organizations* (OPOs) seeking to place donated organs for transplantation.

Organ allocation is the main and hefty responsibility of UNOS. For assistance it has divided the country into 11 organ procurement regions. Within each region, OPOs operate according to agreed distribution and sharing criteria, providing organ recovery services to transplant hospitals. The regions have more than one OPO, and each OPO operates in an exclusive designated donation service area within the region, working with transplant centers within that service area.

OPOs become involved when a patient is identified as a potential donor of organs and tissue. The hospital of the potential donor contacts its OPO, which then coordinates the donation process.

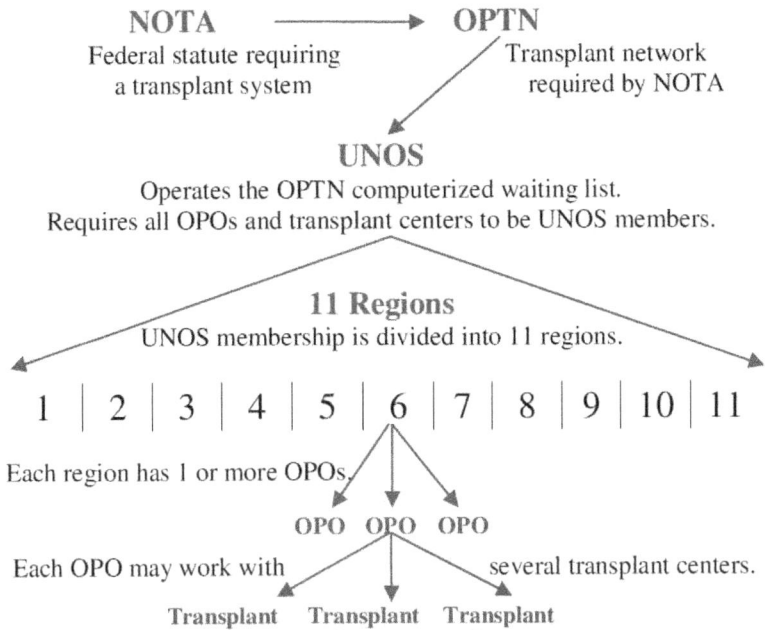

NOTA $\longrightarrow$ OPTN
Federal statute requiring   Transplant network
a transplant system   required by NOTA

UNOS
Operates the OPTN computerized waiting list.
Requires all OPOs and transplant centers to be UNOS members.

11 Regions
UNOS membership is divided into 11 regions.

1 | 2 | 3 | 4 | 5 | 6 | 7 | 8 | 9 | 10 | 11

Each region has 1 or more OPOs.

OPO   OPO   OPO

Each OPO may work with   several transplant centers.

Transplant   Transplant   Transplant
Center   Center   Center

The above diagram illustrates the national transplant deceased organ donor system. As an example, we (your authors) live in Indiana, which is part of Region 10, along with Michigan and Ohio. Region 10 is represented by six OPOs. The Indiana OPO (IOPO) assists the four transplant centers located in the Indiana donation service area, including Indiana University Hospital.

All U.S. transplant centers and OPOs must be members of the OPTN to receive Medicare funds, and they are linked to the OPTN computer network. Every patient waiting for a solid organ is registered with UNOS and included in the OPTN computer network.

When a deceased donor is identified, the OPO enters the donor's height, weight, and blood type into the UNOS computer. The computer quickly provides a list of suitable candidates, in order of matching priority, to receive the organ. The computer eliminates candidates with blood types incompatible with that of the donor, then ranks the rest of the candidates based on a point system. The kidney allocation point system is described later in this Chapter.

Where the patient lives affects waiting time. For example, Alabama has the longest median wait time of 9.3 years, while the median wait in Kentucky, Utah, or Iowa is less than 1 year. Patients can register at more than one transplant center, meeting the testing requirements of that second center. I considered this, as the average waiting time in a neighboring state was much shorter, but its transplant centers did not have the same outstanding transplant reputation as Indiana University Hospital.

> **Transplant candidates can register at more than one transplant center.**

2. The Long Wait

A total of 10,622 deceased donor kidneys were transplanted in the U.S. in 2010, an increase of 10 percent from 5 years earlier. Despite the donation increase, the wait list for a deceased donor kidney is 8 times longer than it was 5 years ago. OPTN data as of March, 2011, show over 88,000 renal transplant candidates listed for a kidney. The USRDS projects median wait time for those listed in 2010 is 3.6 years.

Blood Type→	A	AB	B	O
Wait Time in Years→	1.9	1.3	4+	4+

The median wait time varies by blood type, with the longest wait for those with blood types B or O. Candidates who are "sensitized" may wait 5 or more years for a kidney or never receive one. (We discuss "sensitized" later.)

> **The average deceased donor is age 45 to 59, and most are white.**

Race also has an impact on the wait. Of the patients placed on the kidney-only wait list in 2003, 69 percent of white patients had received a kidney after 5 years compared to 59 percent of non-whites. The USRDS projects the wait time for patients listed in 2010 will range from 2.3 years for whites to 3.7 years for African-Americans.

RECENT RESEARCH ➔ Scientists analyzing data found that access to kidney transplantation is not equal for all patients. Blacks are less likely than whites to be placed on the waiting list. They are 57% less likely if they also are from poor neighborhoods. Disparities in wait time also exist among UNOS regions, ranging from 1 year to 10 years.

Journal of the American Society of Nephrology
April 2009

The transplant format does not discriminate because of race. African-Americans have twice the rate of kidney failure as whites and locate living donations less frequently. Also, blacks are more likely to be sensitized or have blood type B, making it less likely they will match a potential donor. Thus, they tend to wait longer.

Many waiting for a deceased donor kidney become inactive listings because of cardiovascular disease, cancer, or other intervening illnesses that occur while on dialysis. Also, because of the long wait, the likelihood of dying while on the waiting list approaches 40 percent. Death while waiting is greatest for older dialysis patients, with about half of those age 60 or older projected to die before receiving an organ from a deceased donor. Given the anticipated lengthy wait for newly listed transplant candidates, it is no surprise that 45 percent of waiting patients have designated a willingness to accept an inferior or expanded criteria donor (ECD) kidney, hoping to receive a deceased donor kidney more quickly (ECD is discussed later).

1 in 4 transplant recipients received dialysis for 5 or more years before transplantation.

B. Types of Deceased Donors

Efforts to obtain consent for organ donation begin only after a patient's attending physician has declared the patient dead or after deciding the catastrophically injured patient cannot live. The potential recipient's attending physician is not involved in the organ donation process. Deceased donors are divided into groups:

❖ **Donation after brain death**. Most deceased organ donors are brain dead following severe brain injury. While brain-dead donors are dead, their hearts continue to pump and maintain circulation, making it possible for surgeons to begin removing the donated organs soon after circulation has stopped. Artificial support systems maintain circulation to facilitate organ donation. This translates into healthier organs for transplantation. A brain-dead donor may provide two kidneys, a pancreas, heart, liver, small intestines, tissues, and corneas.

The diagnosis of brain death requires irrefutable evidence that the injury is irreversible, and there is an absence of blood flow through the brain and absence of cerebral and brainstem function. Brain death and a coma or persistent vegetative state are not the same. A person in a vegetative state or coma has remaining brain function.

❖ **Donation after cardiac death**∗. After cardiac death, blood no longer circulates through the deceased individual's organs. Organs with no blood circulation are referred to as "ischemic," and rapid cell death occurs. Blood begins coagulating in the organs, damaging them and making them less desirable or even unusable for transplantation.

Cardiac death donors fall into two categories.

- **Uncontrolled donors** – These donors are pulseless after failed attempts to resuscitate. Ischemia begins immediately upon the death. Some trauma centers attempt to minimize the ischemia by cooling the organs intra-venously until the family is informed of the death and can consent to donation. Upon consent, the organs are removed quickly.

- **Controlled donors** – These donors are comatose, irreversibly brain damaged and respirator-dependent, but not brain dead by strict definition. The family decides to withdraw life support and

---

∗ We use the terms *brain death* and *cardiac death* because the terms are understandable. Medical professionals prefer the terms *death determined by neurologic criteria* and *death determined by cardiorespiratory criteria.*

only then is approached by an OPO representative regarding consent to organ donation.

Donations after cardiac death are associated with an increased rate of delayed **graft** function. However, long-term graft function and survival are similar to those from brain-dead donors. A graft is the name for an organ once it is transplanted.

Before the acceptance of brain-death criteria, all deceased donor kidneys were recovered from patients with cardiac death. After acceptance of brain death and the resulting better organs, the use of donations after cardiac death decreased. The severe organ shortage has revived such donations. As of 2007, all OPOs and transplant centers must develop and comply with protocols to facilitate recovery of organs from donors after cardiac death.

> The USRDS reports that 1 in 9 deceased donor transplants is a donation after cardiac death.

❖ **ECD Donors**. As of 2009, deceased donor kidneys are categorized as being either standard criteria donor kidneys (SCD) or expanded criteria donor kidneys (ECD). Kidneys donated after brain death are SCD. An ECD kidney is a substandard kidney from a deceased donor at least age 60 or from a deceased donor 50 to 59 years of age with at least two of these criteria:

- cerebral vascular accident (stroke or aneurysm) as cause of death

- hypertension at any time during life

- creatinine level greater than 1.5 mg/dL

UNOS permits transplant candidates to indicate their willingness to accept an ECD kidney. When one becomes available, it first is offered to a

> ECD kidneys account for 22% of deceased donor transplants.
> 2010 Annual Data Report, USRDS

125

patient on the transplant waiting list who has agreed to accept an ECD kidney and knows the risks associated with the graft.

An ECD kidney is not perfect, and the recipient has an increased risk of loss of the graft. However, survival with an ECD kidney is better than with dialysis. Accepting an ECD kidney also reduces the waiting time for the willing candidate.

RECENT RESEARCH → Researchers looked at the graft survival outcomes for patients who received either a single kidney or both kidneys from ECD donors from 2000 to 2008. Over 56% of the dual ECD kidneys failed to function immediately, while 39% of the single kidneys had delayed function. At five years, 89% of the dual kidneys still functioned versus 78% of the single ECD kidneys.

Transplantation Proceedings, 2010

Those most likely to accept an ECD kidney are usually age 60 or older, younger than 60 but with diabetes or heart disease, or they are intolerant of dialysis.

❖ **Double Kidney**. Kidneys from adult donors are offered individually unless the deceased donor has signs of CKD (high creatinine level, long-standing hypertension, or diabetes) and is age 60 or older. The recipient may receive both of the donor's kidneys to better the chance of an increased GFR for the recipient.

If the deceased donor is a young child, both small kidneys may go to one recipient. Recent research suggests this may not be necessary.

RECENT RESEARCH → Adult recipients who received a single kidney from very young deceased donors did just as well as those receiving both kidneys, so long as the donor weighed over about 70 pounds. The single kidney grows larger over time and increases function.

American Journal of Transplantation, 2009

C. Becoming a Listed Candidate

Qualifying for the deceased donor transplant waiting list is not simply a matter of having poor kidney function. The testing to become a candidate is thorough to increase the odds of survival for both the recipient and the transplanted kidney.

1. Early Referral is Important

Early referral to a transplant center is important for the patient with advancing CKD. As kidney disease progresses, the patient's overall health declines from uremic complications and the rising likelihood of cardiovascular complications. This inevitable increase in negative health effects decreases post-transplant survival. Also, earlier referral raises the possibility that the patient will locate a willing living donor.

Ideally, the nephrologist refers a patient to a transplant center when the nephrologist is sure the patient is headed toward end stage. With the results of successive blood and urine tests, the nephrologist can estimate the rate of decline in kidney function and refer as the patient approaches Stage IV of CKD, or when GFR is less than 30mL/min.

RECENT RESEARCH → Compared to veteran MDs, recent medical school grads are more likely to refer CKD patients for kidney transplantation before the patient requires dialysis.
American Society of Nephrology, August, 2009

The USRDS reports that patients referred to a nephrologist at least a year before dialysis have lower death and disease rates. Those patients also are more likely to have preemptive transplantation, which is transplantation before dialysis. Preemptive transplantation improves both patient and graft survival rates by 20 to 30 percent, compared to the survival rates for patients receiving a graft after being on dialysis for more than six months. Unfortunately, 53 percent of patients with CKD are not referred to a nephrologist until just before dialysis. Early referral is not possible for up to 50 percent of patients who do not become aware of their CKD until it has reached end stage.

The UNOS deceased donor kidney allocation program currently in place allows transplant candidates to accrue points on the waiting list when GFR is estimated at 20mL/min or less (this is late Stage IV of CKD and before the need for dialysis). Yet, less than 5 percent of patients added to the waiting list are pre-dialysis, making preemptive transplantation infrequent.

> **Of the 385,000 patients on dialysis in the U.S., only about 20 percent are on the transplant waiting list.**

Dialysis centers must be associated with a transplant center, and all of their Medicare patients legally are entitled to referral to a transplant center. But again, this is late referral.

Studies suggest that the longer a patient is on dialysis before the transplant, the less time the transplanted kidney will last. This emphasizes the need for rapid referral to a transplant program. Also, the longer the patient is on dialysis while waiting for a transplant, the less likely the patient is to receive a transplant because of ensuing health problems arising during dialysis. Only about half of dialysis patients ultimately qualify for a transplant because of poor health that results during the time on dialysis.

2. Testing

A patient referred to a transplant center for evaluation must qualify psychologically and medically for inclusion on the transplant waiting list. Few absolute contraindications exist for referral and ultimate transplant surgery. Transplant centers may impose their own standards, usually based on overall health status.

> **Patients over age 50 are the fastest growing segment of the transplant waiting list.**

A common reason to decline referral is that the patient's condition is so poor that the patient will not survive with a transplant for more than 2 years (*e.g.*, incurable cancer or severe heart disease). Individuals may be excluded because of cardiovascular disease, smoking, obesity, incurable infectious diseases, cancer, mental illness, or ongoing substance abuse.

I was assigned a transplant coordinator to assist with the waiting list qualification process. "Transplant coordinator" is the term transplant centers apply to the medical staff person who arranges all testing for qualification, and who continues to coordinate testing for the term a patient is waitlisted. Concurrently, my nephrologist insisted I have the veins of my arms mapped, a simple ultrasound test, as preparation for surgical placement of the AV fistula for hemodialysis. He also arranged for me to attend a two-hour workshop to learn about hemodialysis and peritoneal dialysis--a sobering day.

The transplant coordinator scheduled a series of medical tests to assess both my short-term and long-term survival prospects following surgery. We discuss the testing required for transplantation in Chapter 13. This same testing applies for qualification for the waiting list.

The qualification process for both the waiting list and transplantation surgery begins with an informational conference. My conference included my transplant coordinator and a transplant surgeon who presented to me my odds of survival with a transplanted kidney compared to

> **I was surprised to learn the transplanted kidney would be placed into my lower abdomen, on the front side.**

dialysis, as well as the odds of survival of the graft itself. Survival odds were better if I could locate a living donor. The surgeon explained the surgical approach, risks, recovery process, and the need for ongoing monitoring of immuno-suppressants. This conference was aimed, in part, at assuring I was informed sufficiently to give the required consent to the testing and surgery.

Each transplant center has its own testing requirements. The medical tests used for my qualification on the waiting list and for transplant surgery included some or all of the following:

- physical exam and medical history;
- kidney function tests;
- cardiovascular exam;
- routine lab tests, including blood count and liver function tests;

- blood and tissue typing;

- panel reactive antibodies (PRA) to determine the antibodies in the blood that may react to a transplanted organ;

- blood tests for active viral infections like hepatitis B and C, human immunodeficiency virus (HIV), Epstein-Barr virus (EBV), syphilis, and cytomegalovirus (CMV).

Singer Natalie Cole received a deceased-donor kidney in May 2009 after beginning dialysis in September 2008.

While I waited for a transplant, I would have further tests to assess whether my health status remained stable. The process is structured and strict.

A patient's "health intelligence," or ability to understand basic health information, impacts that patient's likelihood of being listed for and then receiving a donated kidney. Qualifying for transplantation requires keeping numerous appointments and preparing for often cumbersome testing. Likewise, after transplantation the patient must be able to adhere to strict medication and test schedules and follow overall good health practices. The ability of the patient to obtain and understand health information and to make appropriate health decisions becomes critical in the process.

RECENT STUDY →

A 2009 study revealed that those with poor health intelligence have more difficulty understanding written health material, processing oral instructions, and navigating the healthcare system than those of sufficient health literacy. Those with poor health intelligence were 78% less likely to be referred for transplant evaluation than the more intelligent. If referred, it took 3.6 months for them to qualify for listing instead of the average 2.1 months.

Clinical Journal of the American Society of Nephrology, 2009

3. Remaining on the Wait List

Waiting time currently begins on the date a recipient is listed on the UNOS waiting list, but not until GFR is estimated at 20mL per minute or less, late Stage IV of CKD. This GFR limitation does not apply to patients younger than age 18. UNOS has proposed a change in the allocation system so that time

> **Over 6% of those on the waiting list die each year, an average of 17 waiting patients per day.**

spent on dialysis determines wait time. That way, those qualifying for the wait list early, perhaps months before dialysis, are not favored.

Once on the waiting list, a patient stays on the list by complying with all additional listing requirements and remaining in good health. Patients on the waiting list often become "inactive," because a new health issue has developed while on dialysis. Changes in health will impact wait time. The wait is difficult for those on dialysis who often suffer infections, heart and vessel problems, and hospitalizations. All these occurrences affect immediate availability for transplant surgery.

D. What is a Match?

The donor kidney and the patient must be matched before transplantation can occur. The matching is important to assure the patient's immune system will accept the new kidney rather than reject it.

The immune system is extremely complex and involves cells, tissues, organs and body processes, all aimed at self-protection. Your immune system's job is to protect your body from disease by identifying and killing any invading agent, whether that is bacteria, viruses, parasitic worms, cancer cells, or foreign tissue. To function properly, the immune system is highly evolved to distinguish between self and non-self. If non-self enters your body, your immune system recognizes the invader is non-self and attacks to destroy.

Humans would not survive long without the protection of an immune system to defend against invading bacteria and viruses, foreign cells, and even your own cells that become cancerous. At the same time, when a donor kidney is placed into your body, the immune system detects the graft as non-self. The immune system is so extremely adept at protecting the body from invaders, it will begin destroying the non-self transplanted kidney soon after it is grafted into the recipient. The attack nearly always can be controlled with today's powerful immunosuppressant drugs.

If the donor-kidney tissue is similar to the recipient's tissue, an immune system attack can be avoided altogether and the graft will last longer. Three primary factors are important in matching a donor organ to a patient needing that organ.

1. Blood Type

The most important matching factor is blood type. Your blood type must be compatible with the donor's blood type. While a total of 30 human blood group systems are now recognized by the International Society of Blood Transfusion, the ABO system is the most important.

The ABO system contains four blood types: A, B, AB or O. Two genetically-based antigens and two antibodies are responsible for the ABO blood types.

Percent in Population	ABO Type	Antigen A	Antigen B	Antibody anti-A	Antibody anti-B
40%	A	✓	–	–	✓
12%	B	–	✓	✓	–
43%	O	–	–	✓	✓
5%	AB	✓	✓	–	–

For example, those with type B blood, like your authors, have the antigen B on the surface of their blood cells. We do not produce B antibodies because those antibodies would lock onto our B antigens and destroy our own B blood cells. Our immune systems, however, do produce A antibodies. If A blood were injected into us, our A antibodies would attack the A antigens to destroy the "invading" blood.

The same principle applies to transplanted organs. If a person with type B blood receives a non-matching kidney from someone with type A blood, the recipient's A antibodies

132

would see the non-matching A antigens as foreign and swiftly attack the kidney until it dies.

2. HLA Typing

The potential match between the recipient's tissue and the donor's tissue uses a method called **Human Leukocyte Antigen** (HLA). Our immune system uses HLAs to differentiate self from non-self cells. Any cell with your HLAs on its surface is self and seen as belonging to you. Any cell displaying some other HLA type is non-self and is an invader.

> **With immuno-suppressant drugs, HLA matching is a relatively minor predictor of transplant outcome.**

HLA looks primarily at 6 antigens carried on the surface of your white blood cells. You inherit three of the HLAs from each of your parents, as did a prospective donor. The 6 HLAs analyzed are:

- HLA Class I antigens = HLA-A, HLA-B, HLA-C.

- HLA Class II antigens = HLA-DP, HLA-DQ, HLA-DR.

Because these 6 antigens are highly reactive with your immune system, the closest possible match between recipient and donor means the markers of "self" are similar or identical, making the immune system less apt to attack the transplant. Family members who wish to donate a kidney are more likely to have a complete match.

> **UNOS provides a list of HLAs that can be entered through its computer, UNet.**

We each have numerous HLA proteins within each class of HLAs. For example, there are 767 different HLA-A proteins and 2121 HLA-DR proteins. It is unlikely that any transplant candidate and donor (unless identical twins) will match at all HLA levels. For transplant matching purposes, the greater the number of HLA matches, the higher the probability the transplanted graft will survive longer than it otherwise would. If the recipient's immune system recognizes non-matching HLA antigens of the donor graft as foreign, they will attack the graft over time.

3. Cross-Matching Antigens

> **The USRDS reports that sensitized patients tend to wait twice as long for a kidney.**

If the potential kidney recipient had received foreign tissue in the past, perhaps from a blood transfusion or a previously transplanted organ, that exposure will have caused the recipient's immune system to create antibodies against the foreign tissue. The antibodies created after these "sensitizing" events are called alloantibodies.

When this **sensitized** patient receives a donor kidney, the alloantibodies might attack that graft as soon as it is transplanted. This immediate alloantibody attack of the kidney right after the transplant is called hyper-acute rejection and usually results in loss of the transplanted kidney.

To prevent this waste of a kidney, each potential transplant recipient receives a **panel reactive antibody** (PRA) test to check the level of sensitization resulting from prior exposure to foreign antigens. A negative result means no attack and allows the surgery to proceed. A positive crossmatch means an attack occurred and is a strong indicator against transplant.

The PRA test combines the transplant candidate's blood serum with samples of dozens of other individuals. The number of reactions (clumping) is counted. Each clumping is an attack by your antibodies to the antigens in the blood sample.

The PRA score is given as a percentage, which ranges from 0 to 99. The score represents the percentage of the U.S. population that cause your alloantibodies to react. Patients with a high PRA (75%, for example) are less likely to receive a kidney transplant because of the high probability of immediate rejection. If the patient has had past transfusions, the PRA test can show a sensitivity to most of the comparison samples.

When a potential deceased donor is identified, a cross match is performed specific to the recipient with that donor. A six-of-six HLA match with no PRA reactivity is the best match, but not common. Five-of-six and four-of-six are the most common matches. With powerful immuno-suppressant therapy, less than perfect matches do not prevent transplantation.

> **Antibodies can come and go. So while the patient waits for a deceased donor kidney, the patient's blood is tested regularly for PRA.**

In some situations, the alloantibodies of sensitized patients are removed from the body by plasmapheresis (plaz-muh-fuh-REE-siss), a process of circulating the blood through a machine similar to dialysis. The plasma or liquid part of the blood that contains the antibodies is removed, while the red and white blood cells and platelets remain. The patient receives substitute plasma.

E. The Kidney Allocation Point System

Because of the wide gap between kidney supply and demand, a major responsibility of UNOS is fair allocation of kidneys among patients waiting to receive them. UNOS has developed a complex point system that is designed to balance fairness with efficiency.

First, patients are categorized by blood group. The blood groups O and B have the greatest wait time for a kidney, currently about 5 years, and even longer in some states. In many cases, patients with blood types A and AB receive a kidney within a few months of being on the waiting list.

> **UNOS allocates kidneys first locally, then regionally, then nationally.**

Allocation of kidneys within each blood group is based on the UNOS point system. The more points a waiting patient has, the greater the likelihood of receiving a deceased donor kidney. The patient accumulates points based on:

Waiting time. Waiting begins when the candidate is placed on the waiting list and when estimated GFR is 20 mL/min or less. For candidates younger than age 18, waiting time begins with placement on the waiting list, regardless of level of kidney function. One point is assigned to the candidate waiting for the longest period, with fractions of points assigned proportionately to all other candidates. An additional point is assigned for each full year of waiting time. Points are calculated separately for each geographic (local, regional, national) level of kidney allocation.

UNOS Point System as of 2010

Relevant Factor	Points
Time on UNOS computer (per year of waiting time)	1
Zero HLA-DR mismatches (a perfect match)	2
One HLA-DR mismatch	1
Less than 80% PRA/ negative cross-match	4
Child recipient (for donor under age 35)	4
Past organ donor	4

Quality of antigen mismatch. Points are assigned to a candidate based on the number of HLA mismatches between the candidate's antigens and the donor's antigens at the donor-recipient (DR) locus. UNOS assigns two points if there are no donor-recipient mismatches, and one point if there is one DR mismatch.

Sensitized/PRA value. The calculated PRA value is the percentage of donors expected to have one or more unacceptable antigens indicated on the waiting list for the candidate. The transplant center determines the candidate's PRA-specific antibodies and lists them on the waiting list.

Children. Children under age 11 receive 4 points, and those ages 11 to 17 receive 3 points for allocation of kidneys from donors with zero antigen mismatches. Kidneys from donors younger than age 35 are offered first to children, regardless of the number of points an older matching candidate may have accumulated. Exceptions are adult candidates assigned 4 points for PRA level of 80% or greater who otherwise rank higher than all other listed candidates.

Prior donations. A candidate who previously donated a kidney or other organ in the U.S. receives 4 points.

The kidney allocation system has existed for 24 years and has not kept pace with current trends in medicine. UNOS's Kidney Transplantation Committee is reviewing this allocation system, because it does not always result in the best matches--an important factor in graft survival. For example, a 35-year-old deceased donor kidney might end up in a 70-year-old man with heart problems who realistically will not use it as long as would a younger recipient.

The current allocation system also fails to consider the quality of the deceased donor kidney. All non-ECD organs are assumed to be the same quality. But, quality varies based on obvious factors of donor age, cause of death, presence of diabetes, hypertension and renal function.

RECENT STUDY → Scientists looked at 14 donor/transplant factors such as donor age, race, history of diabetes or diabetes, creatinine level, cause of death, ischemic time, and effect on graft survival after transplantation. The fewer negative factors, the better the graft survival rate. *Transplantation,* 2009

UNOS standards also require that ABO type O kidneys are only transplanted into ABO type O recipients, and all zero antigen mismatched kidneys (perfect matches) must be offered for transplant to the perfectly matched recipient. These requirements often necessitate that the organs are shared throughout the U.S; that may mean shipping a kidney outside of the area where it is obtained, delaying the surgery and making delayed graft function more likely.

A kidney stays healthy outside the body for 48-72 hours.

F. Deceased Organ Becomes Available

Nationwide donation consent ratios have increased over the last 5 years to 65%

Hospitals are required by the Center for Medicare and Medicaid Services (CMS) to identify and refer all potential organ donors to their local OPO. Hospitals are to identify and refer patients in imminent death, those requiring mechanical ventilation who may be brain-dead, or patients who will be withdrawn from life support pursuant to a family decision. Organ

137

donation is not discussed with family members until after the patient is declared dead, unless the family initiates the conversation.

After consent to donation is confirmed, the OPO conducts a medical and social history of the potential donor to determine if the organs are suitable for transplantation. Not all potential deceased donors are suitable. If the donor has HIV or active malignancy, the donor is excluded. OPOs and transplant centers differ as to other exclusion criteria.

Some will exclude for the presence of certain potentially transmissible infectious diseases, while others will not. There isa balance between the risks associated with the particular donation and the risks of continuing with dialysis.

If the OPO determines the organ/tissue donation is appropriate, the OPO:

- Makes contact with the donor's family to discuss donation and also coordinates the process with the hospital staff;
- Ensures the donation decision is based on informed consent;
- Manages the clinical care of the donor once consent is finalized;
- Begins the process of evaluating all potential organs for transplant;
- Enters the donor information into the UNOS network to find matches for each organ;

While 90% of Americans support organ donation, at least 40% of transplantable organs are buried or cremated.

- Coordinates the organ recovery process with the various surgery teams;
- Provides follow-up information to the donor family and donating hospital regarding the donation outcomes; and
- Maintains the identities of the organ donor and organ recipient in confidence, unless later mutual consent to

disclosure is obtained from the donor family and the transplant recipient.

Organ donations are regulated by each state within the guidelines of NOTA. And, all states have adopted some version of the Uniform Anatomical Gift Act (UAGA), which governs organ donations. However, the anatomical gift laws are hardly "uniform".*

The UAGA adheres to an "opt-in" principle, requiring that the deceased donor or someone acting on the donor's behalf makes some affirmative statement to donate. Many states encourage donation by allowing consent on the driver's license or donor cards. If no consent is given during the life, the UAGA allows a relative or agent to consent to donation following the death. Our "opt-in" system is contrary to the "opt-out" system of European countries, where individuals are deemed to be donors unless they or someone on the individual's behalf opts out.

From the moment the donor family consents to the release of the donor's body for organ or tissue donation, the OPO receives all bills associated with the donation process. Neither the donor's family nor the donor hospital is responsible for any recovery expenses. The cost is absorbed by the transplant center, the recipient's insurance, or Medicare.

When a kidney becomes available, the UNOS team considers several factors in selecting the recipient. The OPO will access the UNOS computerized organ matching system to identify a match for the organ. The UNOS computer includes each recipient's:

- blood type and tissue type
- time on waiting list
- distance between donor and recipient
- blood antibody levels (high levels mean a higher risk of rejection)

---

* UAGA was last amended in 2006. Some states still cling to the prior 1968 and 1987 versions of UAGA that fail to comport with changes in federal law adopted after 1987. Both prior versions also are inconsistent with the policy to encourage donations. Those states adopting the 2006 version may have modified the act in diverse ways.

- whether recipient is a child
- whether body sizes of recipient and donor are similar

The computer identifies the top-ranked matching recipient, and the local procurement coordinator contacts that recipient's transplant center to offer the organ. The transplant center surgeon determines whether the organ is suitable for the selected patient in view of the patient's current health and medical history. If the organ is turned down, the transplant center of the next listed patient is quickly contacted, until the kidney is placed.

Once the organ is accepted, the OPO makes arrangements for transportation of the organ, and the transplant surgery is scheduled. Generally, standard kidneys are first offered locally based on the donor's location and according to the UNOS point system. Then, a kidney is offered to a potential candidate within the same procurement region, and then nationally, based on the point system and factoring in transportation time.

G. Survival

Chapter 12 of this Guide discusses the post-transplant survival facts for both the kidney recipient and the transplanted kidney itself. Data show that graft and patient survival are better in those receiving a living donor kidney. However, a deceased donor kidney clearly is better than dialysis, both as to patient survival and quality of life. The chart below, but also provides an appropriate summary of graft survival rates for those with a transplanted kidney or on dialysis.

Survival Rates

Time Lapsed	With Living Graft	With Deceased Graft	On Dialysis
1 year	95%	89%	77%
3 years	88%	78%	62%
5 years	80%	67%	39%
10 years	58%	40%	---

Kidney transplantation cannot exist without kidney donors. During 2010, the U.S. performed 8,887 deceased donor and 5,207 living donor transplantations. As of February, 2011, kidneys from deceased donors outpace those from living donors nearly 2 to 1.

The staggering number of patients with end-stage CKD waiting for a transplant relative to the number of available kidneys to transplant requires the continuing development of effective mechanisms to identify potential deceased donors. Concurrently, the lengthy wait for a kidney and the excessive health burden of dialysis necessitate more patient involvement in self-care to preserve health during this fragile time and to remain eligible for transplantation. That is the subject of KidneyStep 3.

12.

LIVING DONOR

I am your author who donated one of my kidneys to save my mother--your other author. Donating was not a decision I made lightly. I secretly wrestled with the donation concept since Mom's diagnosis of Alport's syndrome.

Mom talked little about her condition and never about her intentions. I believed she likely would reject dialysis, with its severe lifestyle restrictions and numerous associated health complications. I knew that she would neither request that my sister or I donate a kidney nor accept one from us if we volunteered. My sister had offered several times, and each time Mom refused.

A. Important Considerations

Originally, I had not offered my kidney and had much to consider as I contemplated the idea. I am a single mother of two young sons, and at the time, was only recently employed. My concerns, common among many prospective donors, were:

❖ What does donating a kidney mean to my long-term survival?

❖ What was the possibility of side effects or even death from the surgery?

❖ Would my employer permit a several-week leave of absence to accommodate the time needed for the required pre-donation health tests and then for the surgery and recovery?

❖ What are the potential financial burdens associated with donating?

❖ Could I obtain both health and life insurance after donation?

❖ Could I safely become pregnant in the future?

Mom had finished necessary tests for inclusion on the disturbingly long transplant wait list for a deceased-donor kidney. During the evaluation process, she was assigned a "transplant coordinator" at the transplant center. I decided to telephone that coordinator and just talk, without Mom's knowledge. Kathy Carnes, Mom's transplant coordinator at Indiana University Hospital, agreed to meet with me immediately and discreetly. In her exceptionally kind way, Nurse Carnes addressed most of my concerns and offered assistance where she could. I learned the following, applicable to many donors:

Long-term Impact. Research indicates that donating a kidney has little impact on long-term health and survival. See Section F of this chapter.

The Surgical Risk. Death or disability resulting from the surgery was unlikely, but as with any surgery, was still a possibility. National statistics reveal 3 to 4 deaths per 10,000 **nephrectomies** (surgical removal of kidneys for any cause).

Other risks of surgery included bleeding, injury to organs adjacent to the kidney being removed, wound infection, and urinary tract infection from the catheter. Those complications occur between 10 percent and 30 percent of the time. Post-operative pain is a certainty.

Financial Issues. I would have no medical expenses from donating. The recipient's medical insurance, the transplant center, and/or Medicare cover all costs associated with the pre-donation screening, the surgery, and the recovery. If the transplant recipient has inadequate health insurance, Medicare covers the donation costs, recipient and donor ages notwithstanding. The donor's family is not responsible for any medical expenses.

> **Federal legislation is pending to provide a tax credit of up to $5,000 for unreimbursed donation expenses.**

Medical insurance does not cover out-of-pocket costs such as transportation to and from the hospital, loss of income, or child care. While it is illegal to be paid to donate an organ, federal law has an exception for "reasonable payments for travel, housing and lost wages" incurred in the donation process.

Donors with financial need can obtain reimbursement of up to $6,000 for these legitimate non-medical expenses from the National Living Donor Assistance Center (NLDAC). Also, the Transplant Recipients International Organization (TRIO) has arranged with United Airlines for free air travel for donors for the transplant procedure. Some states will provide a tax credit to the donor for such costs. See KidneySteps.com for a list of such states and to link to NLDAC and TRIO.

Employment Leave. Pursuant to Federal Statute 5 U.S.C. §6327, federal employees and many state employees may use up to 30 days of paid leave each calendar year to serve as an organ donor. Generally, other donors must use vacation or sick leave for donation.

Future Insurability. Kidney donation typically causes neither higher insurance rates nor inability to obtain health or life insurance. While the recipient's health insurance will cover the donor's related medical expenses for up to one year post surgery, donors must rely on their own insurance if they have subsequent related medical problems (not a common occurrence). Some insurers have denied coverage to donors, reasoning that the donation was elective or a pre-existing condition. The 2010 Health Care Act, though, prevents denial of insurance coverage based on preexisting conditions as of 2014.

The transplant coordinator can assist in educating an insurance company if an insurability issue arises post-donation. The American Foundation for Donation and Transplantation operates the Living Organ Donors Network (LODN), which offers life, health, and disability insurance to kidney donors if the donor's transplant center is enrolled in the LODN Registry. You may link to the LODN site at KidneySteps.com.

Pregnancy. Most evidence suggests that donating a kidney does not cause health problems to the donor mother or the baby in a future pregnancy. However, experts recommend waiting at least 6 months to a year after a donation to allow the remaining kidney to obtain its maximum new growth (hypertrophy), which it will do to compensate for the loss of the other kidney. Also, experts recommend obtaining early prenatal care to screen for high blood pressure and to monitor kidney function.

In a 2008 study of 2025 women who had donated a kidney (the largest study to date), 459 subsequent pregnancies occurred. The researchers concluded that these women did not face increased hypertension, diabetes, risk of miscarriage, or premature births when compared to women who had never donated.

Presented at American Society of Nephrology
Annual Meeting, Nov. 2008

A 2009 study of 1085 living donors showed fetal and maternal pregnancies after donation were similar to those of the general population but were somewhat inferior to the donors' pre-donation pregnancy outcomes when they were younger.

American Society of Transplantation, Dec. 2009

Special Precautions. Kidney donors continue to live normal lives after the surgery. However, certain precautions are prudent. A donor should avoid high protein diets or protein supplements, which can stress the kidneys by contributing to hyperfiltration injury.

Hyperfiltration is an exaggerated increase in GFR commonly occurring after ingestion of a protein load, which can damage the glomeruli.

Long-term use of NSAIDs and related pain relievers can injure the single kidney, just as they can injure the kidneys of a non-donor. I was told to avoid over-the-counter pain relievers, including Motrin and ibuprofen, as well as allergy medications and decongestants.

Because the single kidney grows larger and heavier than normal, it is more vulnerable to injury. The American Academy of Pediatrics, American Academy of Family Physicians, and the Medical Society of Sports Medicine all recommend that people with one kidney avoid sports that involve a higher risk of heavy contact or collision, such as boxing, field hockey, football, ice hockey, lacrosse, martial arts, rodeo, soccer, and wrestling.

B. About Living Donations

The first living donation occurred in 1954 when a twin donated his kidney to his brother. Rejection is not an issue between identical twins, so the recipient brother recovered successfully. The donor brother remains alive, well over 50 years later. Since 1954, advances in immunosuppressive therapy now allow virtually all related and unrelated individuals to be considered as donors.

1. Categories of Living Donors

Living donations are categorized as:

- **Living related**: The living donor directs the donated kidney to a specific recipient who is a blood relative--a parent, child or sibling, for example. I wanted to direct my kidney to my mother.

> **Over the last 10 years, 75% of living kidney donations were living-related. Such donations have decreased 18% over the last 5 years.**

- **Living unrelated**: The living donor directs the donated kidney to a specific recipient who is not a blood relative--a spouse, friend or neighbor, for example. Mom's husband wanted to donate his kidney to Mom but was rejected as a donor because of age and hypertension.

- **Living non-directed**: The living donor donates but does not direct the kidney to a specific recipient. This is an "anonymous" or "Good Samaritan" donation, where donor and recipient may not know one another. The compatible recipient is selected from the transplant waiting list. Some transplant centers will not allow these Good Samaritan transplants for fear the arrangement involves illegal compensation. This skepticism about the motives of altruistic donors may not be justified. Public surveys in the U.S. report that up to 50 percent of adults are willing, in principle, to donate a kidney to a stranger.

- **Paired exchange:** Paired exchange involves two donor-and-recipient pairs who are not compatible as pairs but who are when interchanged.

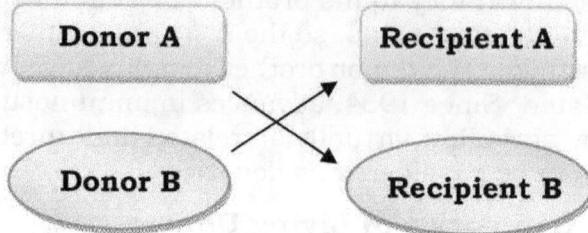

Mom's husband also could not donate a kidney because his blood type A does not match Mom's B type. A paired exchange makes donation possible in such mismatched cases. Some transplant centers initially refused to participate in paired donations for fear that the "trade" of organs violated the "no compensation" prohibition of federal law. In December 2007, the law was revised to clarify "that kidney paired donation does not involve the transfer of a human organ for valuable consideration." The change in the law should dramatically increase the paired exchange process. As of 2010, OPTN is coordinating a national project to facilitate paired donations.

> **Paired donations rose 125% between 2006-2009, but made up only 4.6% of transplants performed in 2009.**

- **Chains.** Another type of donation involves a series of donations and transplantations prompted by a single donor. In 2008, UNOS, the national organization responsible for allocating donated organs for transplant, revised its published policies to permit chain donations.

In one instance, a 29-year-old Michigan man donated his kidney, which led to 13 transplants. A chain begins when a donated kidney that does not match an intended recipient is given to a compatible recipient who also has a non-matching donor. That second donor then gives to another matching recipient, who also has a non-matching donor, and so on. If the chain is broken because no paired donor exists, a Good Samaritan donor can bridge the gap to keep the chain moving.

The problem is locating quickly a potential donor and matching recipient to prevent the chain from breaking. A national mechanism for chain matching has only recently been developed.

2. Why Living Donors?

The number of kidney transplants each year cannot keep pace with the growth in the number of patients developing kidney failure. According to OPTN[*] data as of June 2011, 88,988 individuals are awaiting a kidney. In contrast, during 2010, only 16,898 transplants occurred. The expanding waiting list and the shortage of deceased donors emphasize the importance of living donors in the transplant process.

Graft Survival Rates

After transplant	Living donor	Deceased donor
1 year	95%	89%
3 years	88%	78%
5 years	80%	67%
10 years	58%	40%

Kidneys from living donors are favored. Living donor kidneys are healthier and survive longer than grafts from deceased donors. These **grafts**, as transplanted kidneys are called, function better, as illustrated by OPTN data for kidney transplants from 1997 through 2010.

It is projected that individuals receiving a living donor kidney and surviving the first year have a 50 percent chance of surviving with it for 24.8 years, compared to 12.6 years for those receiving a deceased kidney donation.

The best graft survival rates are from identical living kidney donations (twins), and then donations from well-matched siblings. However, graft survival from living donors, well matched or not, is better than a deceased donor kidney.

---

[*] Congress established the Organ Procurement and Transplantation Network (OPTN) in 1984 as part of the National Organ Transplant Act. The United Network for Organ Sharing (UNOS) administers OPTN to collect data relating to organ transplants.

Living-kidney recipients also often take lower doses of immunosuppressants.

3. Donor Characteristics

During 2010, 5,209 living-donor transplants were performed in the U.S., accounting for over one-third of the total kidney transplants. Despite recent drops in donations, the total number of living donations over the last 10 years has nearly doubled. That increase relates to greater public awareness of the need for living donors; the increased graft survival rates (no donor wants the donated kidney to last only a short time); advances in immunosuppressant drugs; and the refinement in surgery techniques that make donation less arduous for the donor.

> **Studies find that where the transplant center meets with the patient's family and friends, living donations increase.**
> *American Society of Nephrology*
> October, 2009

OPTN Data from January 1, 1988 through October 31, 2010, show that the 104,247 living donors in the U.S. over the last 22 years have had the following characteristics:

58 % were female **42 % were male**	**45 % had type O blood** **38 % type A** **13 % type B** **4 % type AB**
71 % were white **13 % black** **12 % Hispanic** **3 % Asian**	**45 % were between** **ages 35 and 49** **35%, ages 18-34** **19%, ages 50-64**

Over the last 22 years, donors gave kidneys to the following family members:

15 % to a child	33 % to a full-blood sibling
16 % to a parent	10 % to a spouse

4. Purchase of Organs

The characteristics of donors in other countries vary significantly, in part depending on whether the country permits the purchase of organs. The United States prohibits organ compensation. In 1983, during a Congressional hearing, an overzealous doctor, Barry Jacobs (who had created his own for-profit company called International Kidney Exchange Ltd.) proposed using third-world citizens' kidneys in exchange for money. Congress reacted strongly. Tennessee congressman Al Gore vigorously attacked the purchase concept. Shortly thereafter, Congress passed the National Organ Transplant Act, which made it illegal to purchase organs:

> **National Organ Transplant Act, 42 USC§ 274e(a)—**
> **Prohibition of organ purchases.**
> It shall be unlawful for any person to knowingly acquire, receive, or otherwise transfer any human organ for valuable consideration for use in human transplantation if the transplant affects inter-state commerce.

The penalty for violating the Act is a fine of up to $50,000 and imprisonment of up to 5 years. Each state also has statutes prohibiting the purchase of body organs. Most states have adapted the Uniform Anatomical Gift Act, originally passed by Congress in 1968 and revised in 2006.

My mother and I disagree about the purchase issue. I support the prohibition against purchasing organs, because a purchase undermines the significance of the donation I wished to make. Since my mother needed a donated kidney, she was more inclined to see both the pros and cons of the organ-sale issue.

PROS:

• Financial incentives and a regulated compensation structure would encourage donations, so more donors would become available at a time when they are desperately needed. Some of the over 93,000 people currently waiting for a kidney have waited for five or more years. The median wait time is projected to reach up to 7 years for those listed in 2010. Many patients die while waiting for a kidney that never comes.

The World Health Organization estimates that up to 10% of organ transplants involve an illegal sale.

• The newest anti-rejection drugs reduce the importance of tissue matching. Almost anyone can donate to anyone else. Thus, worldwide matches through the Internet could easily be arranged in a legal and controlled manner. Internet websites exist for people seeking a kidney donor.

• Studies show that the donor's long-term health is not compromised by donating a kidney. Also, those receiving a living donor kidney have fewer rejection episodes and live longer than those receiving a deceased donor kidney. So, a person could choose to make a profit without long-term personal harm while also providing a life-saving advantage to the purchaser.

CONS:

• Wealthier kidney recipients can afford to buy organs. Unless the purchase process were properly regulated, poor individuals who suffer kidney failure would be left with dialysis or the lengthy wait to receive the inferior deceased-donor kidney because of lack of financial bargaining ability.

• The desperately poor could easily be coerced into selling a kidney. In some countries, kidneys have been sold for only a few dollars. Several states were con-cerned about the potential of compensation, and as a result, have outlawed anonymous donations. Yet, altruistic people exist who want to donate without receiving compensation in return.

- The sale of body organs is illegal throughout the developed world and prohibited by international transplantation organizations on ethical grounds. It is unethical to exploit vulnerable populations.

Despite the ethical debate regarding compensation, it remains that the exchange of money for a kidney in the United States is both a federal and a state crime.

> **The recent Declaration of Istanbul on Organ Trafficking and Transplant Tourism (created by medical leaders worldwide) is designed to end sales of organs.**
> See KidneySteps.com to link to this Declaration.

C. Informed Consent

Informed consent arguably is the most critical aspect to living kidney donation. Living donation is not designed to advance the donor's health, but rather to benefit the recipient. The living-donation process challenges basic medical ethics tenet of *primum non nocere,* "first, do no harm." Obtaining a donor's informed consent to donation and the surgery is imperative for medical and legal reasons. A donor must be fully informed of the possible risks and alternatives and then freely give consent.

1. Elements of Informed Consent

The OPTN has yet to standardize informed consent language or requirements for living donors. A steering committee consisting of the National Kidney Foundation, the American Societies of Transplantation, Transplant Surgeons, and Nephrology, and representatives of the transplant community, created recommended practice guidelines for the well-being of the live organ donor. The committee concluded that the person who gives consent to be a live organ donor should be:

"...competent, willing to donate, free of coercion, medically and psychosocially suitable, fully informed of the risks and benefits as a donor, and fully informed of the risks, benefits, and alternative treatment available to the recipient. The benefits to both donor and recipient must outweigh the risk associated with the donation and transplantation of the living organ."

These elements of informed consent are utilized in most transplant centers. Additionally, transplant centers must obtain informed consent to receive Medicare and Medicaid reimbursement for the transplants the centers perform. The elements of informed consent are applied as follows:

Competency. Competency is a legal concept requiring that the donor be an adult with decision-making capacity. Young donors (in their late teens or early 20's) require careful evaluation to explore both their maturity and understanding of the donation process and that they are not subjected to family pressure to donate.

Courts have permitted children and incapacitated adults to donate kidneys where the donor's relationship with the recipient is very close, so that both parties mutually benefit.

Willing to Donate/ Free from Coercion. The decision to donate is completely voluntary, and the donor can change his/her mind at any point, even when entering the surgery room. The donation decision is to remain free of pressure from others.

As of 2009, transplant centers must provide an independent advocate that is not part of the team caring for the recipient; this advocate independently assists and supports the donor. If the donor does not want to donate, the advocate can champion on the donor's behalf.

Certainly, I received no pressure to donate. I had told no family member that I was thinking about donating. I knew that once I made the commitment to donate, it would be

154

extremely difficult to change that decision. So, I continued with my secrecy until I had the facts I needed to be informed.

Medically/Psychosocially Suitable. A potential donor is carefully evaluated on medical and psychological grounds to ensure that the donor is fit for surgery and has no disease that could bring undue risk or the likelihood of a poor outcome for either the donor or recipient. The psychological assessment is to ensure the donor gives informed consent and is not coerced or bribed.

You may chat with kidney donors at KidneySteps.com

Risks and Benefits to Donor and Recipient. I used the Internet, textbooks, and doctor consultations to study and better understand the risks of living kidney donation for both my mother and me. I also conferred with prior donors.

Alternative Treatments. If no donation occurs, the individual with ESRD can usually continue to live on dialysis and can wait for a kidney from a deceased donor.

2. Recipient's "Health Intelligence"

One kidney transplant recipient at IU Hospital celebrated 32 years with her transplanted kidney.

I love every organ in my body, and I was particular about the type of person to receive my precious kidney. I wanted it to go to someone who also would cherish it by taking good care of it. I could expect my kidney to survive another fifty or so years if kept in me. However, that same lifespan for the kidney, once donated, is not realistic. But, with proper care, the transplanted kidney could function 20 years or more.

For the kidney to survive after transplantation, the recipient requires the "health intelligence" to adhere to a careful schedule of testing and medication. The recipient must also follow good health practices, including strict control of blood pressure, blood sugars and lipid levels, and, maintaining sound eating and exercising habits.

RECENT STUDY →

CKD patients' ability to understand basic health information impacts likelihood of receiving a transplant and surviving with it. Those with poor health literacy are 78% less likely to be referred for transplantation.

Clinical Journal of the American Society of Nephropathy, 2009

I knew my mother had the health intelligence to comply with these necessities and to understand the interplay of her habits with her wellbeing. Also, I knew that she would love and care for my kidney.

3. The Offer

The day arrived when I offered my kidney to my mother. Her GFR was down to 11 mL/min, and she was menacingly close to needing dialysis to survive. I wanted to provide a preemptive donation, one that allowed her to have transplant surgery before facing dialysis. Preemptive transplantation results in a better functioning graft and a better long-term survival for the recipient.

I arranged to meet with Mom over a glass of wine, and, hoping to soften her, I began my approach. I stressed that I had fully and completely explored the medical consequences of donating my kidney and that I wanted to donate not only to save her life, but also to keep her in my family's life. Making this gift would enhance my sense of purpose.

Despite my heartfelt and well-prepared presentation, Mom refused my kidney. In her matter-of-fact way, she stated: "I did not give birth to you to harvest your organs for my own use."

OPTN data show that **25,748 preemptive transplants occurred between October 1987 and February 2009.**

Mom may be stubborn, but so am I. I had an alternate plan, and back to the transplant coordinator I went to discuss a paired exchange. I knew Mom would not refuse a kidney donated from a stranger. Her problem was taking one from her own child.

My plan was to donate my kidney to an unknown transplant candidate. Mom would receive another donor's kidney. The complication was that Mom and I likely were a good match. We both have blood type B. A paired exchange ordinarily does not involve donors and recipients all of whom match. I was certain the transplant coordinator could work this out, though. The need for kidneys is substantial, and creativity in pairing is crucial to encourage donations.

*Interview: **Kathy Carnes*** *(Transplant Coordinator) "Jennifer's decision to donate changed my bias about a child donating to a parent. Being a parent myself, I had to agree with Vicki's decision to refuse a kidney from her healthy, beautiful daughter. Then Jennifer presented the idea of a "paired donation," which I completely supported. She was self-educated, and well-informed about donation. She could, and likely would, give her kidney to a stranger if her mother did not accept it. My mindset changed, and I then understood the joy a child could receive from this donation. I owe Jennifer a big "thank you."*

I approached Mom again, telling her I would donate to a stranger if she continued to refuse my kidney. As I hoped, she was completely undone and passionately attempted to dissuade me. I will skip over our conversations, tears, and pleading, and simply relay that Mom is realistic and was forced to accept my kidney (no law prohibits coercion of the recipient by the donor). She knew she would care for the donated organ better than a stranger would, and the good match increased the chance of survival for my kidney and for her. Also, Mom finally realized that I would enjoy the psychological gain from seeing her benefit from my altruism and knowing that I had saved a life.

The transplant was on, and I was excited. Mom felt over-whelming gratitude and guilt. We all ignored her feelings of guilt. She, quite literally, could "live" with that.

D. Pre-Donation Testing

The medical evaluation involved in living kidney donation will vary among transplant centers, with only some components mandated by UNOS. The process begins with a determination of blood type and a socioeconomic/psychiatric evaluation. It then moves into a medical evaluation of kidney function and cardiovascular status, and a search for the presence of infectious diseases and malignancies. The overall goal of the exam is to assure the donor is both suitable and healthy.

> I was physically in shape. I run, lift weights and eat wholesome food. I follow KidneySteps 4 and 5.
> So, I could easily endure surgery and had excellent odds of a quick and full recovery.

1. Psychosocial Evaluation

> I also updated my Will, power of attorney, and healthcare directives before surgery.

The psychosocial evaluation was performed early in my process. The psychologist explored my motivation for donating, looked for any hints of coercion or payment, and assessed my level of understanding of the living donation process and its risks. She searched for indications of psychiatric problems or undue stress in my life that might impair my ability to donate or recover from surgery. She inquired about my social support to assist me after surgery. The exam was aimed, in part, at fulfilling the tenet of informed consent, as many aspects of the conversation involved the elements comprising consent.

In 2007, UNOS made recommendations to standardize the psychosocial assessment, but those recommendations remain unapproved. You may link to the UNOS recommendations at KidneySteps.com if you would like to review the likely evaluation subjects.

2. Medical Evaluation

The medical exam began with blood pressure, height, weight, body mass index (BMI) calculation, and questions about my personal medical history, including my history of use of prescription or recreational drugs, smoking, alcohol, and any past kidney or urinary tract issues. The exam also required:

A. BLOOD TESTS

Mandatory laboratory evaluation included a determination of my blood type for compatibility and cross-matching with the potential recipient, and HLA tissue typing (revisit Chapter 11). I recall being startled when the lab technician drew 17 vials of blood. The hospital also checked other important health indicators, such as:

- Blood count and clotting time (important during and following surgery)

- Fasting blood glucose test (for evidence of diabetes)

- Comprehensive metabolic panel (checking for albumin, electrolyte balance, and cholesterol, among other things)

- Viral serologies (for evidence of hepatitis B and C, HIV, syphilis, tuberculosis, Epstein-Barr virus, herpes simplex, cytomegalovirus (CMV), viral infections that could be transferred in the donation process)

- Pregnancy (if male, a prostate-specific antigen)

B. RENAL TESTS

My kidney function tests included a urinalysis, two separate 24-hour urine clearance tests, blood tests, and a CT scan with contrast (see Chapter 8 regarding these tests). Because Alport's syndrome is a hereditary disease, it was important to determine whether I was affected, too. I had neither proteinuria nor hematuria, which would have eliminated me as a donor. My GFR was well above the 80 ml/min lower limit for donating.

The CT scan not only confirmed the healthy status of my kidneys, but also provided information for surgery. The scan identified the number of renal arteries and veins, kidney size, how the kidneys drain, and any abnormalities. Both of my kidneys were healthy, and the surgeons selected my left kidney for donation. The left kidney is preferred because it has a longer renal vein, making connection in the recipient easier.

> I remember the flushing sensation in my body as the dye flowed through during the CT scan.
> I also thought I had urinated during the test, a common but false feeling caused by the dye.

C. OTHER TESTS

I had several of the following tests:

- electrocardiogram (EKG) for heart function

- chest X-ray for evidence of lung disease

- Pap smear and mammogram (for women age 40 or older)

> I was pleased to receive the most thorough medical exam of my life at no cost to me.

- PPD skin test (for tuberculosis)

- colonoscopy (for donors over age 50)

While none of my tests revealed health irregularities, abnormal results would necessitate additional testing or even elimination as a donor. The kidney donor must be a healthy individual, with suitable cardiac and pulmonary sufficiency. Also, both kidneys of the donor must function well so each person is left with a healthy kidney. The screening process is strict for the protection of both donor and recipient.

E. The Surgery and Post-Surgery

1. The Big Day

On the morning of the surgery, after I was weighed, signed additional consents and changed to a gown, I walked into a cold surgery room already staffed with several medical personnel. I hopped onto the surgery table, and a flurry of activity began. One person wrapped compression bands around each leg to aid my circulation and help prevent clots. Another taped my arms for insertion of an IV and anesthetic. I was anesthetized almost immediately. I was catheterized to collect my urine, and my entire abdominal area was shaved.

I had chosen laporoscopic surgery (as do most donors) rather than open surgery. The traditional open surgery requires an incision of about 10 inches that cuts through the abdominal muscles to remove the kidney. Laparoscopic surgery, as opposed to open surgery, means less pain, a cosmetic incision, a shorter hospital stay and faster recovery.

About 75% of kidney removals in the U.S are performed laparoscopically.

Laparoscopic nephrectomy, which began in 1995, involved making a 3-inch horizontal incision below my navel, matching my prior C-section incision from the birth of my second son. The surgeon also made 3 small holes under my ribs to insert instruments, including a laparoscope which contains a miniature camera for viewing the kidney removal on a video monitor. Carbon dioxide gas was inserted into my abdomen to expand it for easier movement by the surgeon. After the kidney and its connecting renal vessels and ureter were removed, they were placed in a frozen saline slush, and the renal arteries flushed with a cold solution.

Advances such as laparoscopic surgery, which led to a decrease in pain and scarring and to a swift recovery, have the potential to boost donor numbers. Another advance occurred in 2009 at the Johns Hopkins Medical Center, where a healthy kidney was removed through the donor's vagina. Surgery requiring only one entry point at the navel is yet an additional advance. Neither technique was available to me in 2008.

An experimental technique called chimerism is being developed but is not widely used. The donor first donates bone marrow to the recipient to minimize the need for anti-rejection drugs; the donor's bone marrow changes the recipient's bone marrow. Sometime later, the donor's kidney is transplanted. The success of such an approach remains unclear.

2. Post-Surgery

Post-surgical recovery was faster for me than for Mom, but I experienced more pain. For much of my 1½-day hospital stay, I remained on a morphine pump and an IV for hydration and nourishment. The anesthesia during surgery slows the intestinal tract for a short period. However, I had liquids the night following the surgery and solids the next day. Pneumonia is always a post-surgical risk, and I was to breathe deeply into a device to exercise my lungs. While not painful in the least, the task was annoying.

The surgery was on Good Friday, and I went home early Sunday morning. Other than the pain, which lasted until the abdominal gas dissipated, I suffered no complications and was up walking the day after surgery. I was told not to lift anything over 5 pounds for six weeks to avoid hernias. I took it easy for a couple of weeks but was back to my hectic schedule after that.

While I experienced no depression following surgery, research suggests that over 10 percent of donors are prescribed antidepressants after donating. Relationships with family members can change, particularly if the donation was to a relative.

F. Living With One Kidney

Medical research on the long-term consequences to living donors using a large number of kidney-donor subjects is only now developing. Current research is positive.

1. Kidney Function / Mortality

Within days after donating a kidney, the remaining kidney increases its filtering capacity, and the glomerular filtration rate (GFR) escalates to about 75 percent of pre-donation value. Over the next several months, the single kidney grows in size to accommodate the extra filtering burden on it. This growth is called hypertrophy.

At long-term follow-up, the kidney donors may exhibit:

- increased proteinuria, along with decreased GFR
- increased blood pressure

Proteinuria/GFR. Immediately following surgery, the donor's GFR is reduced by about 50 percent but increases in a few weeks. Just like individuals with two kidneys, kidney donors show a GFR loss per decade of 4 to 5 mL/minute.

A large 2006 review of 5048 living donors conducted by the Donor Nephrectomy Outcomes Research Network (DONOR) evidenced that 7 years after donation, the average GFR of the kidney donor's remaining kidney was 86 mL/min (slightly lower than normal), and the average urine protein was about 150 mg/per day (slightly higher than normal). Additional studies also suggest that urinary protein in donors is higher compared with non-donors a decade after donation, and that increases over time. Nonetheless, this increase in protein and slight decrease in GFR are not associated with any higher than normal risk of kidney disease.

Hypertension. The incidence of hypertension in the donating population is similar to that in the general, two-kidney population. In the DONOR review referred to above, the 7-year follow-up indicated that donors may experience a 5-mmHg increase in blood pressure over the average within 5 to 10 years after donation, a clinically insignificant finding.

No kidney disease. Several large follow-up studies report the incidence of ESRD in donors is the same as in non-donors. The UNOS database also records similar results. In a 2009 follow-up study of 3688 donors, some of whom donated 35 years earlier, only 11 had developed ESRD. This translates into a rate of 180 cases per 1 million persons per year. The rate in the general population is 268 cases per 1 million persons per year. Thus, the donor rate of ESRD was lower than that of the general population! Could it be that donors take better care of themselves for better health? On the next page is a 2010 study:

RECENT STUDY ➔

Researchers at Johns Hopkins University examined the outcomes of 80,347 live kidney donors in the U.S. between April 1, 1994 and March 31, 2009. The researchers found that long-term mortality for the kidney donors was similar to or lower than mortality for the general population comparison group.

JAMA, March 2010

Likewise, in a much smaller and earlier follow-up of 400 donors 20 years later, researchers found an 85 percent survival rate compared to a 66 percent rate in a similar group of non-donors.

In the reference section for this chapter, we cite several more donor outcome studies. While the study results are positive for donor outcomes, more research is needed regarding the effects of the increased proteinuria in donors and any associated risks of cardiovascular disease.

2. Bottom Line

Living kidney donation, based on current research, has no apparent adverse effect on the donor's long-term survival. In fact, living donors tend to be healthier than the general population and live longer as a result. Nearly all (96 percent) of kidney donors would donate again and report a higher quality of life and a greater sense of self-worth and self-esteem.

More recently, transplant centers have lowered the medical criteria for accepting living donors who have some medical abnormalities such as high blood pressure, high lipid levels or obesity. This expansion of the living donor criteria may result in long-term health risks for those particular donors. Following KidneySteps 4 and 5 is particularly important for them.

G. Critical Reflections

I remain pleased with my decision to donate a kidney. That said, I observe flaws in the current donor system.

Donors and GFR. I note with dismay that the National Kidney Foundation recommends a diagnosis of CKD simply because a person has a consistently lower GFR of 60 or less, even in the absence of other markers of kidney damage. Living kidney donors often have GFR's hovering in this area, have no other indicators of kidney malfunction, and live normal, healthy lives without suffering any of the progressions of CKD. In this respect, the National Kidney Foundation Guidelines are inappropriate and may lead to faulty labeling of donors as having a chronic disease that they really do not have.

National Donor Registry. Currently, the U.S. lacks adequate long-term follow-up of kidney donors. We are rather ignored following our recovery from surgery.

Over 100,000 U.S. individuals have undergone nephrectomy for donation over the last 22 years, making donors a significant group of available study subjects for valuable data on long-term donation effects. Yet, few adequate studies of national trends in living donor outcomes exist, and most of those include small samples of donors or cover short time periods. While a registry for transplant recipients is mandated by UNOS, no mandated registry exists for donors. Medical centers have extracted living kidneys for over 50 years. Yet, only some of them routinely follow the long-term impact on the relatively small number of donors from those centers.

Surgery Follow Up. Few transplant centers systematically follow the post-transplant renal function of donors. After release from the hospital following surgery, I had two follow-up visits with the surgeon, both within 3 months of surgery. After that, I was "released" from the transplant center with no long-term follow-up tests of function. In sharp contrast, the transplant center monitors Mom, the recipient, closely for life, with significant lab tests and regular doctor visits.

UNOS has recently implemented a requirement for transplant centers to report all living donor deaths and significant medical events and to follow up with donors for 2 years post-surgery. Yet, UNOS also indicates that medical centers lose track of 40 percent of living donors after only six months post-surgery and another 40 percent after one year.

The National Kidney Foundation launched a Living Donor Council in 2010 to advocate for actual and potential donors.

A stated purpose of this new council is to identify unmet needs of donors and advocate for necessary change. Certainly, mandating a donor registry and long-term follow-up of donor outcomes are important and unmet needs.

H. A Final Word

Donating an organ and saving another person's life have substantially altered my focus and self-perception. The act of donating also sets a positive example for my children, and I have assisted others who contemplate an organ donation. As a result of the donation experience, I have left my profession as an elementary school teacher and am completing an accelerated nursing degree. I plan to practice nursing at a transplant center, helping both recipients and donors.

My mother notes that the donation act itself helps define who I am and states clearly the depth of my character. Moms can be overly complimentary to their children, but maybe she has something there. I recognize my strength and resilience as reflected in my donation decision. If asked to describe myself, I reply that I am a mother, a soon-to-be nurse, and a living kidney donor. The picture of me is not complete without adding that last point.

13.
KIDNEY TRANSPLANTATION

This chapter begins at the time your author with CKD entered Stage V or end-stage renal disease (ESRD). My inherited kidney disease was relentless, finally succeeding in destroying nearly all kidney function.

My nephrologist noted my continuing energy, ability to work full time, and lack of physical complaints. He credited my eating and exercise habits (see KidneySteps 4 and 5) as my edge over most others with ESRD. I showed no evidence of heart disease; my blood pressure was easily controlled; I needed no special diet restrictions because blood chemicals typically impacted by diet remained in their normal ranges; and, I had few outward symptoms of kidney failure.

Yet, I soon would exhibit the effects of uremia as toxins accumulated in my body because of my kidneys' progressive inability to eliminate them. Already, I evidenced hyperparathyroidism resulting from my debilitated kidneys' failure to manufacture adequate calcitriol, the active form of vitamin D. I faced three undesirable choices:

1. Begin Dialysis, either hemodialysis or peritoneal. As explained in Chapter 10, dialysis is time-consuming, restrictive, and physically difficult. The average dialysis patient lives slightly under 6 years, often only after repeated hospitalizations for infections, blood clots, and other dialysis complications. However, the average dialysis patient is older than I and usually has co-existing health issues. Still, the prospect of dialysis was dismally off-putting. I had only a few months, at best, before I would need it.

2. Wait for a Kidney.
A transplanted kidney would function much like my old ones did before they deteriorated. I began the necessary testing to qualify for inclusion on the UNOS transplant waiting list to receive a kidney from a deceased donor. Unfortunately, the number of available

> **As of February, 2011, OPTN reports that 87,795 people are waiting for a kidney, but only 16,898 received one in 2010.**

kidneys to transplant is significantly less than the number of people waiting for one. The USRDS' 2010 Annual Data Report states that 1 in 5 patients dies waiting for a deceased-donor kidney, and the median wait time is nearly 3 years and growing. Those with my rather rare blood type B can wait over 4 years.

3. Choose Death. Death is a disturbing but obvious option. I could choose death at any time by refusing dialysis. The effects of uremia are relatively swift, and pain controllable. Heart failure results quickly.

Of the three options, kidney transplantation was the easy choice with the greatest potential for restoring a healthy, productive life.

A. Transplantation, Generally

1. A Treatment, Not a Cure

Patients who receive a transplanted kidney, whether from a living or a deceased donor, usually survive years longer with the transplanted organ (called a "graft" once implanted) and have a better quality of life compared to patients on dialysis. Life with the graft approaches "normal," and the recipient generally has more energy and fewer complications than on dialysis. This appears true regardless of age, race, gender, or cause of CKD. Accordingly, transplantation is the preferable treatment for ESRD.

Transplantation, though, is a medical treatment for ESRD and not a cure. As the transplant patient progresses to end stage, the patient is exposed to the adverse consequences of CKD, such as cardiovascular disease, bone deterioration, or metabolic imbalances. These concurrent health issues may remain as problems even after transplantation. The anti-rejection and other drugs the recipient must take have associated side effects, even to the transplanted kidney itself. Most importantly, the recipient after transplant still has CKD with some of its effects, such as high blood pressure, which must be controlled. The regular exams and tests required for transplant recipients will not reflect perfect health. Blood tests reveal I remain in Stage II of CKD with a GFR in the 60's, despite successful surgery and a well-functioning graft.

That said, life after a transplant is normal in most respects. A transplant recipient can eat, work, play, and live with only minor modifications. The recipient must accommodate the use of anti-rejection drugs and the resulting increased risks for infection and cancer because of the drugs' suppression of the immune system.

Kidney Transplantation

Pros	Cons
• Post-transplant diet generally is normal • Patient is not restricted by dialysis • Patient feels and looks normal • Life expectancy is longer than with dialysis	• The wait for a deceased-donor transplant can be years • Transplant surgery carries the risks of major surgery • Some grafts fail, sometimes more than once • 90% of transplant patients have high blood pressure • Patient must take immuno-suppressant drugs for life, and these drugs have side effects.

2. Who Cannot Have Transplant Surgery?

Not all patients are suitable for transplantation. Generally, few restrictions apply to preclude the patient from a referral to a transplant center. The most common reason preventing referral is that the patient's overall health is so poor, the patient is unlikely to survive more than 2 years, even with a transplant. Such patients include those with incurable cancer or severe cardiovascular disease or who are severely debilitated.

The type of kidney disease itself and the risk that it might recur in the graft do not prohibit transplantation. Focal segmental glomerulosclerosis (FSGS) is the most

No age limit exists for transplantation. The USRDS reports that people over 50 comprise the fastest growing segment of the waiting list and receive 55% of transplanted kidneys.

common kidney disease to cause loss of the transplanted graft. The recurrence risk of FSGS is up to 30 percent in the first transplanted kidney and at least 50 percent in the second.

Type 1 diabetics may experience graft failure after transplantation. These patients are candidates for pancreas transplantation. The transplanted pancreas generally prevents the recurrence of diabetic nephropathy, but also increases the risk of complications from the transplant itself.

A recent observational study of post-transplant biopsies of transplanted kidneys confirmed that glomerulonephritis is the third most common cause of graft failure; but long-term graft survival remains good. Other forms of CKD, such as sickle cell nephropathy, reduce the risk of graft survival but do not necessarily preclude transplant surgery.

B. Evaluation for Transplant Surgery

Once the patient is referred to a transplant center, the patient is evaluated to determine suitability for surgery. Patients actively listed on the deceased-donor waiting list have been evaluated for transplantation suitability, with periodic additional evaluations to address new issues arising during dialysis that might impair transplant suitability. Patients who have a prospective living donor also require the same stringent evaluation. UNOS has not imposed uniform guidelines for valuating transplant candidates.* The evaluation process differs from one center to another. My experience was as follows:

1. Education and Consent

Patient education regarding ESRD options is an essential aspect of the transplant evaluation process. The patient must determine that a transplant is appropriate for the patient's own well-being. All potential transplant patients are asked to attend an informational session, accompanied by family and friends. The meeting I attended covered the following topics:

- The risks of the surgery and its potential complications

---

*Guidelines for patient referral and management of transplant-eligible patients are proposed by the Clinical Practice Committee of the American Society of Transplantation.

- Side effects of, and risks caused by, the immuno-suppressant drugs

- A comparison of the relative benefits of living donor and deceased donor transplantations

- Graft survival rates

- Transplantation survival compared to life with dialysis

This information assisted me in providing informed consent to the pre-surgery evaluation process and the surgery itself. The Center for Medicare Services requires that this formal consent process is made available to all potential kidney transplant patients.

2. Medical Evaluation

Once the patient and nephrologist decide transplantation is an appropriate option, the medical evaluation for the upcoming surgery proceeds. The evaluation is aimed at assessing the patient's chances of recovering from surgery, maximizing short- and long-term survival, and assessing the likely impact of transplantation on quality of life. Thus, the evaluation includes medical and psychosocial issues.

History/Physical Exam. The customary initial exam by the patient's nephrologist includes:

- A detailed medical history of the transplant candidate to determine the cause of the underlying renal disease, if not already known. This might include 24-hour urine, blood, and imaging tests. Revisit Chapter 8 for kidney function tests.

- A cardiovascular and infectious disease history, including family history.

- Laboratory studies, including blood count and chemistry.

- Compatibility testing for blood type (A/B/O), human leukocyte antigens (HLA), and for panel reactive antibodies (PRA)--tests important for matching recipient and donor. Revisit Chapter 11 for the matching elements.

The candidate also is evaluated for certain risk factors that specifically impact post-surgery graft and patient survival:

Cancer. The kidney transplant recipient is carefully screened for cancer with a physical exam, chest x-ray, colonoscopy (if over age 50), mammogram, pelvic exam and Pap smear (if female), prostate exam (if male), and blood tests. The immuno-suppressants a transplant recipient must take post-surgery favor the growth of malignant tumors.

> **The overall recurrence rate for cancer treated before transplantation is about 25%.**

So, the patient has a better chance for survival if any pre-surgery malignancy is treated before transplantation. Many transplant centers require a disease-free interval between cancer treatment and transplant surgery.

> **Many transplant centers require patients to stop smoking before transplant surgery.**

Patient Interview: *Bill, age 75, began dialysis a few months ago when transplant surgery was postponed because of his prostate cancer. Bill tells us he must wait at least another year to ensure the cancer does not recur before he can receive a kidney from his daughter.*

Infections. Immunosuppressants greatly increase the risk of life-threatening infections. The prospective transplant recipient is screened and treated for active infections prior to surgery, including influenza, pneumococcus, tuberculosis, Epstein-Barr virus, syphilis, and cytomegalovirus (CMV). The presence of human immunodeficiency virus (HIV) does not preclude a transplant, and some transplant centers show positive results in graft survival in HIV patients.

Cardiovascular disease. Patients with CKD, including kidney transplant patients, are high-risk for cardiovascular disease (CVD). CVD causes nearly half of deaths in patients who die within 30 days after transplantation. CVD also is the major cause of death for all transplant recipients. Thus, candidates undergo a stress test to assess cardiac health prior to surgery. Patients who have suffered heart attack or stroke may be unable to undergo transplant surgery. Following surgery, recipients must carefully monitor blood pressure, cholesterol, and blood sugar (if diabetic). They must also abstain from smoking. Proper diet and exercise are critical in avoiding CVD.

Patient Interview: *Nate was waiting for a kidney transplant when he developed prostate cancer. Nate said the cancer was treated 6 months ago, and he must remain cancer-free for another 18 months before he is eligible for transplantation surgery. In the interim, he is beginning nocturnal dialysis.*

Obesity. Some transplant centers will not perform kidney transplantation on obese patients (with a body mass index (BMI) exceeding 39 kg/m²). Obesity carries an increased risk of post-operative complications, wound infections, type 2 diabetes, graft failure, and death.

Bone Disorders. CKD patients nearing end stage suffer from bone disorders, often including hyperparathyroidism and dialysis-related bone disease. Transplantation is the best treatment, although elevated parathyroid hormone (PTH) levels may continue post-transplantation. To minimize bone damage during the pre-transplant period, the patient requires treatment with a vitamin D analog.

Older Patients. As of February 2011, nearly 20 percent of those waiting for a kidney transplant are age 65 or older. Of transplants performed in 2009, 1 in 6 transplants were in patients 65 and older. Elderly transplantations have increased over the years, and

> **Only about 5% of dialysis patients older than 65 years are on the transplant waiting list.**

the trend is continuing. Just as in younger patients receiving a transplant, the elderly survive longer than those on dialysis. This is true even though older transplant patients have a greater risk of death from cardiovascular disease in the first months after the surgery.

Because older patients with their limited life expectancies may not benefit from the transplant as long as would a younger recipient, particularly after spending years on the deceased-donor waiting list, some transplant centers

173

encourage them to accept an ECD kidney. Revisit Chapter 11 regarding ECD kidneys.

Liver Disease. Liver failure is an important cause of disease and death after kidney transplantation. Therefore, candidates are screened carefully for liver diseases, such as hepatitis B and C. The presence of these liver infections requires treatment before transplantation.

3. Psychosocial

The transplant candidate is screened for cognitive and psychological impairments that may interfere with the ability to give informed consent to the surgery or to adhere to immunosuppressant therapy and medical follow-up requirements. A transplant recipient must schedule lab tests on a continuous basis for the life of the graft and carefully follow a strict immunosuppressant dosage schedule. Individuals who are unable to adhere to these strict requirements cannot receive the graft. Failure to adhere to treatment recommendations is a major cause of graft rejection. Indicators of adherence inability often are evident even before surgery.

> *Patient Interview:* *Marcus, a 6-year dialysis patient in his 30's, was removed as a transplant candidate because he repeatedly "failed to show up for my required testing" for inclusion on the transplant wait list, he told us.*

During the initial transplant assessment, the psychologist/ sociologist attempts to determine how the patient copes with difficulties. The patient requires the emotional strength and social support to accept the importance of the patient's own conduct (adherence to strict drug and blood test schedules post-surgery) for graft and patient survival. Signs of avoidance, depression, mood disorders, or distortion can result in non-adherence.

> **Depression is associated with a threefold increase in non-adherence to drug/testing schedules.**

If all tests are acceptable to the surgeon and the transplant center, and if a matching kidney is available, the surgery can proceed.

C. The Transplant Surgery

My kidney transplant surgery, which was typical, proceeded as follows:

❖ I arrived at the transplant center at 5:00 am on Good Friday. After changing to a hospital gown, I was weighed, asked to sign consent forms, and questioned by medical staff, including the anesthesiologist and surgeon.

❖ In the surgery room, a whirl of activity ensued. My legs were wrapped with compression cuffs to discourage clot formation. Both arms were taped for intravenous administration of antibiotics and immunosuppressant drugs given during surgery, saline solution, and anesthetic. (I apparently annoyed the staff by bombarding them with questions during this initial activity, and a resident injected the anesthesia "to quiet me," he said.)

The renal artery, renal vein, and ureter of the donated kidney are connected, or grafted, to the recipient's leg artery and vein and to the bladder. Thus, the transplanted kidney is called a "graft."

❖ After I was unconscious, my abdominal and pubic area were shaved, a central line was inserted into the jugular vein of my neck (for the numerous blood draws and drug infusions over the next two days), a gastric tube was inserted down my esophagus, a ventilation tube was inserted into my trachea, and a catheter was placed in my bladder to collect urine.

❖ My daughter, the donor, was in an adjacent operating room. Her nephrectomy procedure started before my surgery. Timing was important so that as soon as her kidney was removed and prepared, her surgeon could deliver it to my surgeon to slip into my pelvic area (lower abdomen).

❖ The transplant surgery lasted about 2½ hours. The surgeon made a diagonal incision beginning at a center point in the abdomen just above my pubic hair line and angling up and to the right about 6 inches. The surgeon placed the donated kidney into the lower, right abdominal cavity, outside of the peritoneum. My failed kidneys were not removed.

❖ Not only did I receive the graft, but also its connected vessels and ureter. The renal artery of the donor kidney (previously branching from the abdominal aorta of the donor) is connected to the external iliac artery in the recipient. The renal vein of the donor kidney (previously draining to the inferior vena cava in the donor) is joined onto the external iliac vein in the recipient. The iliac vessels carry blood to and from the legs.

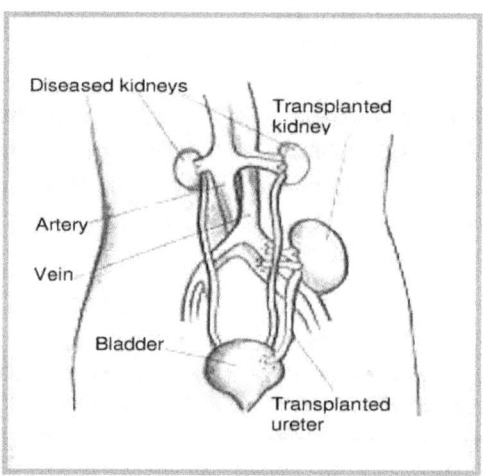

❖ The final step is connecting the ureter from the donor kidney to the recipient's bladder. A stent is inserted in the connection of ureter to bladder to keep the connection open as it heals. This stent is removed 3 to 4 weeks later in an easy and quick outpatient process. The bladder is drained with a catheter for a couple of days following the surgery to allow the ureter connection to heal.

❖ Depending on its quality, the donor kidney may begin working during the surgery or may take up to a few weeks to make urine. About 80 percent of deceased donor kidneys and 95 percent of living donor kidneys function immediately, as mine did. If the transplanted kidney fails to work immediately, the patient may undergo a short trial of dialysis.

> **At the Indiana University Hospital transplant center, 90% of deceased donor grafts and 99% of living donor grafts function immediately.**

❖ My hospital stay was another 2 days, but can be several weeks for some patients, depending on how well the graft is functioning. During this stay, my urine volume was continually measured. The surgeon kept a close watch on my serum creatinine. Proteinuria is an early marker of graft damage.

After the surgery, recovery is often swift, as was mine. The nurses monitored my urine production carefully and drew blood for chemical studies every 12 hours to identify quickly any dysfunction of the kidney and the effectiveness of the anti-rejection drugs. After just a few days, my blood chemistries showed a marked change in fluid and chemical status because of the well-functioning graft. Good graft function is almost uniform with living donors. Kidneys from deceased donors can take days to weeks to function properly.

D. Following Surgery[*]

1. Immediate Post-Surgery Complications

Immediate complications are common following surgery, and might include:

---

[*] The National Kidney Foundation sponsors the Kidney Disease Improving Global Outcomes (K/DIGO) initiative, which has developed and recently revised guidelines on the monitoring, management and treatment of kidney transplant recipients. The K/DIGO Guidelines are based on the most recent and best information available. You may view the K/DIGO Guidelines at: http://www.kdigo.org/clinical_practice_guidelines/kdigo_guideline_for_care_ktr.php

Delayed Graft Function. With delayed graft function, the patient requires dialysis following transplantation and until the graft functions. The delay in function occurs in about 3 percent of living-donor grafts. Kidneys from deceased donors, particularly those from older donors or those that have prolonged storage time, are slow to function 21 percent of the time. In most cases though, the graft performs within a couple of weeks.

Rejection. Rejection is triggered when the kidney recipient's immune system detects the transplanted kidney as a foreign object and activates antibodies, primarily T-cells, to destroy the invader. This early attack injures the graft and is called **acute rejection**. Acute rejection occurs in 10 percent of patients during the first 60 days after transplantation.

Beginning during the surgery and then for as long as the graft survives, the patient receives powerful **immuno-suppressant drugs** (anti-rejection drugs) to suppress the body's immune system, lessening the odds of attack on the graft. The current immunosuppressive therapies are effective in blocking T-cell activity, and most acute rejection episodes are prevented or reversed. These drugs are so effective that over 90 percent of transplant patients still have the organ a year later.

Sometimes, though, rejection of the transplanted kidney still occurs. Rejection does not necessarily mean loss of the organ, but does require additional treatment and medication adjustments. If the rejection episode cannot be reversed with a different mix of immunosuppressant drugs, the patient loses the graft and returns to dialysis.

Infection. Infections occur commonly, in part, because of the suppressed immune system caused by the large doses of anti-rejection drugs given during and following surgery. The patient should always report any symptoms of post-transplant infection to the transplant coordinator, such as:

- fever over 100°F (38° C)
- flu-like symptoms (chills, nausea, vomiting, diarrhea)
- coughing with yellow or green mucus
- changes in urine

- changes in pulse rate, shortness of breath, blood pressure

Thrombosis. Renal artery thrombosis (a clot in the artery to the graft) occasionally is seen in patients with clot tendencies or atherosclerosis. Thrombosis most often occurs in the 2 to 3 days following surgery. Because the clot stops blood flow to the transplanted kidney, the graft is lost. Thrombosis can occur in the renal vein leading from the kidney, also resulting in loss of the organ.

> **Following surgery, 15% of transplant patients are hospitalized for cardiovascular issues, and 20% of those for heart failure.**

Kidney transplant recipients also have a moderate risk of deep vein thrombosis, which can cause life-threatening pulmonary embolism. These clots are generally treated with anticoagulants.

Renal Artery Stenosis. Transplant stenosis (TRAS) occurs in up to 10 percent of recipients. TRAS is a narrowing of the renal artery carrying blood to the kidney, which harms the kidney.

Ureter Obstruction and Leaks. The newly connected ureter can become obstructed from swelling, compression, clots, and stones. If obstructed too long, urine backs up into the kidney and damages it.

Urine leaks can occur at the point where the donor ureter is connected to the recipient's bladder. Any leaks usually appear in the first 3 days following surgery and generally are treated without additional surgery.

2. First Few Months

The recipient is monitored closely during the first 3 months after surgery, a particularly vulnerable period for the graft. Monitoring continues on a less stringent schedule after that. While transplant centers differ on the monitoring approach, here is my experience:

❖ Two times each week, I reported to the transplant center for "clinic" that included blood draws, urinalysis, and physical exam. The lab results reflected kidney function, blood levels of immuno-suppressants, white and red blood cell counts, levels of blood lipids and other chemicals that could be affected by the immunosuppres-sants, and imbalances in electro-lytes. The doctor made adjust-ments in medication based on the clinic results.

> **Over the first few weeks, my immuno-suppressants dosages were reduced in response to the blood tests.**

❖ At home, I was to weigh myself daily (rapid weight gain may result from water retention, a sign of faulty graft function), monitor my temperature to catch infections early, and measure blood pressure. I was to report immediately any irregularities.

❖ Exercise was important. I began walking the day following surgery, and daily thereafter, increasing speed and time. Within a couple of weeks, I was walking briskly for 30 minutes every day.

❖ For 6 months after surgery, I took antibiotic and antiviral drugs to compensate for my suppressed immune system as it adjusted. Immunosuppressant drugs, twice daily forever, are mandatory. If I become too ill to take the drugs orally, I will need hospitalization for administration.

The frequency of visits and blood tests decreases over time, depending on graft function and any co-existing medical conditions. A transplanted kidney can increase its function, reaching a level of function that is about 40 percent greater than a normal level for a single kidney. Sometime during the first few months following surgery, the recipient's creatinine level will become stable, and a baseline is deter-mined. For example, my creatinine level jumped from .9 to 1.3 during the first weeks following surgery and finally stabilized at .9 to 1.0, where it has remained. Now, if the level were to rise, it could indicate graft dysfunction.

Kidney graft dysfunction is defined as an increase in serum creatinine of 15 percent from baseline. Such increase might necessitate a biopsy to determine the cause of the graft distress. Besides rejection, the increased creatinine level might indicate a toxicity caused by the immunosuppressants, which is not uncommon and still signals kidney harm.

The first year following a transplant is a critical year. Hospitalizations in the first year are relatively high, at 41 percent, primarily for rejection episodes, infections, and cardiovascular issues. If the patient survives that year with the transplanted kidney still functioning, the graft is likely to function several more years.

3. Immunosuppressants

A transplant recipient must take immunosuppressant drugs daily for as long as the graft functions. Immuno-suppressants weaken the immune system by diminishing the ability of the immune cells to function.

The most common immunosuppressant format today, used by three-fourths of kidney transplant recipients (and the one recommended in the K/DIGO Guidelines), is a cocktail of tacrolimus and mycophenolate. A minority of patients may instead take the drugs cyclosporine, serolimus, or azathioprine. Patients may also receive prednisone, for a week following surgery.

The immunosuppressants are powerful, which is necessary in preventing kidney rejection. However, the drugs impact the entire body, causing varying side effects dependent upon the drug and upon the transplant recipient's response to the drug. Cyclosporine can

Ruth Tucker received the first U.S. kidney transplant in 1950 at age 44. She received no immunosuppressant therapy, and her body quickly rejected the kidney.

be physically disfiguring, causing an overgrowth of the gums and hirsutism (excess hair) on the face and body. Tacrolimus' side effects include insulin resistance, and about 22 percent of patients taking tacrolimus develop insulin-dependent diabetes.

Prednisone, a steroid drug, has serious side effects and is less commonly prescribed. Prednisone alone usually is inadequate to prevent rejection of a transplanted kidney. When other non-steroid immunosuppressant agents are used, lower doses of prednisone are needed.

The three most commonly used immunosuppressants can have the following side effects:

Tacrolimus	High blood pressure, high cholesterol, insulin resistance, acne, unwanted hair loss, diarrhea/ constipation headache tremors changes in renal function
Mycophenolate	Anxiety, headache, abdominal pain, gastric reflux, diarrhea, trouble sleeping, cough, weakness, tumors, anemia, high blood pressure
Prednisone corticosteroids	Puffy, moon face, weight gain, glucose intolerance, diabetes, bone loss/fractures, muscle weakness, high cholesterol, cataracts, severe acne, hypertension

All these drugs cause increased susceptibility to infection and, over time, increased risk of cancers. As the likelihood of rejection of the graft decreases, the dosages and number of drugs are reduced, so side effects diminish. A recipient can expect monitoring of the blood level of drugs on an ongoing basis. An excessive level of any of these drugs is toxic, and too little a dosage results in graft rejection.

E. Long-Term Survival

A distinction is made between the death or loss of the transplanted kidney and the death of the recipient. Loss of the graft does not mean the death of the recipient, who can continueto survive on dialysis and even have a second transplant surgery. In 2009, 12 percent of the trans-plantations were performed on previous recipients.

1. Causes of Death of the Graft

While short-term survival of the transplanted kidney is surprisingly high (90 percent of grafts surviving the first year), long-term graft survival remains problematic. For example, at 5 years, only 69 percent of deceased-donor grafts and 82 percent of grafts from living donors survive.

> **Rejection of the graft after the first year often stems from patient failure to take anti-rejection drugs as prescribed.**

The leading cause of graft loss is the death of the graft recipient, most often because of cardio-vascular disease. Transplant recipients with hypertension, diabetes, or poor graft function have the greatest risk of cardiovascular death.

The second most common cause of graft loss is graft nephropathy, or disease within the graft, destroying it over a period of months or years. Causes of graft harm include:

> **Transplanted kidneys almost always show CNI toxicity over time.**

The immunosuppressant drugs: The immunosuppressant drugs can harm the graft. Tacrolimus, used in over 75 percent of transplant patients, is in a class of drugs known as calcineurin inhibitors (CNIs). Over time, CNIs become toxic to the graft, causing elevated creatinine levels.

A biopsy of the kidney will show a striped pattern of damage to the glomeruli and tubules. The offending drugs may be discontinued or the dosage reduced to help lessen the damage.

Infections: BK polyomavirus or cytomegalovirus (CMV) are common viruses that rarely cause harm in a healthy two-kidney person; however, the viruses may threaten the kidney of a transplant recipient. My daughter carries an antibody for CMV, indicating she had been exposed to the virus at some point in her life. Her immune system responded to the virus, forming antibodies to prevent further CMV infections. But the CMV virus continues to lie dormant in the organs of the infected person.

When the CMV-exposed organ was transplanted into me, the dormant virus tagged along. I had never been exposed to the virus and had no fighting antibodies specific to it. Thus, the likelihood of developing the CMV infection is increased. Without a strong immune response, a CMV infection could damage the graft. Regular lab tests include a blood test for evidence of a CMV infection. When caught early, treatment can lessen damage to the graft.

Recurrent kidney disease: The cause of the original kidney failure can damage the graft. Diabetics who fail to control glucose levels can destroy the graft over time. Certain glomerular diseases can recur, such as FSGS or sickle cell nephropathy.

Uncontrolled hypertension: Hypertension is seen in up to 80 percent of transplant recipients, which threatens long-term graft survival. The recipient must be aggressive in monitoring blood pressure and taking sufficient medication to control hypertension. The National Heart, Lung and Blood Institute recommends blood pressure targets below 130/80 mmHg for transplant recipients.

2. Causes of Death of the Recipients

According to the 2010 Annual Data Report of the USRDS, the leading causes of death in kidney transplant recipients are cardiovascular disease, infections, and malignancy.

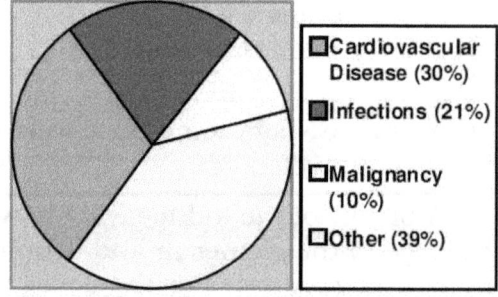

Cardiovascular Disease (30%)

Infections (21%)

Malignancy (10%)

Other (39%)

A. CARDIOVASCULAR DISEASE

Despite transplantation, the graft recipient continues to have kidney disease. As with any patient with CKD, cardiovascular disease is the leading cause of death, including for those with a transplanted kidney. Over 30 percent of transplant recipients die from cardiovascular events.

Several factors increase the risk of cardiovascular disease, including proteinuria, hypertension, high lipid levels, and diabetes. The use of immunosuppressants increases the

184

> **As many as 60% of transplant patients are obese at the time of transplantation.**

likelihood of developing such risk factors. Those drugs, in different combinations and at varying doses, can damage the graft, resulting in proteinuria, hypertension, and increased lipid and glucose levels. Being African-American, over age 60, obese, or diabetic also increases the likelihood of cardiovascular death from these combined effects.

New onset diabetes after transplantation (NODAT) also increases the risk of cardiovascular events and death. NODAT is estimated to occur in 9 percent of patients at 3 months post-transplantation, and 16 percent at 1 year, with the greatest risk of occurrence in the first 6 months. According to the 2010 Annual Data Report of the USRDS, over 40 percent of recipients have evidence of NODAT by the end of the third year after transplantation. The immunosuppresssant drugs raise the likelihood of developing NODAT, as these drugs can cause increased blood glucose levels and insulin resistance.

Anemia is also common in transplant recipients, occurring in about 30 percent of them, and increasing cardiovascular death risk. Anemia can be the result of insufficient erythropoietin production by the graft (revisit Chapter 6 regarding EPO); the drugs used (including certain blood pressure medications and the immunosuppressants); or even viral infections.

B. INFECTIONS

Post-transplant, the recipient's risk of infection increases, because of the drug-suppressed immune system. Infections can be carried to the recipient by the donor kidney or otherwise contracted by the recipient.

Donor-derived infections might include HIV, hepatitis C virus, West Nile virus, tuberculosis, or even cancer. The potential for transmission of deadly infections from donor to recipient has prompted the Centers for Disease Control and Prevention (CDC) to

> **Viral infections are most common during the first year after transplantation.**

announce plans to develop and operate a Transplantation Sentinel Network to detect and prevent transmission of diseases from donors to recipients.

For the first 6 or so months following transplantation, the recipient receives anti-bacterial, antiviral, and sometimes anti-fungal drugs to minimize the risk of infections while the recipient's newly suppressed immune system adjusts and immunosuppressant drug dosages are stabilized. Additionally, recipients are cautioned to avoid crowds when possible, wash hands often, and stay away from others with obvious illness. These are precautions that should last a lifetime.

C. MALIGNANCY

The incidence of malignancy after kidney transplantation is rising, and affects about 10 percent of recipients in the first 3 years following surgery. The 3 most common cancers impacting transplant recipients are:

- nonmelanoma skin cancer

- Kaposi's sarcoma—a malignant tumor caused by a herpes virus

- non-Hodgkins lymphoma—a cancer that begins in the lymphocytes of the immune system

When compared to the general population, the risk for development of one of these cancers is 20 times higher in the transplant recipient. Resulting death also is higher in the recipient, and relates to the drug-suppressed immune system. An important goal is finding the balance between sufficient immunosuppressant drug dosage and cancer risk.

F. Long-Term Care

For both the graft and the recipient to survive after transplantation, the recipient requires the "health intelligence" to adhere to a careful schedule of testing and medication, and to follow good health practices. The last page of this Chapter is a checklist for living a long life with your graft.

G. The Costs

You may wish to revisit Chapter 10, Part E on paying for ESRD, including transplantation. Each year, about 16,000 kidney transplants are performed, and Medicare is the primary payer for most of these. Recipients, no matter the age, are eligible for Medicare coverage for 36 months following transplant, including coverage for the costs of immuno-suppressants. Transplant recipients must take immuno-suppressant drugs for as long as a transplanted kidney functions, and these drugs can cost $1500 per month.

In 1999, Congress passed a law that restricts Medicare from paying for these necessary drugs for more than the 36 months if the recipient is under age 65. Seventy-five percent of patients with end-stage renal disease rely solely on Medicare coverage following transplant. If a person cannot show ability to pay for immunosuppressants following the 36 months, this impacts qualification as a transplant candidate. It wastes a donated kidney when patients without insurance cannot afford the drugs to prevent rejection of the graft.

On the other hand, Medicare pays for dialysis for nearly 400,000 patients, not just for 3 years but until they die. Medicare currently spends over $77,000 per person annually for hemodialysis treatments, in addition to the costs associated with these critically ill patients who, on average, have two hospitalizations a year from infections, strokes, heart attacks, and other complications of dialysis. In total, Medicare pays about $150,000 per year per dialysis patient, which is much more than the average $26,600 a year to maintain a patient after transplant.

In March 2009, bills were introduced in the Senate (S565) and the House (HR1458) to extend Medicare coverage of the drugs for as long as the patient has a functioning transplant. The bill was not passed as part of the 2010 healthcare package. Dialysis is currently using $17 billion yearly of Medicare funds and total care of these patients, which is over 10 percent of the entire Medicare budget. Promoting transplants and transplant maintenance would be much less burdensome to the Medicare budget.

H. Final Thoughts

Patient Interview (your author with CKD): The day following the transplant surgery, Dr. Milgrom, a favorite surgeon, asked me how my daughter was doing after her nephrectomy. My guilt raw, I replied, "I wish I knew for certain what the loss of a kidney cost her." Dr. Milgrom's response remains with me. "Well, it cost her something," he said. "She was born with two kidneys. But, look what she received!"

Dr. Milgrom was referring not only to my daughter's saving my life, but also to the resulting pride and expanded sense of purpose she would feel. In making the donation decision and insisting upon completing the act, she tested the depths of her own character, realizing a strength few exhibit. Her heroic act will define her forever.

I took tests at age 21 to donate a kidney to my own mother. I was greatly relieved when the nephrologist rejected me as a donor, coincidentally, because I was pregnant with my future kidney donor. If my daughter likewise had been rejected as a donor, she would have felt significant disappointment rather than the relief I had known. My daughter displayed a unique strength and love. She is amazing.

Daily Checklist

☐	**Brush and floss.**
	Good mouth and gum health lowers risks of infection and cardiovascular disease
☐	**Take immunosuppressants.**
	Don't skip doses, take exactly as prescribed.
☐	**Eat to live.**
	Eating properly increases your longevity. Follow KidneyStep 4.
☐	**Walk 30 minutes.**
	Working out benefits your heart, kidneys, weight and brain. Follow KidneyStep 5.
☐	**Wash hands often.**
	Avoid crowds and infectious situations.
☐	**Check blood pressure.**
	Hypertension damages the graft and increases cardiovascular risk.
☐	**Drink water.**
	Drink 3 to 4 quarts of liquids each day. Water and unsweetened tea are best
☐	**Take 1000 mg calcium and 1000 IU vitamin D.**
	Both boost bone density and vitamin D does even more for good health.
☐	**Monitor glucose.** (If diabetic).
☐	**Take no drugs other than what your nephrologist prescribes.**
	Even aspirin can hurt the graft.

Tests & Shots

Adhere to lab test schedule.
Tests monitor graft health and your health.

Influenza vaccination.
Once a year.

Pneumonia vaccination.
Once every 5 years.

PSA test. (if male)
Every year.

Mammogram. (if female)
Every year after age 50.

Cervical exam. (if female)
Every year after age 50.

Colonoscopy.
Every 5 years beginning at 50.

Stress test. Once a year. (You are a high risk for cardiovascular disease).

Know Your Numbers

- **Blood pressure** (120/80)
- **Blood cholesterol** (<200)
- **HDL level** (> 45)
- **LDL level** (< 90)
- **Fasting blood sugar** (< 95)
- **Vitamin D blood level** (>40 ng/L)

KIDNEYSTEP 3

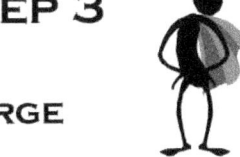

TAKE CHARGE

KidneyStep 3 encourages you to monitor and manage your health conditions and become active in your care. By doing so, you might avoid the progression of kidney disease. You will learn how to command the best treatment if you have CKD so you retain health and survive longer. If you advance to the later stages of kidney disease, self-management enables you to remain strong and functional on dialysis, and increases the likelihood that you remain healthy enough for transplant surgery.

KidneyStep 3 applies whether you:

- **Have diabetes or high blood pressure.** If you are persistent in your efforts to control these CKD risk factors, you may avoid kidney disease.

- **Have chronic kidney disease.** Your involvement in your own care may help you slow or halt the progression of CKD. Self-care may allow you to avoid heart disease and other complications that so often arise when kidneys malfunction.

- **Are on dialysis.** Your health and survival on dialysis are fragile. Your daily actions will determine how well and how long you live.

- **Have a transplant.** You, your nephrologist, and your transplant center will work together to obtain optimal health for you and the graft.

- **Have a single kidney.** Conscious focus on your own care is important to protect the solitary kidney.

The health benefits of self management and lifestyle changes are well researched. Individuals who become involved in their own care will have fewer symptoms and disease complications. Following KidneyStep 3 (along with KidneySteps 4 and 5) provides the edge you need to avoid or survive CKD, a frightening and devastating disease.

14.

TAKING CHARGE – THE OBVIOUS

The most important factor in avoiding, delaying, or lessening the impact of diabetes, hypertension, or kidney disease is not your doctor--it is you. Your physician has several hundred patients and cannot control your everyday actions or identify all of your health issues without your conscientious involvement. You are responsible for monitoring your day-to-day health status and modifying your behavior to improve that status. The more actively you manage your health conditions, the better you will do.

This Chapter highlights several factors you can control for improved health and to preserve kidney function. Committing to take charge of these lifestyle factors can make a substantial difference in your well-being and kidney status:

Manage the Obvious

Become responsible for your own care Partner with a nephrologist Avoid/control diabetes Monitor/control blood pressure Lose excess weight Reduce cardiovascular disease risks	Make lifestyle changes: Increase physical activity Don't smoke Avoid non-prescribed drugs Eat better to live longer Sleep 7-8 hours

A. Assume Responsibility for Your Own Care

Traditionally, a physician's role in healthcare was to diagnose and prescribe, and the patient's role was to comply with the physician's orders, passively accepting whatever treatment the physician doled out to the patient. This approach is much less effective for chronic diseases, such as kidney disease, diabetes, and cardiovascular disease. Effective control of chronic illness relies heavily on patient involvement and day-to-day self-management of the condition.

Self-management involves becoming informed about your condition; making your own decisions about treatment with the help of your doctor; and, setting your own management goals: what you eat, how you keep fit, and how you will control blood pressure, weight, and glucose levels. Researchers have long known that self-management improves health.

INTERESTING STUDY → Patients with chronic conditions (diabetes, cardiovascular disease, arthritis) were taught self-management skills to manage their health conditions. After 6 months of self-management, the patients demonstrated improved understanding of their illnesses, improved ability to deal with their symptoms, and greater confidence. They also exhibited health-related behaviors.

Australian Health Review, 2008

Self-management may mean that we must develop new ways to cope with illness. Some of us naturally are assertive and easily take control of health conditions and their progressions. Others are reluctant to make lifestyle changes and prefer the sick role, blaming others if they don't get better. Individuals who become active in their own care, though, will change their healthcare path and will regain control over their lives.

The *Joint Commission's 2010 National Patient Safety Goals*∗ encourage patient involvement, because involvement substantially impacts health outcomes and quality of life. These take-charge steps require you to:

- Partner with a doctor familiar with the latest clinical guidelines and standards for CKD.

- Learn what you can about kidney disease and any other co-existing condition you might have so you can ask questions and identify problems that require attention.

- Be your own advocate--understand what is available to treat your condition, and ask your physician about it.

- Work with your doctor to set goals for better management of your condition

---

∗ The Joint Commission is sponsored by the U.S. Department of Health & Human Services.

- Develop an appropriate food plan and ask to see a nutritional dietitian for special situations, such as diabetes, late-stage CKD, or dialysis.

- Understand your medications, the importance of them, and the side effects.

- Keep a health diary to remind you of your medications, appointments, and lab results.

Research illustrates that patients who take an active part in their own care have fewer disease complications, report fewer symptoms, and live longer.

- Take responsibility for your own health, including life-style changes (e.g., exercising, eating differently, quitting smoking).

Your involvement is essential for quality care. You are an "expert" on your situation, and only you know your own preferences and tolerances.

B. Partner with a Nephrologist

Can't we just trust that our family doctors will provide us with the best treatment if we are threatened by or have CKD? Unfortunately, the answer is "no." Common sense tells us that no one doctor has all the answers, and some doctors may even have embarrassing gaps in knowledge. We cannot rely on the notion that "doctor knows best." Primary-care physicians, in particular, are unable to keep up with the flood of research on every condition they see. They are unlikely to be well-trained in the area of nephrology.

If you are threatened by or have kidney disease, you are more likely to receive appropriate treatment from a physician specifically trained to treat the disease and the associated risks and complications. Such a physician is a **nephrologist**. Nephrologists have several functions in the diagnosis and care of patients at any stage of CKD, which can be a life-threatening condition. They determine the cause of the CKD, recommend specific therapy and treatment to slow progression, and identify and treat kidney disease-related complications.

The National Kidney Foundation (NKF) recommends referral to a nephrologist no later than Stage Four of CKD. Earlier is better though, because heart and blood vessel disease associated with CKD can begin well before Stage Four, and because some kidney damage can be stopped if caught and treated in earlier stages.

According to the NKF in a comment aimed at non-nephrologists, CKD is "underdiagnosed" and "undertreated" in the U.S. "This leads to lost opportunities for prevention of complications and worse outcomes for patients with chronic kidney disease."

Most people threatened by CKD never see a nephrologist for evaluation and treatment until just before reaching end stage, when it is too late to intervene meaningfully in the progression of the disease. The deteriorating patient remains under the "care" of the general practitioner, and the statistics indicate that this delay in referral to a nephrologist is seriously detrimental to the patient. Late referral to a nephrologist also is associated with a higher risk of death after starting dialysis.

RECENT RESEARCH →

Researchers analyzed data of more than 30,000 U.S. patients starting dialysis and evaluated the quality of patient care before their CKD progressed to ESRD and how that care affected dialysis outcome. Half the patients received at least 6 months of predialysis care from a nephrologist. For those patients, the chances of surviving dialysis in the first year were 50% higher than for the patients not receiving nephrologist care.

Clinical Journal of the American Society of Nephrology, 2009

According to the data analyzed and reported by the U.S. Renal Data System (USRDS),* the current treatment of individuals at risk of (or with) CKD is woefully inadequate in many important respects, primarily because the patient is

---

* The USRDS is an arm of the National Institutes of Health, National Institute of Diabetes and Digestive and Kidney Diseases. It continually collects data relating specifically to kidney disease, reports the data, and comments on trends evidenced by the data.

not seeing a nephrologist. Here are just some of the criticisms stated in the 2009 Annual Data Report of the USRDS, along with our translation of the criticisms:

USRDS Criticism:	Translation:
"Recognition of CKD, even in those who reach ESRD, is slow, and referral [to a nephrologist] is generally late. Use of diagnostic tests to track the degree of kidney failure progression and the risk factors for cardiovascular disease is also low...".	• Doctors fail to screen at-risk patients for kidney disease, even though early detection can slow or halt its progression. • Doctors delay referring CKD patients to nephrologists for better care. • Doctors fail to test CKD patients for signs of heart and vessel disease, a common killer of those with CKD.
Despite information on the use of prescription medications, "management of risk factors such as hypertension and cardiovascular disease in CKD patients is characterized by poor control of blood pressure and lipid levels."	• Doctors fail to prescribe appropriate drugs to control high blood pressure and high cholesterol in CKD patients.
"The CKD population carries a high burden of disease, and treatment and control lag behind recommended practices."	• Treatment of those with CKD is inferior to recommended medical practices.
"While 80 percent of adults with CKD Stages 4-5 have hypertension, only 20 percent are being adequately managed..."	• Doctors fail to treat hypertension aggressively in most CKD patients.

These statements of the USRDS suggest that general practitioners too often fail to intervene with proper treatment of patients with CKD and even miss diagnosing CKD and its associated diseases. Consequently, people with potential or actual kidney disease must educate themselves and become actively involved in their own care. Patients must insist upon early referral to a nephrologist, when intervention can prevent continuing damage to the kidneys or can address coexisting complications.

C. Diabetes--the Key is Control

You know from prior chapters that diabetes is the leading cause of kidney disease, which in patients with diabetes is called diabetic nephropathy. Self-management of the conditions leading to the diabetes can prevent kidney disease in the first place, or it can stop any further kidney decline if kidney damage already exists.

> **According to the CDC, diabetes is the seventh leading cause of death in the U.S.**

The number of Americans who have prediabetes or diagnosed diabetes is a startling 105 million, nearly 1/3 of the entire U.S. population. Seventy-five percent of diabetic adults also have hypertension, compounding the threat to the kidneys. About half of all diabetics develop CKD.

Recall from Chapter 9 that excess glucose levels damage the glomeruli of the kidneys, scarring and eventually destroying them. Microalbuminuria is an early sign of kidney damage. Blood tests can identify whether you have prediabetes or diabetes.

1. Address the Possibility of Diabetes

The American Diabetes Association (ADA) sets out known risk factors for prediabetes and type 2 diabetes. If you have any of these symptoms of prediabetes and diabetes, see your doctor for further testing.

- **Overweight.** Having a body mass index (BMI) of 25 or higher is the best known risk factor for diabetes. The more excess weight you have, the more resistant your cells become to insulin, causing blood glucose levels to rise.

- **Abdominal Fat.** Abdominal fat, even if you appear thin, boosts diabetes risk. It is this visceral belly fat that hinders insulin processing. The single biggest risk factor for prediabetes is having a waistline of 40 inches or more (if male) or 35 inches or more (if female).

- **Relative with Diabetes.** Whether it is genetic or environmental, diabetes tends to run in families.

- **Little Exercise.** Individuals who are not physically active substantially increase their odds of diabetes.

> **A large waist doubles your risk of cardiovascular disease and kidney disease.**
> *Vascular Health Risk Management* **2009**

- **High Blood Pressure.** High blood pressure and diabetes are related. In a recent study of 38,000 midlife women followed for 10 years, researchers found that hypertension doubled the risk of developing diabetes, regardless of BMI. The risk of diabetes rose if blood pressure increased over time--even if it stayed under the hypertension threshold.

- **High Levels of Blood Fats.** Patients with diabetes often have increased cholesterol, triglycerides, and LDLs.

- **Vascular Disease.** Excess blood glucose damages small vessels feeding nerves in the extremities, causing loss of sensation.

- **Increased Thirst.** Excess blood glucose draws water from cells, causing excessive thirst. The resulting increase in fluid intake also causes excess urination.

- **Slow-healing Cuts and Frequent Infection.** Excess glucose interferes with the body's ability to heal and fight infection.

> **The CDC estimates that 40% of adults ages 40 to 74 have prediabetes, the precursor to diabetes; and, 2 out of 3 Americans over age 65 are prediabetic.**

Prediabetes can be prevented from progressing to diabetes and CKD, if caught early. According to researchers, primary care physicians are not diagnosing and treating prediabetes early enough, and patients are not recognizing the signs of prediabetes.

Researchers examined whether 1402 people with prediabetes were adopting preventive measures to avoid diabetes, such as modest weight loss and increased physical activity. Approximately half reported that they had tried to lose weight or had increased exercise over the last year, and only one-third had been advised by healthcare professionals about helpful behaviors. A mere 7.3 percent of prediabetics were told they had the condition, and less than half with prediabetes reported a test for diabetes or high blood sugar in the last year.

American Journal of Preventive Medicine, 2010

A simple blood test can determine whether you have prediabetes or diabetes.

2. Control is the Key

You are the key in controlling blood sugar levels and in preventing, arresting, and even reversing CKD associated with diabetes. The NKF states in its *Clinical Practice Guidelines for Diabetes and CKD*:

"The success of strategies to promote glycemic control and minimize progression of CKD depends upon patient self-management, or the ability and willingness of the patient to change and subsequently maintain appropriate behaviors regarding diet, physical activity, medicines, self-monitoring, and medical follow-up visits."

Studies show that blood glycemic control through strict dietary measures, exercise, and stringent adherence to drug regimens prevents the onset of kidney disease. For example, in studies in which "non-diabetic kidneys" were transplanted into diabetic patients, the presence of damaging effects of hyperglycemia (too much blood sugar) eventually harmed the transplanted kidney. In patients who maintained control over

Diabetes increases your odds of stroke and death from heart disease by up to 4 times.

their glucose levels, diabetic nephropathy did not develop in the transplanted kidney.

A landmark study by the Diabetes Prevention Program (DPP) of over 3,200 individuals with prediabetes showed that individuals who made lifestyle changes (e.g., losing weight, exercising, eating a heart-healthy diet) were 58 percent less likely to develop type 2 diabetes than patients not making the lifestyle changes. In a 10-year follow up, most of the DPP participants who made lifestyle changes delayed type 2 diabetes by about four years, compared to the control group. Participants over age 60 halved their 10-year diabetes risk with the lifestyle changes.

A 2010 study showed that diet and exercise work twice as well as drugs in preventing type 2 diabetes.

In another long-term, 10-year follow up to the DPP study, researchers reported that when 4,883 people ages 60 and up combined five positive lifestyle factors--factors within the patients' control--they could reduce diabetes incidence by 80 percent. The health habits were:

- Physical activity
- Healthful diet
- Light or moderate alcohol consumption
- Not smoking
- Avoiding being overweight

Even for those adults without a perfect score on all five lifestyle factors, each additional positive factor reduced diabetes risk by 34 percent. Two key factors--physical activity and a healthy diet--were associated with a 46 percent lower risk of diabetes.

In a recent survey conducted by the Consumer Reports National Research Center of more than 5,000 diabetics, respondents who had successfully managed their diabetes were twice as likely as those who were unsuccessful to have lost weight with control of diet and some exercise. When it comes to winning the battle against diabetes and resulting CKD, a healthful diet and physical activity are essential and are within your control. Whether you are prediabetic or have full-blown diabetes, you owe it to your kidneys, heart, and the rest of your body to begin today to take control of your condition and follow KidneySteps 4 and 5.

D. Monitor and Control Blood Pressure

As discussed in Chapter 9, hypertension is both the second leading cause of kidney disease and a consequence of kidney disease. Up to 94 percent of individuals with CKD have hypertension. Despite strong evidence that high blood pressure is a risk factor for CKD progression, over 80 percent of people with high blood pressure fail to monitor or treat it adequately. What a risk they take!

RECENT RESEARCH → In a study of 300,000 people with no diagnosis of kidney disease, those who had blood pressure readings over 120/80 mmHg were more likely to develop ESRD than those who kept blood pressure down. The risk of ESRD in individuals with blood pressure readings of 210/120 mmHg was 4½ times greater.

International Society of Nephrology, 2010

Blood pressure is easy to measure and, for most of the 80 million U.S. adults with high blood pressure, simple to control with intervention.

1. Monitoring Your Own Blood Pressure

Monitoring your blood pressure is quick and painless and leads to tighter blood pressure control. Your regular, day-to-day pressure readings better predict cardiovascular and kidney disease risk than the occasional reading at the doctor's office. Even a modest and consistent increase in blood pressure is an independent risk factor for the unwanted progression of kidney disease.

One out of three U.S. adults has high blood pressure

A 2007 study published in the journal *Hypertension* suggested that patients who monitor their blood pressure at home are more likely to control high blood pressure and often require less medication to keep the condition in check. These patients may be more motivated to stick to diet and exercise recommendations and to take medication as prescribed.

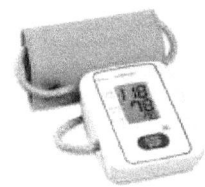 Blood pressure monitors are relatively inexpensive and are widely available at pharmacies and online. The American Heart Association (AHA) recommends an automatic cuff-style model. You place the cuff on your upper arm and press a button, or inflate the cuff with a hand-held pump. The finger and wrist versions are less accurate.

You may take your home monitor with you to your doctor's office every six months or so to assure it is accurate. The doctor will calibrate your home monitor with the office monitor. You do not want faulty information from an inaccurate monitor. The AHA categorizes blood pressure as follows:

Blood Pressure Categories

Category	Systolic (mmHg)	Diastolic (mmHg)
Normal	Less than 120	Less than 80
Pre-hypertension	120-139 OR	80-89
High/Stage 1	140-159 OR	90-99
High/Stage 2	160 or higher OR	100 or higher

I (author with CKD) take blood pressure readings at home morning and evening, as should anyone with kidney disease, diabetes, or cardiovascular issues. Following these AHA guidelines will result in more accurate blood pressure readings:

➤ Wait 30 minutes after exercising, showering, eating, or drinking.

➤ Rest your arm at heart level.

➤ Support your back.

➤ Rest feet on the floor (don't let legs dangle).

➤ Don't talk during the measurement.

➤ Check your pressure in AM and PM.

For adults ages 40 to 70, each increase of systolic pressure of 20 mmHg or diastolic pressure of 10 mmHg above 115/75 doubles the risk of kidney failure as well as heart disease and stroke.

Joint National Committee on Prevention, Detection, Evaluation, and Treatment of High Blood Pressure

Keep a written log of your blood pressure readings. Some monitors will store your measurements or will hook directly to your computer so you can upload and store your readings. The AHA has a free online site at www.heart360.org where you can log your blood pressure, glucose, cholesterol, and other important information in a password-protected system. You can take your log with you when you visit your nephrologist.

2. Take an ACE Inhibitor or ARB

Doctors treating kidney patients or individuals with diabetes, a high risk group for CKD, generally prescribe drugs for high blood pressure that directly interfere with the renin-angiotensin II cycle (revisit Chapter 6). Such drugs are:

❖ Angiotensin converting enzyme (ACE) inhibitors
   - includes lisinopril, quinapril, ramipril
❖ Angiotensin receptor blockers (ARBs)
   - includes candesartan, losartan, valsartan
❖ Renin inhibitors - includes aliskiren

Studies show that these classes of drugs help preserve kidney function, particularly for individuals with diabetes, by decreasing high blood pressure and reducing proteinuria.

> **USRDS reports that only 50 percent of people diagnosed with CKD are being treated with an ACE/ARB/renin inhibitor.**

Current studies suggest that some patients with CKD may slow progression of the disease by combining an ACE inhibitor with an ARB. In a large study called *The Cooperate Study*, progression of kidney disease to end stage was reduced by over half at the 3-year follow-up of patients on the combined drug therapy versus patients taking only an ACE inhibitor or an ARB.

Most recently, researchers are using a renin inhibitor called aliskiren to reduce blood pressure and protect the kidneys. In one study, patients with diabetic nephropathy taking aliskiren for blood pressure control had a reduction in proteinuria of up to 50 percent. The renin inhibitor was less likely to result in excess potassium in the blood of the patient compared to other classes of antihypertensive drugs. This is important because excess potassium can be a life-threatening condition in individuals with CKD.

The bottom line: talk with your physician about an ACE inhibitor, ARB, or renin inhibitor if you are not on one and you have diabetes or kidney disease. Receiving the right antihypertensive drug benefits the kidneys and also helps you avoid cardiovascular disease.

3. Ways to Control Blood Pressure

Important lifestyle changes can reduce the risk of high blood pressure by up to 80 percent.

RECENT RESEARCH → Researchers analyzed data from 83,882 women ages 27 to 44 years who participated in the second NHANES health study, funded by the National Institutes of Health. The women were followed over 14 years. Researchers found six factors associated with up to an 80% reduced risk of developing hypertension:

- BMI>25
- Daily mean of 30 min/day vigorous exercise
- Eating a DASH diet
- Modest alcohol intake
- Analgesic use less than once per week
- Intake of 400 mcg/day of folic acid

JAMA, 2009

In light of recent research, both the AHA and the American Society of Hypertension (ASH) recommend the following lifestyle changes to control your high blood pressure:

1. *Watch your weight.* In the above study, BMI alone was the most powerful predictor of hypertension. Aim for a BMI of less than 25 kg/m². Recent studies show that even a modest weight loss has an impact. Losing as little as 10 pounds can reduce blood pressure in people with hypertension and can also prevent hypertension in the overweight. Losing additional weight can have an even more dramatic effect on blood pressure.

The DASH diet is similar to the recommended diet of MyPyramid.

205

2. *Eat a DASH-like diet.* Eating a balanced diet is a proven strategy to lower blood pressure. Researchers in a large study, called the DASH (Dietary Approach to Stop Hypertension) study, followed individuals on three different diets. One diet was the typical American diet: low in fruits, vegetables, and dairy and high in fat, saturated fat, and cholesterol. A second diet was rich in fruits and vegetables. The third, the DASH diet, was a balanced diet that was lower in saturated fat, cholesterol, and sweets, and high in whole grains, fruits, vegetables, and low-fat dairy. Those on the DASH diet experienced a significant reduction in blood pressure. (The eating plan set out in KidneyStep 4 is based on the DASH diet.)

3. *Avoid salty foods.* If the DASH diet is accompanied by a reduced salt intake, the impact on blood pressure is even more significant (See Chapter 15 for salt discussion).

4. *Limit alcohol.* Reducing alcohol consumption helps reduce blood pressure. The ADA and the ASH recommend no more than 2 drinks per day for men and 1 drink per day for women.

5. *Take your blood pressure medications* (see above).

6. *Be physically active.* Regular physical activity can lower blood pressure, even if weight loss has not occurred. (See KidneyStep 5.)

7. *Avoid/limit painkillers.* Take aspirin and other over-the-counter painkillers only occasionally.

E. Lose the Fat -- It's Dangerous

Despite the irrefutable evidence that excess pounds are dangerous, one in three Americans is obese, and two out of every three U.S. adults is overweight or obese:

RECENT RESEARCH → Researchers analyzed height and weight measurements from 5555 adults as part of the NHANES health study. The prevalence of abdominal obesity was 37.8 percent for men and 55.8 percent for women.

International Journal of Obesity, 2010

Obesity predisposes individuals to insulin resistance, type 2 diabetes, heart disease, hypertension, and a host of other ailments. Overwhelming evidence establishes that

> **Individuals who are obese are twice as likely to have hypertension compared to healthy weight individuals.**

excess weight is a risk factor for the progression of CKD. Losing excess weight can improve kidney health, cardiovascular health, and diabetes.

RECENT RESEARCH →

Researchers examined trials that included 522 obese and overweight subjects and compared their levels of proteinuria before and after weight loss intervention. Weight loss by any method resulted in a significant decrease in proteinuria.

Nephrology Dialysis Transplantation, April 2010

Similarly, in another recent study:

RECENT RESEARCH →

Researchers pooled data from 13 studies that examined weight loss and its impact on kidney function. They found that adults with CKD who lost weight through diet and exercise reduced their proteinuria. The researchers also found that weight loss may prevent additional decline in kidney function in obese adults with CKD.

Clinical Journal of the American Society of Nephrology
September 2009

How fat is too fat? A body fat content of 18.5 to 24.9 percent of body weight is normal. Anything over that is overweight or even obese.

> **For a BMI calculator, go to the National Heart, Lung and Blood Institute website, www.nhlbisupport.com/bmi**

According to the CDC, the calculation of true fatness is the body mass index (BMI), a measure of your weight to height. To estimate BMI, multiply your weight by 705, and then divide that number by your height in inches squared:

$$BMI = \frac{Weight\ (lbs) \times 705}{Height\ (inches)^2}$$

An adult with a BMI between 25 to 29.9 is overweight. If BMI exceeds 29.9, the adult is obese. For example, to have a BMI between 19 and 24, a 5-foot 4-inch individual should weigh between 110 and 140 pounds. A six-foot person should weigh between 140 and 177 to maintain a normal BMI less than 25.

BMI	Weight Status
Below 18.5	Underweight
18.5 – 24.9	Normal
25.0 – 29.9	Overweight
30.0 -39.9	Obese
40.0 or above	Morbidly Obese

Fat is particularly unhealthy if the fat is in your abdominal area. Large, rounded bellies are associated with cardiovascular disease and kidney disease.

RECENT STUDY → Scientists looked at 350,000 people and found that a large waist doubles the risk of dying prematurely, even if BMI is normal.

New England Journal of Medicine, November 2008

Measure your waist. It should be 35 inches or less for women and 40 inches or less for men. To measure, place the tape measure just above the hip bones and exhale.

Metabolic syndrome is a combination of undesirable conditions linked to excess weight and diabetes. The poor health conditions that often occur together include:

- **Excess abdominal fat**. Do you have a waistline of 35 inches or more (if female) or 40 inches or more (if male)?

- **Elevated blood pressure**. Do you have higher than normal blood pressure--130/85 mmHg or higher?

- **Abnormal cholesterol levels**. Are your triglycerides 150 mg/dL or higher? Is your HDL cholesterol less than 50 mg/dL?

- **High fasting blood glucose level**. Is your normal fasting blood sugar 100 mg/dL or higher?

208

The AHA estimates 35 percent of U.S. adults suffer from metabolic syndrome. If you have a combination of any three of the above, you are said to have metabolic syndrome and are at a substantially higher risk of developing diabetes, heart disease, and CKD.

Obesity and metabolic syndrome are disproportionately concentrated among the poorest and least educated individuals. In the U.S., blacks are 50 percent more likely to be obese than are whites, and Hispanics 20 percent more likely. Further, nearly 20 percent of American children are obese, which increases their risk of diabetes and CKD.

6% of adults fall into the morbidly obese category, with a BMI exceeding 39.

Shedding excess weight through diet, exercise, and even surgery, if necessary, is shown to improve kidney function in some people with CKD. It can also ward off decline in kidney function; improve control of diabetes; lower blood pressure and cholesterol levels; and reduce the risk of heart disease.

F. Reduce your Cardiovascular Disease Risk

Nearly anything that is good for the heart is good for the kidneys. Controlling your blood glucose levels if you have diabetes, blood pressure, and weight protects the kidneys and the cardiovascular system. As stressed repeatedly in this Guide, cardiovascular disease (CVD) and CKD are intertwined; one increases the risk of the other. Even a small amount of protein in the urine increases the odds of CVD. Likewise, CVD risk factors raise the odds of CKD.

The AHA has identified 7 health factors key to a healthy heart. The AHA seven are:

- You have never smoked, or you quit more than one year ago.

- Your BMI is less than 25.

You may assess your own 10-year risk of a heart attack at http:/ /hp2010.nhlbhin. net/atpiii/ CALCULATOR.asp **or link to the site at KidneySteps.com.**

- You engage in physical activity at least 150 minutes (moderate intensity) or 75 minutes (vigorous intensity) each week.

- Your diet includes the key components (fruits, vegetables, grains).

- Your total cholesterol is less than 200 mg/dL.

- Your blood pressure is below 120/80 mmHg.

- Your fasting blood glucose is less than 100 mg/dL.

The AHA reports that only five percent of Americans meet all of the criteria for maintaining a healthy heart. Over 25 percent of Americans age 50 or older have at least two risk factors for CVD, such as high blood pressure, elevated cholesterol level, or an elevated blood sugar level. Over 90 percent of the individuals with CKD also have cardiovascular disease risk factors.

Studies show that blood pressure medication reduces heart attack risk up to 27%.

According to the Framingham Heart Study, a federal study of heart disease in Framingham, Massachusetts, a 50-year-old with none of the cardiovascular disease risk factors has only a 5 percent (for men) to 8 percent (for women) chance over the next 45 years of having a heart attack. If that individual has just a single risk factor, such as high cholesterol, the chance of a heart attack jumps to 30 percent (for women) and 50 percent (for men).

Controlling all the risk factors for CVD will extend your life expectancy and the life of your kidneys and cardio-vascular system.

G. Lifestyle Changes

You may have noticed that similar recommendations for optimal health apply whether the recommendations are aimed at kidney health, heart health, blood pressure control, or control of diabetes. The body is an interconnection of organs and systems. Poor health of one organ/system impacts the health of other organs/systems. The numerous studies on prevention and control of disease, including CKD, diabetes, and cardiovascular disease, all emphasize the importance of the following lifestyle factors.

1. Exercise

If there is a fountain of youth--a life-expectancy extender-- it is exercise. Physical activity is instrumental in maintaining good health, not only to avoid or repair cardiovascular disease and diabetes, but also to prevent, halt, or slow kidney disease. Higher urinary protein predicts future CKD, hypertension, and cardiovascular disease. Exercise reduces proteinuria, the primary sign of kidney damage, in many with CKD. As just one of numerous studies shows:

INTERESTING RESEARCH ➔ Twenty patients with CKD were assigned to a 12-week regular aquatic exercise group or to a sedentary (no exercise) group. Proteinuria decreased by 50 percent in the exercise group, while there was no change in the sedentary group.

International Journal of Rehabilitation Research,
2003

Likewise, lack of exercise is linked to increased mortality rates in those with CKD, according to a 2009 study.

RECENT RESEARCH ➔ A study of 15,368 adults followed for 7 to 9 years found a lack of physical activity increased the odds of death by up to 56% in CKD individuals compared to individuals without CKD. The data suggest that physical activity gives the CKD population a survival benefit.

Clinical Journal of the American Society of Nephrology
2009

What's more, if you have diabetes and want to improve or even eliminate it, dieting without exercise may be insufficient. Researchers analyzed data on 14,528 people from the National Health and Nutritional Examination Survey III (NHANES) health study and found dieting alone was inadequate to stave off diabetes. It also was important to have good muscle mass and strength from exercise.

KidneyStep 5 presents an appropriate physical activity program for both beginners new to exercise and for the more advanced.

2. No Smoking

Nearly 25 percent of U.S. adults smoke, and studies show a strong association between smoking and impaired kidney function,

Within 1 year of quitting smoking, heart attack risk is cut in half.

as well as progression of kidney disease. In a large Australian study of 11,000 apparently healthy people, smoking was significantly associated with damaged kidney function. Likewise, a Swedish study compared 926 CKD

Smokers are 2 to 3 times more likely to die from heart disease than non-smokers, reports the AHA. Add CKD to that, and the risk of death is more than doubled again.

patients with 998 control patients who did not have CKD. Heavy long-term smokers had the fastest progression of CKD.

Tobacco is a killer. Smoking not only hastens the progression of kidney disease, but also increases the likelihood of protein in the urine, which is the key sign of distressed kidneys. Smokers progress to ESRD or kidney failure **TWICE** as fast as non-smokers. Tobacco, whether smoked, chewed, or taken in second-hand, will kill.

Smoking's impact on health issues is multiple:

❖ The nicotine in tobacco raises blood pressure, which damages the kidneys.

❖ Tobacco use substantially increases odds of coronary heart disease, heart attack, stroke, and CKD.

Nicotine is a poisonous chemical used to kill insects (and you).

❖ Tobacco use increases odds of lung cancer by 20 times.

❖ Your smoke hurts those around you, causing them lung and cardiovascular diseases.

3. Limit Use of Medication

As presented in Chapter 9, many common drugs pose risks to kidneys, particularly to aging kidneys or otherwise damaged kidneys. The effect on the kidneys is magnified in older people because of the naturally declining kidney function with age. Decreased kidney function slows the elimination of many medications, allowing medication levels to become toxic. Common, over-the-counter pain medications, such as aspirin and ibuprofen, are among ones that become concentrated in the kidneys over time, damaging the glomeruli.

We follow a simple rule to avoid harm to the kidneys caused by many common drugstore medications. We take no drug, including pain relievers, cold medicines, or antihistamines, without physician approval. Basically, that means we take only an occasional Tylenol tablet or the drugs prescribed by a doctor who is knowledgeable about the impact of drugs on kidney function. This precaution best protects the kidneys from the inadvertent damage caused by many common drugs.

4. Eat Better to Live Longer

What you choose to put into your mouth is important. Besides creating unattractive weight, poor eating results in poor health, and your cardiovascular system is particularly responsive to your food choices. Low-quality food contains bad fats, excess sugar and salt, and toxic preservatives. The bad substances clog blood vessels, making them unnaturally rigid and causing the heart to work harder to move blood through those rigid vessels. Remember the glomeruli--the tiny capillaries that are the filters of your kidneys? Those tiny capillaries are part of that circulatory system and are impacted by diet. It is damage to those capillaries that results in kidney disease.

KidneyStep 4 sets out important eating principles: eat vegetables, fruits, low-fat dairy, high-fiber, and whole grains. Avoid refined foods, excess fats, and sweetened products.

5. Sleep--It's Healthful

A good night's sleep is about more than feeling energetic the next morning. The body needs sleep for cell repair and growth. If you sleep the 7 to 9 hours per night the experts advise, you will protect your heart and kidneys and have other health benefits. Researchers have found the following:

Lower blood pressure. Not getting enough sleep is a risk factor for high blood pressure. Researchers analyzed data for 1,741 adults who slept an average of less than 5 hours nightly. These insomniacs were five times more likely to have high blood pressure than adults who averaged more than six hours nightly. Also, a 2009 study reported that for every one-hour reduction in sleep, the risk of hypertension increased 37 percent.

> **When deprived of sleep too long, people become fatigued, suffer illness and can even die.**

A trimmer waist. People who averaged 7 to 9 hours of sleep per night had an average BMI of 24.8--almost 2 points lower than the average BMI of individuals who slept less.

Lower diabetes risk. People who sleep less than 5 hours a night on average are 3 times likelier to have diabetes, compared with those without insomnia who slept more than 6 hours.

Make it a point to indulge in some sleep, but don't go overboard. Studies suggest that those who sleep excessively--napping more than 3 hours per day or sleeping more than 9 to 10 hours every 24 hours--are over twice as likely to die from cardiovascular disease.

> **The risk of high blood pressure among people sleeping less than 5 hours per night was 500 times greater than for those logging more than 6 hours.**
> *Archives of Internal Medicine.* 2009

15.

CONTROL INTERNAL CULPRITS

Cardiovascular and bone diseases are common, co-existing problems in individuals with chronic kidney disease (CKD), often resulting in disability and death. The potential impact of these concurrent diseases begins in the early stages of CKD as the damaged kidneys become unable to maintain the proper balance of critical **electrolytes** (ee-LEK-troh-lites) or chemicals in the blood. Electrolyte imbalances become more pronounced as kidney function deteriorates. Blood tests identify these imbalances for appropriate intervention to delay or prevent heart, blood vessel, bone diseases, and early death.

A. Monitor and Control Imbalances

Electrolytes are chemicals responsible for heartbeat, nerve cell responses, brain function, muscle movements, and numerous other actions involved in living. We commonly refer to electrolytes in chemical terms. You may see them by chemical notation on your lab reports. You will want to become familiar with the chemical notation and the normal blood level of each chemical (see chart).

Electrolyte Blood Levels

Electrolyte	Chemical Notation	Normal Blood Balance	Daily Amount to Eat
Sodium	**Na^+**	135 – 145 mg/dL	Less than 1500 mg.
Potassium	**K^+**	3.5 – 5.1 mEq/L	4700 mg.* or more
Calcium	**Ca^{2+}**	8.5 – 10.5 mg/dL	1000- 1200 mg.
Phosphates	**PO_4^{-3}**	2.4-4.1 mg/dL	700 mg.*
CO_2 (Bicarbonates)	**CO_2^-**	20-29 mEq/L	Doctor determines

---

* As kidney disease progresses, your nephrologist may advise you to restrict your intake of potassium and phosphorus.

Our bodies require a perfect balance of these chemicals to function properly. Ailing kidneys cannot control electrolyte balance. Too little or too much of any of the electrolytes for too long may result in death.

1. Sodium

Sodium (Na⁺) is found abundantly in your blood and in the fluid surrounding your cells. Most of the sodium you consume is from salt (sodium chloride); but, additives in packaged, canned, or frozen foods also contain salt in other forms, such as sodium phosphate, sodium carbonate, or sodium bicarbonate (baking soda).

> Researchers found that decreasing salt intake to less than a teaspoon a day lowered risk of stroke by 23%.

You need salt to live. Its two components, sodium and chloride, are essential for numerous body functions, including fluid balance and muscle movement. Even if you ate no salt whatsoever, you would still receive what you need, the equivalent of one-third of a teaspoon (500 mg.) per day, naturally from meat, fruits, vegetables, and grains.

Most Americans eat a surprising 3500 to 7000 mg. of salt each day--several times the maximum 1500 mg. recommended by the American Society of Hypertension for blacks, people ages 40 and over, and individuals with high blood pressure, diabetes, or kidney disease. These groups together comprise about 70 percent of the U.S. population. As of 2010, the American Heart Association (AHA), the CDC, and the National Academy of Sciences recommend the same 1500 mg. limit for everyone else.

Healthy kidneys eliminate excess sodium eaten and maintain the amount of sodium in the body at a precise level. Nephrons in your kidneys control sodium levels by filtering out the excess into the urine. When your body needs more sodium, your kidneys will reduce the amount they filter from the blood.

When kidney function declines, the damaged kidneys cannot efficiently remove excess sodium. Initially, undamaged nephrons excrete more than their share of sodium in an attempt to maintain proper sodium balance.

216

Eventually, though, the excess sodium is not removed and may lead to salt-induced hypertension, heart attacks, or strokes.

Physiology Basics:

Excess sodium draws water from your cells and into your blood and the spaces around the cells. You may notice edema or swelling of your hands, feet, or face caused by the excess water in the blood and tissues. This excess water also causes shortness of breath, a rise in blood pressure, and excessive work for your heart. At the same time, your cells become dehydrated. The dehydrated cells cannot function properly; you begin to feel fatigue, irritability, and confusion. Eventually, seizures and coma will result if the condition is not corrected.

The relationship between excess sodium intake and hypertension is well established. Remember the DASH study mentioned in Chapter 14 and its positive effect on blood pressure? A follow-up (the DASH-Sodium study) investigated whether reducing the amount of salt in three different diets could help lower blood pressure. It did. The biggest pressure reduction occurred in the subjects who followed the DASH diet while limiting salt intake to 1500 mg. daily. In those subjects, 84 percent achieved blood pressure control.

Substantially limiting salt intake can improve not just blood pressure, but also kidney function. Consistent experimental evidence links "increased salt exposure with kidney tissue damage," according to a 2006 report in the *American Journal of Nephrology*. Likewise, a 2009 study showed that a reduction in salt intake results in "significant reductions in urinary albumin and albumin/creatinine ratio," as well as a reduction of high blood pressure:

RECENT RESEARCH → People with stubborn high blood pressure (would not budge even with multiple hypertensive drugs) reduced their blood pressure by slashing sodium intake to just 1,150 mg/day. The low-salt diet also lowered the protein in urine (indicating improved kidney function) and reduced cardiovascular and osteoporosis risks. *Hypertension, Journal of the American Heart Association, 2009*

Experts, including the AHA, promote a lifestyle approach to lowering blood pressure, including following a DASH-like diet with low sodium intake. The American Dietetic Association released a 2009 position paper on diet and blood pressure, promoting the health advantages of a vegetarian diet in reducing blood pressure. The beneficial components of the DASH diet and plant-based diets include potassium, magnesium, antioxidants, good fats, and fiber. We address salt reduction and the DASH diet in more detail in KidneyStep 4.

2. Potassium

Potassium (K⁺) is important for several body functions:

- Potassium is necessary for fluid balance. About 95 percent of the potassium in your body is inside your cells, with the rest in the fluid outside the cells, including in your blood. The potassium inside the cells helps balance sodium that is outside the cells to maintain pressure and water balance in the body.

> **Potassium helps reduce the risk of kidney stones by causing the body to excrete citrate, a compound that leads to stones.**

- Potassium is important for nerve and cell function. It assists your muscles in contraction (including heartbeat) and in nerve impulse conduction.

- Potassium helps maintain blood pressure. It signals the kidneys to excrete excess sodium from the body. A diet with plentiful potassium (lots of fruits, vegetables, grains, and nuts) is shown to help lower blood pressure.

- Potassium aids in bone health. It helps keep the bone-building minerals, calcium, and phosphorrus, from being lost from the bones and excreted by the kidneys.

According to the *2010 Dietary Guidelines for Americans*, adults should consume 4700 mg. of potassium daily, but the average American diet contains only about 2300 mg. per day. Potassium is commonly found in fruits and vegetables. The

Dietary Guidelines recommend at least 7 servings of fruits and vegetables each day to meet potassium needs. The average American eats less than 4 servings per day.

Potassium-Rich Foods

Fruits	Vegetables	Other
Apricot	Beans	Bran products
Banana	Beets	Chocolate milk
Cantaloupe	Broccoli	Molasses
Grapefruit	Brussels Sprouts	Nuts
Honeydew	Cabbage	Seeds
Kiwi	Carrots	Peanut Butter
Mango	Greens	Yogurt
Oranges	Lentils	
Papaya	Potatoes	
Prunes	Squash	
Raisins		

If your kidneys function relatively well, you can consume as many potassium-rich foods as you want without any known danger from excess potassium. Any excess potassium is excreted by the kidneys into your urine.

However, as kidney disease progresses, the ability of the nephrons to excrete potassium decreases. Initially, the still-functioning nephrons will increase the amount of potassium they excrete to compensate for the loss of other nephrons. As the kidneys' filtration ability declines, the damaged kidneys are unable to remove the excess potassium from the blood, causing **hyperkalemia** (high-per-kuh-LEE-mee-yuh).

A patient with progressive CKD should have regular blood tests to measure blood potassium levels. A normal level is reported as 3.5 to 5.1 microequivalents per liter (mEq/L). Anything outside of normal limits is dangerous.

When left untreated, hyperkalemia can cause irregular heartbeats, heart failure, and death. To compensate, a patient with failing kidneys must restrict dietary potassium to maintain serum potassium levels within normal limits. This is particularly important for dialysis patients who have little or no remaining kidney function.

3. Calcium, Phosphorus, Vitamin D

A. CALCIUM

Calcium is the most abundant mineral in your body, located primarily in bones and teeth. Calcium has several functions:

- Calcium works with phosphorus to provide strength and structure to your bones and teeth. Calcium makes up almost 40 percent of the weight of your bones. You need an adequate dietary supply of calcium to maintain bone mass.

- About one percent of calcium is in your blood, muscles, and tissues. Calcium is needed to dilate and contract blood vessels, assist with blood clotting, and help your nervous system transmit messages.

Calcium Food Sources (mg.)

Milk (1 c.)	306
Yogurt (1 c.)	419
Cheese (1½oz.)	300
Broccoli (1 c.)	62
Kale (1 c.)	94
Canned salmon w/bones(3 oz.)	250

- Studies suggest that calcium from a heart healthy diet, the DASH diet for example, can help lower blood pressure.

- Some research suggests that diets inadequate in calcium stimulate fat production and storage, which increase the risk for obesity.

The Department of Agriculture recommends that adults get 1,000 to 1,200 milligrams of calcium daily, depending upon age. Most adults consume less than 800 mg. daily.

If the diet is low in calcium or the kidneys are impaired and cannot maintain a proper balance of calcium in the blood, calcium leaves bones to correct improper levels. If this leaching of calcium from the bones continues, the bones become less dense, brittle, and weak. Osteoporosis and bone fractures can result.

B. PHOSPHORUS

Phosphorus is the second most abundant mineral in the body. About 85 percent of phosphorus is located in your bones, with the remainder in your cells and blood.

Phosphorus has several important functions:

- Phosphorus works with calcium for building and maintaining bones and teeth. Phosphorus also helps form your cells' membranes.

- Phosphorus helps store energy generated from the metabolism of carbohydrates, protein, and fat from food.

- If your blood becomes too acidic, phosphorus helps neutralize it, bringing it back into balance so tissues are not damaged.

- Phosphorus is part of the structure of your DNA, your genetic code.

Phosphorus Food Sources (mg.)

Raisin bran cereal (1 c.)	**259**
Cheese (1 oz.)	**161**
Corn (1 c.)	**169**
Milk (1 c.)	**232**
Yogurt (1 c.)	**331**
Chicken breast (3 oz.)	**194**

Adults need about 700 mg. of phosphorus daily. On average, Americans consume over 1000 mg. daily.

As with all electrolytes, phosphorus must exist in the body at a precise level. Healthy kidneys maintain the perfect balance of phosphorus by excreting excess phosphorus into the urine. As kidneys deteriorate, they fail to maintain a phosphorus balance, leaving too much in the blood.

Consistently high phosphorus levels can accelerate the loss of calcium from bones, increasing the risk of osteoporosis. In a recent study, dialysis patients who took a phosphate binder to reduce phosphorus levels in the blood appeared to reduce their risk of death up to 30 percent in the first 90 days of treatment.

When phosphorus comes from sources such as soft drinks that lack calcium, the phosphorus binds to calcium present in the blood, keeping it from being adequately absorbed.

> **Researchers saw a two-fold increase in odds of faster than normal decline in kidney function in people drinking 2 or more colas per day.**
> *American Society of Nephrology, 2009*

C. VITAMIN D

Vitamin D is neither a mineral nor an electrolyte, but we mention it because of its important role in regulating calcium and phosphorus. Calcium, phosphorus, and vitamin D work together to build and maintain bones. You will recall from prior Chapters that the ultraviolet rays of the sun convert a compound in your skin to a previtamin D form, which is then converted to an inactive form of vitamin D in your blood. As your blood flows through the kidneys, the kidneys convert the inactive form of vitamin D to the active form called calcitriol (see Chapter 6).

Calcitriol acts as a hormone, stimulating the intestines to absorb calcium and phosphorus from your diet, thereby helping to maintain healthy levels of these minerals in your blood and bones. Calcitriol also signals your kidneys to decrease the amount of calcium excreted in the urine. These actions help maintain the appropriate level of calcium in your blood for critical nerve, muscle (including the heart), and cell activities.

As kidney function declines, the damaged kidneys are unable to convert vitamin D from food and sunlight to calcitriol. Without this active form of vitamin D, the kidney patient cannot absorb adequate calcium and phosphorus into the blood and bones, and bones may become brittle and weak.

Even in individuals without CKD, vitamin D deficiency is prevalent. Experts estimate that nearly 80 percent of U.S.

adults are deficient in vitamin D, which results in increased blood pressure and arterial inflammation.

Scientists followed nearly 28,000 patients ages 50 and older with no history of heart disease. They found that patients with very low levels of vitamin D were 77% more likely to die, 45% more likely to develop coronary artery disease, and 78% more likely to have a stroke than patients with normal vitamin D levels. They were also twice as likely to develop heart failure.
Intermountain Medical Center, 2009

It is easy to test for and remedy a deficiency. Your doctor can order a vitamin D analysis, measuring 1,25-dihydroxy vitamin D concentration in the blood. Optimal levels exceed 30 ng/ml, but levels of 50 ng/ml or higher are better. If your level is low, you can:

- Get 10 to 15 minutes of sunlight per day (without sunscreen). If you live north of a line between Atlanta and Los Angeles, the winter sun is too weak to give you the dose you require for adequate vitamin D.

- Eat vitamin D-rich foods (salmon, tuna, fortified juice, or milk).

- Take a vitamin D3 supplement.

Scientists link a deficiency in vitamin D with a host of health problems, including heart disease, cancer, and auto-immune ailments.

For CKD patients, a regular vitamin D pill is unlikely to help with a deficiency, as kidneys may be unable to convert vitamin D to calcitriol. Your nephrologist will prescribe a vitamin D analog that equates to calcitriol.

D. INTERACTION OF CALCIUM, PHOSPHORUS, AND VITAMIN D AS KIDNEYS FAIL

In patients with CKD making inadequate calcitriol, the blood levels of calcium and phosphorus become erratic--the calcium level becomes too low, and the phosphorus level rises too high. When blood levels of calcium drop, four pea-sized, tiny glands in your neck, the parathyroid glands, release the parathyroid hormone (PTH). PTH works with calcitriol to cause calcium to leave your bones and enter the blood.

As CKD worsens, the parathyroid glands enlarge and overwork, producing excess PTH, a condition called **hyperparathyroidism**. Excess PTH accelerates withdrawal of calcium from the bones and deposits it into the blood in an attempt to increase blood calcium to balance the excess phosphorus. Too much PTH in the blood removes too much calcium from the bones, and over time weakens bones. The calcium can end up in blood vessels where it does not belong, damaging the heart and vessels. High PTH can cause:

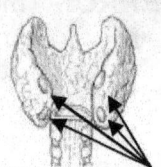

(Back of Thyroid Gland)

Parathyroid Glands

- Heart and vessel problems
- Weak bones, bone pain, skeletal abnormalities
- Anemia
- Nerve damage
- Itching

Renal osteodystrophy (REE-null OS-tee-yoh-DISS-truff-ee) occurs when kidneys fail to maintain proper levels of calcium and phosphorus in the blood, and too much calcium is lost from the bones. It is common in those with CKD and affects 90 percent of those on dialysis. If renal osteodystrophy is not treated, the bones become thin and weak, and the person may feel bone or joint pain and suffer bone fractures.

To diagnose renal osteodystrophy, your nephrologist will check the levels of calcium, phosphorus, PTH, and calcitriol in your blood. Normal levels of each are:

Normal Blood Level

Calcium	8.5 - 10.5
Phosphorus	2.4-4.1 mg/dL
Vitamin D	above 30 ng/ml
PTH	10-55 pg/ml

Treating renal osteodystrophy involves controlling PTH levels. A diet change and medication usually are effective. In extreme cases, the parathyroid glands are surgically removed. If kidneys are not making adequate calcitriol, a synthetic prescription form is taken by pill or injection. Diet changes include reducing potassium intake (*e.g.,* limiting milk, cheese, beans, peas, nuts) to about 400 mg. per day to reduce the leaching of calcium from bones. Exercise also increases bone strength.

4. Bicarbonates

Blood has an acid-base or pH status that is kept in the narrow range of 7.35 to 7.45 for cells to function properly. Even small changes in blood pH can be harmful or even fatal. The lower the pH number, the more acidic the blood. With a blood pH below 7.35, a condition called **acidosis** sets in, which can result in a coma. A blood pH above 7.45, known as **alkalosis,** can result in convulsions.

> **The blood of a person with normal kidney function is slightly alkaline (more base than acid).**

As your body's cells metabolize food to make energy, they release acidic wastes such as ammonia and urea that disrupt the acid-base balance, making blood too acidic. Normal kidneys regulate the acid balance, getting rid of the excess. When a person has CKD, the kidneys fail to eliminate acid from the blood, and acidosis results. Acidosis causes the body to lose protein, leaving the body undernourished and fatigued. Chronic acidity also leads to bone disease and accelerates kidney damage.

A blood test can measure your acid-base status by measuring the concentration of carbon dioxide (CO_2) in your blood. The CO_2 in your blood is in the form of bicarbonate. The lower the CO_2 concentration, the more acidic the body fluids.

Most patients with CKD develop acidosis, but sodium bicarbonate (or "baking soda") easily corrects this condition. Sodium bicarbonate is available in Tums and other antacids. Your nephrologist will determine the proper dosage.

RECENT RESEARCH → Sodium bicarbonate supplements significantly slowed the loss of kidney function and improved the health status of those with advanced CKD in a 2-year study. Creatinine clearance declined at a rate that was two-thirds slower than that of similar patients, and progression to ESRD occurred less often in those given sodium bicarbonate.

Journal of the American Society of Nephrology, 2009

B. Keep Cholesterol in Check

Cholesterol (koh-LESS-ter-all) is a waxy, fat-like substance that is vital to human health. Your cells need cholesterol for proper cell membrane function. Your body uses it to make bile acids, hormones, and vitamin D, among other essential chemicals. However, your liver is able to manufacture all the cholesterol you need. Any extra cholesterol accumulates in artery walls, forming plaque. Plaque narrows these blood vessels, making them less flexible. This condition is **atherosclerosis** (ATH-eh-roh-skleh-ROH-siz), often called hardening of the arteries.

> **A 2010 study of 25,000 patients found that about 50% of the time, doctors fail to set proper cholesterol goals for patients, thereby under-treating high cholesterol.**
> March 2010

If excess plaque builds up in the arteries of the heart (your coronary arteries), the heart muscle suffers, and coronary heart disease may result. A blood test will measure your total cholesterol, which is the sum of all cholesterol in your blood. It should be below 200 mg/dL.

Fatty cholesterol and blood, just like oil and water, do not mix. Thus, cholesterol travels through your blood in packets called **lipoproteins** (LIH-poh-PRO-teenz), with proteins on the outside and the cholesterol inside. When you have a cholesterol blood test, the lab measures two main types of lipoproteins:

- **Low density lipoprotein**, LDL, is the bad cholesterol that carries fatty cholesterol to your body tissues. Most cholesterol in your blood is LDL. An optimal LDL level is less than 100 milligrams per deciliter of blood. That is a little less than one-half cup in your entire bloodstream.

- **High density lipoprotein**, HDL, is the good cholesterol that carries cholesterol away from your tissues to your liver for removal. While an HDL reading of 40 mg/dL is normal, you prefer a reading of over 60 mg/dL, according to the

National Heart, Lung and Blood Institute's
National Cholesterol Education Program.

Triglycerides are the most common form of fat in your blood. Triglycerides are made up of mostly saturated fatty acids called **saturated fats,** whereas those that contain mostly unsaturated fatty acids are **unsaturated fats.** We will address these fats in KidneyStep 4. A fasting blood test shows your "fasting triglyceride" level, which should be below 150 mg/dL.

This chart summarizes the different lipids and their normal levels.

Lipids and Levels

Type of Lipid	Normal Level	Borderline	Undesirable
Total Cholesterol	Less than 200	200-240	above 240
Low-density lipoprotein (LDL) bad cholesterol	Less than 100	130-159	160-189 or above
High-density lipoprotein (HDL) good cholesterol	Above 40 (60 or above is great!)	35-39	below 35
Triglycerides	Below 150	151-199	above 200

Excess lipids in the blood, **hyperlipidemia** (high-per-lip-eh-DEE-mee-yuh), is common in patients with CKD, especially in those with nephrotic syndrome. Studies suggest that hyperlipidemia not only is a risk factor for cardiovascular diseases, but also may enhance the rate of kidney disease progression.

Because cardiovascular disease is so common a killer of patients with CKD, lipid control is a goal of treatment for people with kidney disease. According to the National Heart, Lung and Blood Institute, proven ways to lower total cholesterol, triglycerides, and LDLs include:

- Getting 30 minutes of physical activity daily.
  This also helps raise HDLs (follow KidneyStep 5).

- Limiting saturated fat and adding fiber to your diet (follow the eating plan in KidneyStep 4).

- Losing 10 pounds (if overweight).

- Taking cholesterol-lowering medication, if necessary.

C. Revisiting Diabetes

While we discussed diabetes in previous chapters, we address it again in this self-management section of the Guide because CKD is so often caused by diabetes. Type 2 diabetes is manageable, even preventable. A variety of tests can diagnose prediabetes or diabetes. Among them are:

Fasting Blood Glucose. This is the traditional blood test for diabetes. Blood is drawn after the patient has fasted for at least 8 hours. The 2010 standard guidelines established by the American Diabetes Association (ADA) provide the following regarding fasting blood glucose levels:

2010 ADA Fasting Glucose Levels

Fasting Blood Glucose Level	ADA Designation
<100 mg/dL	Normal
100 to 125 mg/dL	Prediabetes
>125 mg/dL	Diabetes

Recent data suggest a blood glucose reading over 90 milligrams per deciliter requires further evaluation. The CDC reports that one-third of U.S. adults has impaired fasting glucose levels.

Hemoglobin A1c. In contrast to the spot blood tests that measure glucose level only at the moment, the A1c blood test provides a broader picture of blood glucose by averaging blood glucose levels over a 2- to 3-month period. The A1c test measures the amount of glucose that has attached to a portion of the hemoglobin molecule in the blood.

228

ADA Guidelines for A1c

A1c Level	Status
4.5% to 5.9%	Normal
6% to 6.5%	Prediabetes
6.5% or above after 2 separate readings	Diabetes

Hemoglobin is a protein that carries oxygen in your red blood cells. The red blood cells live in the blood for 60 to 90 days. As your blood circulates through your body, glucose in the blood attaches to the hemoglobin, becoming hemoglobin A1c. Normally, hemoglobin A1c makes up about five to six percent of the total hemoglobin in blood. A higher A1c percentage means a greater amount of glucose existed in the blood over the 2- to 3-month period. The ADA standard guidelines on A1c are reflected in the above chart. Recent research suggests A1c results as low as 5.5 percent may signal prediabetes.

Oral Glucose Tolerance Test. In this test, blood is drawn immediately prior to drinking a premixed glucose formula and then again one hour, two hours, and perhaps three hours later to determine the body's ability to regulate blood glucose. The results are compared to the following ADA Guidelines.

ADA Guidelines for Glucose

Blood Sugar	Status
140 mg/dL to 159 mg/dL	Increased risk for diabetes
160mg/dL to 200 mg/dL	High risk for diabetes
Over 200 mg/dL	Full-blown diabetes

Numerous studies have linked hyperglycemia (high blood sugar) with the risk of proteinuria and diabetic nephropathy. As discussed in Chapters 9 and 14, if diabetic nephropathy is identified in its earliest stages, damage to kidneys can be slowed or prevented with strict glycemic control.

D.   Anemia is a Common Problem

1. What is Anemia

Anemia is common in CKD and has a profound impact on the patient. Anemia is a below-normal level of either **hemoglobin** (HEE-muh-globe-in) or **hematocrit** (hee-MATT-oh-krit). Hemoglobin is a protein in red blood cells that carries oxygen to all cells, tissues, and organs throughout the body to enable them to metabolize food for energy. Without oxygen, cells fail to generate enough energy for the muscles and organs (*e.g*, heart and brain) to work properly. Hemoglobin also makes red blood cells red.

> **Hemoglobin is normally about 1/3 the value of the hematocrit.**

Anemia is defined by the World Health Organization as a hemoglobin (Hb) concentration of:

- Less than 13.0 g/dL in adult men and non-menstruating women

- Less than 12.0 g/dL in menstruating women

Hematocrit is the percentage of red blood cells in a blood sample. Anemia is present if hematocrit falls below 37 percent. If you have too few red blood cells, then too little oxygen is carried to the body's cells.

An anemic person tires easily and, because of too little oxygen carried to the body's cells, looks pale and may develop heart problems. Patients with both CKD and anemia have an increased risk of death, stroke, or heart failure. The lack of oxygen makes the heart work harder. Anemia can lead to an increased heart rate and eventually may cause the lower left side of the heart to thicken, making it more difficult for the heart to pump. This condition is called **left ventricular hypertrophy** (LVH) and is evident in 45 percent of renal patients not yet on dialysis. In the CKD patients who need dialysis, up to 80 percent have LVH.

Anemia may begin in the early stages of kidney disease, when the patient is unaware of having CKD, and worsen as kidney function decreases. Nearly all people with ESRD have anemia. The incidence of anemia in those with CKD increases as the estimated glomerular filtration rate (GFR) declines.

Population studies* suggest that the incidence of anemia at each stage of CKD is: ➔

CKD and Anemia

CKD Stage	% with Anemia
I and II	less than 10%
III	20% to 40%
IV	50% to 60%
V	more than 70%

Anemia results when the failing kidneys do not make enough of the hormone erythropoietin (EPO). As explained in Chapter 6, this hormone stimulates the bone marrow to produce the proper number of red blood cells needed to carry oxygen to all of your organs. As kidney function decreases, EPO deficiency increases, making anemia worse. Individuals with CKD may suffer from iron deficiency or poor nutrition, both of which can contribute to anemia.

> **In diabetes, anemia hastens kidney damage.**
> *Diabetes Spectrum,* 2008

2. Iron: An Associated Problem

A **complete blood count** (CBC) blood test will measure your iron level to ensure that it is not contributing to your anemia. Iron is an essential component of hemoglobin, necessary in oxygen transport. According to the CDC, iron deficiency is the most common nutritional disorder in the world. If your body is deficient in iron, body stores will be depleted, and iron-deficiency anemia results.

> **Meat, poultry, and fish provide heme iron for hemoglobin.**

---

* Such important studies include the National Health and Nutrition Examination Survey (NHANES) by the National Institutes of Health, and the Prevalence of Anemia in Early Renal Insufficiency (PAERI) study.

The CBC lab results reveal your iron levels in two measurements: your TSAT and serum ferritin.

- The TSAT indicates how much iron is available to make red blood cells. The TSAT score should be between 20 and 50 percent. A TSAT score of less than 16 percent in an anemic patient with CKD evidences an iron deficiency.

- The ferritin level indicates the amount of iron stored in your body. The ferritin score should be no less than 100 micrograms (mcg) per liter(L) of blood and no more than 300 mcg/L.

Many people with CKD need both EPO and iron to correct anemia. If iron levels are too low, EPO alone will not correct the anemia.

3. Treating Anemia

Treatment of anemia in those with CKD appears to increase life expectancy. The *National Kidney Foundation's Kidney Disease Outcomes Quality Initiative* (K/DOQI) *Clinical Practice Guidelines* recommend annual screening for anemia in all patients with any stage of CKD. If anemia is present, further tests are needed to determine the cause of the anemia.

Your nephrologist may prescribe an EPO stimulating agent and iron supplements to help correct anemia. However, recent research suggests that raising the hemoglobin level above 12 g/dL in people with kidney disease increases the risk of heart attack, heart failure, and stroke. The U.S. Food and Drug Administration recommends a target hemoglobin of between 10 and 12 grams per deciliter, particularly when treated with EPO. Thus, you should receive regular blood tests, including a CBC, to monitor your hemoglobin, particularly if you are treated with EPO.

E. Obtain Lab Results

Your laboratory blood test results provide the best measurement of your health status. Even in the later stages of CKD, you may "feel" fine and believe you are doing well. You may not be aware of the extent of your kidney disease or developing cardiovascular disease. If you have diabetes or hypertension, those chronic ailments are silently and continuously destroying the glomeruli of your kidneys. Even a small amount of albumin in your urine substantially increases your risks of heart and vessel disease and raises your risk of early death. Accordingly, it is important to have ongoing lab tests to identify potential or advanced problems for aggressive treatment.

To participate effectively in your treatment, you must know your test results. Obtain a copy of the lab results. Then, find out what those results mean and what you can do to correct any abnormal values.

RECENT STUDY → A study headed by a doctor at Weill Cornell Medical College identified an alarming percentage of patients who never received their abnormal lab test results, which often results in a failure to treat.

Archives of Internal Medicine, 2009

The next page is a record sheet for you to use to keep track of your lab results and compare your results to the normal values/normal limits.

Description/ Normal Level	Date	My Result	Date	My Result	Date	My Result
Sodium (Na) 135-145						
Potassium (K) 3.5 - 5.1						
Phosphates (PO_4) 2.4 – 4.1						
Calcium (Ca) 8.5-10.5						
Carbon dioxide (CO_2)/ 20 - 29						
Vitamin D>30						
Cholesterol< 200						
Triglycerides ≤150						
LDL< 100						
HDL (high is good) > 40						
Hemoglobin (Hgb) 12 - 15						
Hematocrit (Hct) 37-49%						
TSAT 20 - 50%						
Ferritin 100 - 300						
PTH 10 - 55						
Creatinine 0.6 - 1.4						
GFR						
Fasting Glucose < 100						
A1c 4.5 - 5.9						

16.

COPING, DEPRESSION, DEATH

Chronic diseases are ongoing, generally incurable medical conditions that include chronic kidney disease (CKD), diabetes, cardiovascular disease, and cancer, among others. Chronic diseases are the leading cause of disability and death in the U.S. According to the Centers for Disease Control and Prevention (CDC), chronic diseases are a costly public health challenge, accounting for 75 percent of the more than $2 trillion spent yearly on health care. The USRDS reports that CKD alone costs $57.5 billion, 28 percent of Medicare spending annually. An estimated $34 billion, about 6 percent of the entire Medicare budget, is spent solely on dialysis patients.

> **The CDC reports that more than 1 in 10 Americans has 3 or more chronic diseases.**

Our healthcare system is extremely responsive in treating patients with acute medical problems, such as heart attacks, broken bones, infections, etc. However, patients with a chronic disease may see doctor after doctor, without relief. According to a research group at Johns Hopkins University, individuals with a chronic disease, on average, see three different physicians and fill seven prescriptions per year. People with five or more chronic conditions make 12 physician visits each year and fill 50 prescriptions.

> **Most individuals with CKD also have at least one other chronic condition.**

No wonder 50 percent of patients with chronic illnesses are depressed, according to the survey results obtained by the 2009 National Council on Aging. The CDC states that untreated depressive disorders become chronic and are expected to be second only to heart disease in the global burden of overall disease by 2020.

A. Coping with Chronic Disease

Professionals apply 5 (sometimes 7) stages* of acceptance to describe the grieving process an individual goes through when faced with a traumatic event. The grief-evoking event might be a death, some other significant loss, or the discovery that one has an incurable disease. In the case of a diagnosis of chronic illness such as CKD, the grief often is related to the loss of one's own expectation of good health and to the potential loss of self to deterioration and death. If the patient's CKD progresses to end stage, the grief may also stem from the loss of a normal life because of the time restrictions and diet burdens associated with dialysis. The 5 grieving stages, though not always sequential, are described as follows:

1. **Denial.** When diagnosed with CKD (and perhaps associated diseases of diabetes, chronic high blood pressure, cardiovascular), the patient commonly attempts to minimize the psychological impact of the diagnosis. The patient may think of the diagnosis as a mistake or inconsequential, refusing to accept its true significance. This delay allows the patient time to process the difficult news at a manageable pace. The denial stage is often characterized by a lack of crying as the patient refuses to believe the diagnosis is real.

> **As your author with CKD, I was angry with my family doctor, who failed to tell me about my elevated creatinine until after a second blood test 3 years later and after I had lost much of my kidney function.**
> **Lesson:**
> **Get copies of lab reports and ask questions about them.**

---

* In 1969, Dr. Elizabeth Kubler-Ross proposed five stages of acceptance that individuals pass through when facing death. Dr. Kubler-Ross described these stages in her book, "On Death and Dying." These stages are applied in many loss situations, including discovery of a chronic illness. Some commentators include two additional stages, when depression lifts and when the individual begins reconstructing life, working toward acceptance.

A certain amount of denial may be appropriate, to allow the individual to continue with a normal life. In denial, the patient may ignore medical advice, which could result in faster progression of the disease. However, in its later stages, CKD becomes undeniable.

2. **Anger.** Discovering one has a chronic disease, particularly a disease that may well progress to total organ failure, can make one angry. The thought might be, "Why me?" or "It's just not fair." The patient might be angry for getting sick, or for not having taken certain steps to prevent the disease. The patient might be angry at the healthcare system for not diagnosing the disease earlier or because no cure exists for CKD.

Often it is fear that underlies the anger. At initial diagnosis, the patient may know little about the disease. Learning about CKD helps lessen the fear and anger. Eventually anger tends to fade away as the person learns to live with the disease. Too much time in this stage, though, can result in bitterness that alienates family and friends.

3. **Bargaining.** Bargaining is much like denial. In denial, you attempt to forget that you have the disease. In bargaining, you accept that you have the disease, but you convince yourself that it will go away if you just do something differently. The next urine test for protein will be improved, or the next blood test will show a lowered creatinine level.

It is common for patients to follow a special diet in hopes of reversing kidney disease or to start exercising and stop drinking alcohol, actions that are contrary to what they have done in the past. Certainly, these steps might be helpful, and this Guide encourages exercise and good eating habits; but, these changes in behavior may become harmful if the patient chooses them instead of seeking medical treatment. Some alternatives (like herbal treatments) can worsen kidney function.

4. **Depression.** Depression is common in individuals who suffer from chronic illnesses, including CKD, and is a grieving stage often difficult to surmount. On average, 20 percent of CKD patients suffer from depression. The depression can be evident shortly after diagnosis.

Depression often is associated with taking medications. Upon a diagnosis of chronic kidney disease and associated high blood pressure, the need for prescription drugs begins. This sudden reliance on drugs causes feelings of dependence on the medical system, along with a lack of independent control. The feelings of powerlessness and hopelessness can contribute to feelings of depression.

> **The more pills a patient takes, the lower their quality of life. Dialysis patients average 19 pills per day.**
> *Clinical Journal of the American Society of Nephrology, 2009*

As addressed later in this chapter, lingering depression directly contributes to a worsening of chronic disease symptoms and increases the likelihood of developing other chronic diseases, such as cardiovascular disease, obesity, or diabetes. Lingering depression also increases risk of earlier death.

5. **Acceptance.** We eventually may learn to live with our diagnosis of CKD and whatever other diseases we have, even though feelings of loss or sadness linger. Acceptance is knowing that we have CKD, even though we would prefer not having it, and deciding that we will comply with proper treatment recommendations and any necessary lifestyle changes to enjoy a quality life.

B. Depression in CKD

According to the American Association of Kidney Patients, depression is a serious medical issue impacting nearly 30 million Americans every year. While depression rates in the general population are 5 percent, depression in patients with CKD can rise to 50 percent as the disease progresses to end stage.

1. Depression and Kidney Disease

On average, one in five patients at any stage of CKD is depressed. The depression arises from the kidney disease itself, the drugs the patients takes, or both. This rate of depression in CKD is much higher than the rate in the general population or in patients with other diseases. According to the Centers of Medicare, depression rates are:

Depression Rates	
General population	5%
Diabetes	11%
Cardiovascular Diseases	14-16%
CKD	20%

The rates of depression double in people with multiple chronic disorders.

Even in the early stages of CKD and long before end stage and the need for dialysis or transplant, depression is prevalent.

RECENT STUDY → Researchers examined the rate of depression in 272 kidney patients by evaluating them with clinical interviews and applying standards set in the *Diagnostic and Statistical Manual of Mental Disorders, 4th Edition (DSM IV)*. *DSM IV* is considered the gold standard in evaluating depression. Over 21% were depressed. The mean age was 65, and diabetic patients were twice as likely to suffer depression as those without diabetes. Nearly 63% of the patients had at least 3 other medical conditions, and 41% had at least 4 other conditions.

American Journal of Kidney Diseases, September 2009

Depression severely impacts the ability of the patient to take an active role in self-management of the chronic illness. A depressed patient loses the motivation to be proactive, follow diet restrictions, take medications, and have laboratory tests. Researchers in the above study noted that people with diabetes and depression may not adhere to their medications and physicians' advice, which may contribute to CKD development.

Quality of life is particularly affected by dialysis dependence when the patient reaches ESRD. Only 12 percent of dialysis patients continue to work even part-time, and the death rate for dialysis patients is high, with only one-third of the patients surviving six years. The physical difficulty of dialysis adds to the burden of CKD and increases the rate of depression. Dialysis patients diagnosed with depression are nearly twice as likely to be hospitalized or die within a year as their non-depressed counterparts.

RECENT STUDY ➔ Researchers monitored 98 dialysis patients for 14 months. More than 25% were clinically depressed. Over 80% of the depressed patients died or were hospitalized, compared to 43% of the non-depressed patients. Cardiovascular events led to 20% of the hospitalizations. The addition of heart disease or diabetes increased the CKD patients' risk of death or hospitalization by 30% when compared to patients without those coexisting problems. If the patient also had depression, the risk of death or hospitalization was increased by 100%.

Kidney International, 2008

As illustrated by the prior two studies, kidney disease patients commonly have simultaneously existing chronic illnesses, most notably diabetes, hypertension, cardiovascular disease, or lung disease. In its *2010 Annual Data Report,* the USRDS indicated that older individuals with CKD have the following rates of co-existing chronic conditions:

The greater the number of co-existing illnesses the patient has, the greater the odds of depression.

Percentage of CKD patients with co-existing illnesses	
Diabetes	48+%
Hypertension	91+%
Cardiovascular Disease	77%
COPD (lung disease)	25+%
Cancer	19%
Anemia	52%

Each added co-morbidity increases the likelihood of depression, and the depression, in turn, increases the likelihood of early death from the chronic disease. This direct relationship between depression and worsening of chronic disease is particularly evident in CKD patients. Patients with CKD who are diagnosed with depression are twice as likely to be hospitalized, progress to long-term dialysis, or die within a year from their CKD as patients who are not depressed.

RECENT RESEARCH →

Researchers monitored 267 patients with CKD for a year; 56% of the patients had a depression diagnosis based on DSM-IV. Nearly 61% of the depressed CKD patients either died, progressed to long-term dialysis, or were hospitalized within the year, compared to 44% of the patients without depression.

Journal of the American Medical Association, 2010

The American Association of Kidney Patients reports that:

- Depression is associated with worse outcomes for CKD patients.

- Depressed CKD patients are more than twice as likely to be on dialysis, hospitalized, or die within a year.

- Patients with depression are 42 percent more likely to develop diabetes than non-depressed patients. In turn, patients with diabetes are 57 percent more likely to develop depression than those without diabetes.

- Depression among kidney transplant recipients doubles the risk of graft failure, return to dialysis, and death.

2. Depression in Related Diseases

The special interrelationship between depression and disease is evident from research on chronic conditions common in CKD patients:

Researchers analyzed data of 900 patients with heart disease. If the patient also had diabetes and depression, the risk of dying increased by 30%.

Cardiovascular Disease (CVD). Individuals who are depressed develop heart disease twice as often as non-depressed persons. Depressed patients are more likely to smoke and be physically inactive, which is associated with increased mortality, making them vulnerable to coronary artery disease.

Depression is also predictive of stroke. Individuals with depression are twice as likely as those with few depressive symptoms to have a stroke within ten years. Depressed patients who have a stroke are more likely to die than are non-depressed stroke patients.

Depression is as deadly as smoking. In a survey of over 60,000 people over 4 years, the mortality rate was increased to a similar extent in depressed people as in smokers.

Depressive disorders are related to heart attack risk, with depressed patients suffering heart attacks four times more often than patients with no history of depression. After a heart attack, patients are much more likely to experience severe depression.

Diabetes. Depression is twice as prevalent among persons with diabetes than among non-diabetics, and depression makes diabetes worse. Studies show that when diabetics are depressed, their blood sugar is less well-controlled. Compared with their non-depressed peers, patients with diabetes and depression report frequent overeating of sweets and high-fat foods and are less satisfied with their ability to adhere to a diabetic diet.

RECENT STUDY →
In a pooled study involving 820,900 people followed for over 13 years, the researchers found that death rates from various causes were higher in diabetics than non-diabetics. They calculated that a 50-year-old diabetic without heart disease would die six years earlier than someone without the disease.

New England Journal of Medicine, March 2011

Likewise, people with diabetes and depression have higher rates of diabetic complications and fill more prescriptions than those without depression. Health expenditures for persons with diabetes and depression are nearly five times higher than for diabetics without depression.

Treatment of depression is associated with improved glycemic control in diabetics. Yet, less than 25 percent of those with depression are diagnosed and treated. The failure to diagnose and treat the depression so commonly associated with diabetes results in needless suffering and substantial financial loss.

Obesity. In a 2010 analysis, researchers found that obesity was associated with a 50 percent increased risk of developing depression. In turn, depressed, overweight patients had a 56 percent increased risk of becoming obese. When the overweight/obese learn to modify their eating behaviors and dietary choices, they show decreased psychological distress and become more physically active.

3. Detecting/Treating Depression

According to researchers, physicians are likely to miss the depression suffered by their CKD patients. The patient is consulting with the health professional about the CKD. Yet, both the patient and the physician should expect that the patient diagnosed with CKD will exhibit signs of depression--irritability, withdrawal from friends and family, fatigue, pain, mental sluggishness. The untreated depression leads to increased disability and decreased survival rates.

> **Physicians often fail to ask the patient, "How are you coping with your disease?" Patients fail to volunteer their mental and emotional states to the doctor without such encouragement from the doctor.**

The National Kidney Foundation (NKF) suggests that patients with depression take steps to lessen the depression, such as to:

- Be open about your feelings with your family. People who communicate openly about their feelings and complaints need less treatment and report fewer symptoms, including depression symptoms.
- Seek support from other patients in your position.
- Discuss your concerns with a hospital social worker or an outside counselor.

> **Death rates in CKD patients increased among those who believed their treatment was less effective in controlling their disease.**
> *Nephrology Dialysis Transplant, 2009*

243

- Get regular exercise within your limitations. Exercise is a mood lifter, helps you maintain muscle strength, and can improve metabolic impairment that occurs in diabetes, cardiovascular diseases, and CKD.

> **Despite reduced kidney function, many antidepressants are safe for use by patients with CKD.**

- Avoid making your family members feel guilty or directing anger at them about your illness.

- Find out as much as you can about your CKD and your other illnesses. Such knowledge assists you in obtaining the best treatment available and in maintaining a sense of control over your condition.

- Keep involved in daily living. This keeps you connected to living and boosts your self-confidence.

RECENT STUDY → Researchers analyzed data from 40 clinical trials involving more than 3,000 patients with chronic diseases. They found that patients who exercised regularly reported a 20% reduction in anxiety symptoms. *Archives of Internal Medicine, 2010*

The NKF also recommends that the depressed patient obtain professional help if the following occur:

• Depression lasting more than two weeks	• Loss of interest in activities you used to enjoy
• Thoughts of suicide	
• Loss of appetite or increased appetite	• Repeated angry outbursts
	• Drug or alcohol abuse
• Too much or too little sleep	• Inability to make decisions
	• Social isolation

RECENT RESEARCH → Researchers found that older U.S. persons who are socially isolated and lack social support report poorer general health twice as often as older persons satisfied with their social support. *American Journal of Public Health, 2009*

The National Institutes of Mental Health indicate that only 25 percent of all people suffering from depression obtain help. Of the 25 percent treated, 80 percent of them report a significant improvement in their depression.

C. Death - A Choice

When a patient with kidney disease reaches ESRD, death is imminent without a kidney transplant or the application of external life support, which for renal patients is dialysis. The USRDS reports that most patients with ESRD receive dialysis because a donor kidney is not immediately available. Once the patient is on dialysis, the wait for a donor kidney may be years, or a kidney may never become available. Many patients on dialysis have, or develop, other chronic diseases that prevent them from qualifying for transplant surgery, even if a kidney becomes available. Consequently, dialysis becomes permanent, and withdrawal means death.

1. Withdrawal from Dialysis

Depression and withdrawal from dialysis are common among patients with ESRD. Kidney patients are significantly more likely to withdraw from dialysis (with death resulting) than persons in the general population are to commit suicide.

CURRENT RESEARCH → Researchers tracked 465,563 dialysis patients for five years. Their dialysis withdrawal rates were compared with suicide rates in the general population. The researchers found that dialysis withdrawal rates were 24.2 per 100,000 patient/years, while the rate of suicide in the general population was only 1.84.

Journal of the American Medical Association, 2010

In the past, researchers typically referred to withdrawal from dialysis as suicide. Today, though, withdrawal is widely accepted as an end-of-life medical choice, legally available to the patient. The ESRD patient may decide to stop dialysis or any other life support when quality of life is unsatisfactory. In refusing dialysis, a patient is refusing treatment, allowing himself to die rather than committing suicide. Nearly 30 percent of deaths in dialysis patients occur after the cessation of dialysis.

The risk for withdrawal from dialysis is highest in the first three months after dialysis initiation. It remains relatively high for the first year of dialysis, and diminishes steadily over time. Older age and recent hospitalization are stronger predictors of dialysis withdrawal.

> **Patients with ESRD had an 84% higher rate of "suicide" compared with the general U.S. population.**

Several studies have demonstrated that patients who withdraw from dialysis have a high burden of illness, including malnutrition, physical impairment, and a high frequency of other chronic diseases or cancer. The decision to stop dialysis usually occurs because the patient is dying from another illness. The families of the withdrawing patient may be relieved by, and in agreement with, the withdrawal decision. They may view it as a "good death" that has eliminated suffering.

> **Portrait of a Withdrawing Patient**
> - **Older, white, female in first year of dialysis**
>   ***or***
> - **Has had years of dialysis**
> - **High educational level**
> - **Lives alone**
> - **Has multiple illnesses**
> - **Recently hospitalized**
> - **Is otherwise dying**

In contrast, being white or Asian, having alcohol/drug dependence, or having been hospitalized for mental illness are stronger predictors for suicide in the general population. The families of the suicide victim are often shocked by the death. They may see the death as unnecessary and a waste.

For some patients who are frail, bedbound, and otherwise near death, the burden of dialysis and its complications outweigh the benefits. Elderly patients with ESRD often have multiple physical impairments and high rates of depression. This combination of conditions may make it unreasonable to expect dialysis to be beneficial. As one researcher put it:

"When does the prolongation of living turn into the prolongation of dying?"

CURRENT RESEARCH ➔ Researchers studied the outcomes of 3702 U.S. nursing home residents who underwent dialysis between June 1998 and October 2000. The study found poor overall outcomes the first year of dialysis, with 58% of the oldsters on dialysis dying, and 27% having a decreased functional status (ability to feed selves, get dressed, brush teeth, etc.). Only 13% functioned as well as they did before dialysis.

New England Journal of Medicine, 2009

Because of (i) the increasing number of elderly (ages 75 to 84) starting dialysis with a combination of chronic illnesses, (ii) the adverse impact of dialysis on that group of patients, and (iii) the associated high cost, the Institute of Medicine of the National Academies has recommended the development of clinical practice guidelines for "evaluating patients for whom the burdens of renal replacement therapy [dialysis] may outweigh the benefits." Under such guidelines, the

Some researchers suggest that in the elderly with multiple chronic illnesses, kidney failure may be a sign of the natural dying process.

medical staff would discuss "conservative" care with the elderly and ill. "Conservative" treatment does not involve dialysis. Instead, the physician would focus on drugs to decrease the adverse symptoms of kidney failure as the patient dies.

2. Choosing to Forgo Dialysis

A clear gap exists between end-of-life care for CKD patients who have reached the point of needing dialysis and patient preferences. Patients with advanced CKD are often unhappy with the medical decisions made as their disease worsens. They want end-of-life care that considers their own goals and a realistic approach in view of the burdens of dialysis. Researchers surveyed 584 late-stage CKD patients as they approached the need for dialysis between January and April 2008. This is what the researchers learned:

1) These ESRD patients reported they would like their kidney-care team to help them plan for the future in case they become incompetent to make decisions.

2) They wanted help in relieving pain and other symptoms.

3) Sixty-one percent regretted starting dialysis, noting that their decisions reflected physician or family preferences rather than a personal choice.

4) Less than 10 percent of the patients had discussed end-of-life care issues with their kidney specialists.

5) The vast majority of late-stage CKD patients die in hospitals, but more patients wanted to die at home (36.1 percent) or in a hospice facility (29 percent) than in a hospital (only 27 percent).

To help close this gap in physician practice versus patient preference, the Renal Physicians Association and the American Society of Nephrology have developed *Clinical Practice Guidelines on Shared Decision-Making in the Appropriate Initiation of and Withdrawal of Dialysis, Clinical Practice Guidelines Number 2*. These guidelines recommend shared decision-making about dialysis, with patients fully informed, and with appropriate healthcare professionals involved in palliative care to manage the medical, psychosocial, and spiritual aspects of end-of-life care. These *Guidelines* suggest that if the patient is dying, the patient be counseled about terminal care issues rather than urged to initiate dialysis.

The result of not initiating--or withdrawing from--dialysis is death within a short time. In making this decision, the NKF recommends that patients consider the following:

1. **The dialysis treatment**. If the treatment itself is the root of the decision, can the treatment be altered? Can the patient switch from in-center dialysis to

home dialysis? Those on home dialysis live longer and feel better.

2. **Depression**. If depression is driving the withdrawal decision, the depression should be treated.

3. **Religion**. Religious convictions may contribute to the concern some patients have about withdrawing from dialysis. Concerned patients can talk with their religious advisors.

4. **Dying**. After stopping dialysis, the patient will live a few days to a few weeks, depending on whether the patient has any remaining kidney function. The patient's body will fill with fluid and toxins, in part from the food and water the patient continues to consume. The fluid will make breathing difficult. The toxins will cause fatigue, nausea, nerve damage, itching, restless legs, and muscle cramps. Medications can help make the patient comfortable.

   Studies identify the most common physical symptoms patients experience upon withdrawal from dialysis. Some of these symptoms can be controlled with drugs:

Symptom	Frequency
confusion/agitation	70%
pain	55%
dyspnea (breathing difficulty)	48%
nausea	36%
seizures	27%
edema	21%

5. **The money**. Medicare and other insurance continue to cover the costs associated with CKD after the patient stops dialysis for hospice and nursing care.

6. **Restarting dialysis**. If the patient changes his/ her mind about stopping dialysis, the patient can restart. It may be painful at first because of the excessive buildup of waste in the body.

7. **Legal documents**. At some point, the patient will become unable to make medical decisions and will require a trusted individual to take over those decisions. The patient requires the documents to assure the patient's medical wishes are followed (Living Will and Powers of Attorney).

KIDNEYSTEP 4

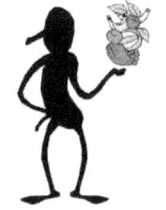

EAT FOR HEALTHY KIDNEYS

For people at risk of (or with) kidney disease, nutrition and lifestyle choices play a critical role in overall health. KidneyStep 4 helps you analyze your eating habits and identify areas where changes will benefit your health.

What you eat will impact your health, vigor, and outcome in kidney disease. Nutrition also plays a critical role in both the prevention and management of many conditions closely associated with kidney disease, including cardiovascular disease, diabetes, and high blood pressure.

KidneyStep 4 looks at why your body needs certain nutrients--including fat, protein, and carbohydrates--and why individuals who care about the health of their kidneys must be particularly careful about food choices. Improving high blood pressure, diabetes, and overall health by making proper dietary changes are the goals of KidneyStep 4. By following the principles in KidneyStep 4, you will see the link between what you eat and how you feel.

17.

POOR NUTRITION LEADS TO POOR HEALTH

Americans eat too much, according to all leading health authorities, including the U.S. Departments of Agriculture and Health and Human Services ("USDA"). Two-thirds of Americans are overweight, and one-third are obese. This obesity epidemic costs billions in associated healthcare expenses from the resulting heart disease, diabetes, hypertension, kidney disease, certain cancers, and numerous other ailments.

Example of Too Many Americans

America is fat, gaining excess weight by eating too many calories that often have little or no nutritional substance--empty, dangerous calories. Individuals of all ages load up on colas, sweets, fat-laden fast foods, packaged snacks, chips, and other convenience store items that hardly qualify as "food." These substances do little more for the body than add weight and contribute to poor health.

Patrick: *"I know you are writing this book, so here is an example for you," Patrick offers. "I was in line behind an obese woman to pay for my gas at a gas station/convenience store. The heavy woman was purchasing a 32-ounce fountain coke and a large bag of potato chips. It was only 9 a.m. She stated to the cashier, as she ripped open her chip bag, that she was tired of going to her doctor with health complaints, only to have him tell her to lose weight."*

Like the misguided lady in the prior example, many Americans "just don't get it." How we look, what we weigh, and our health status are largely related to what we eat. Diets high in fat, sugar, salt, and calories contribute directly to obesity, high blood pressure, diabetes, and CKD. As the indelicate (but accurate) aphorism goes: "Crap in--crap out." KidneyStep 4 is about controlled, healthful eating and avoiding poor food choices that harm your body, shorten your life, and damage your kidneys.

A. America's Weight Issue

The number of overweight or obese adults more than doubled (tripled for some age groups) during the past 40 years. The most recent data indicate that 72 percent of men and 64 percent of women are overweight, with 34 percent of adults now obese. Our weight problem is classified as epidemic by the U.S. Surgeon General and the CDC.

Excess pounds are largely caused by overeating. The eating habits of the typical American differ dramatically from habits 40 years ago. In our current society, most people rarely cook full meals at home, but instead eat pre-packaged or restaurant food. Fast food is readily available at drive-throughs, gas stations, convenience stores, and shopping malls. Much of this food is heavily processed, leaving it devoid of nutritional value.

> **People who live in neighborhoods with readily-available fast food restaurants have a greater incidence of obesity.**
> *Journal of Urban Health,* 2010

Moreover, portion sizes of food have doubled over the past 40 years. "Supersizing" is common. Research shows that the larger the portion size, the more we eat. Research also shows that America's increase in consumption of packaged, processed, and fast foods parallels the gross increase in overweight and obesity and in the rise in chronic disease incidence. The USDA states that eating one or more fast-food meals per week has the strongest association with obesity.

Also contributing to the obesity problem is the sedentary lifestyle of many Americans. We spend our waking hours sitting at work and home, making it difficult to expend enough calories to compensate for excess food consumption. Less than five percent of adults participate in physical activity each day. (Physical exercise is the focus of KidneyStep 5.)

The obesity resulting from excess calorie consumption and inadequate physical activity is estimated to be the leading cause of preventable illness in the U.S. It contributes to the development of CKD, and it increases the risk of developing a number of serious medical conditions associated with CKD, such as:

Obesity Increases Disease Risk

Kidney Disease	Progression of CKD is nearly twice as fast in the obese.
Cardiovascular Disease	Excess weight raises cholesterol and triglycerides, both associated with increased cardiovascular disease and increased risk of stroke.
Hypertension	Two-thirds of high blood pressure cases are attributable to obesity.
Diabetes	Obese individuals are four times more likely to develop diabetes than healthy-weight people.
Cancer	Excess weight is a risk factor for cancers of the uterus, cervix, ovary, breast, gallbladder, colon, rectum, and prostate.

Odds of having excess weight increase as we age. For example, about 67 percent of U.S. adults ages 50 and over are overweight, while only 20 percent of individuals in their 20s suffer a weight problem. We can blame a slowing metabolism and the body's tendency in midlife to lose muscle mass and gain fat that conspire to make it more difficult to maintain a normal weight if we eat as usual. This age-related weight gain contributes to higher risks of morbidity and mortality.

Compounding the age-related weight gain is that many Americans are not starting their 50s with normal weight but enter it carrying extra pounds. A typical woman in her late 40s now weighs 168 pounds, versus 143 pounds in the 1960s. Carrying that extra 25 or more pounds into older age makes attempts to lose weight and avoid diseases that strike later in life more difficult. A recent study found that people in their 60s have more disabilities than in past years when Americans weighed less.

B. You Really Are What You Eat

If you wish to avoid diseases so often associated with aging, your diet choices matter. As shown above, myriad diseases are linked to weight, diseases that increase risk of kidney disease. When it comes to staving off the health problems associated with kidney disease, your diet can be a friend or an enemy.

1. Type 2 Diabetes

Diabetes is not only the leading cause of CKD, but also the seventh leading cause of death in the U.S. One out of 9 adults is expected to have diabetes by 2025, and up to one-half of them develop kidney disease.

Research has repeatedly demonstrated that type 2 diabetes and insulin resistance may be prevented or postponed with diet, exercise, and weight loss. A landmark study by the Diabetes Prevention Program of over 3000 prediabetic individuals showed that those who made lifestyle changes (*e.g.*, losing weight, exercising 2 ½ hours per week, and eating a heart-healthy, plant-based diet) were 58 percent less likely to develop type 2 diabetes than prediabetics not making the lifestyle changes.

The ADA lists 10 Diabetes Superfoods:
- **Beans**
- **Dark green leafy vegetables**
- **Citrus fruit**
- **Sweet potatoes**
- **Berries**
- **Tomatoes**
- **Fish high in omega-3 fatty acids**
- **Whole grains**
- **Nuts**
- **Fat-free milk/ yogurt**

Two main components of diet affect blood sugar levels: calories and types of food. Consuming excess calories puts an individual at risk for elevated blood glucose levels. Excess calories often come from foods with a high glycemic index (high fructose corn syrup or other sugar, white rice, white bread, any food with refined flours and grains). High glycemic foods convert quickly into glucose.

The quick release of glucose into the blood triggers large amounts of insulin. Over time, high insulin levels may cause insulin receptors in cells to become less sensitive to the hormone, so the hormone fails to work as well. As the

Reducing high blood glucose lowers the risk of kidney disease by 50 percent.

receptors lose sensitivity to insulin, more glucose stays in the blood (and spills into the urine). In response to high glucose levels, the pancreas labors to make more insulin and can become exhausted in this vicious cycle. This results in insulin resistance, a precursor to diabetes.

Sugar consumption is particularly threatening to diabetics. The American Diabetes Association (ADA) recommends that people at risk of or with diabetes avoid sweetened drinks--a primary source of significant sugar in the American diet. Here is an example of why:

RECENT STUDY → Researchers examined 11 studies, assessing sugar-sweetened drink intake and risk of type 2 diabetes and metabolic syndrome. Participants who drank 1 or 2 sugared drinks per day had a 26% greater risk of developing diabetes and a 20% greater risk of metabolic syndrome compared to participants drinking less than 1 serving per month. *Diabetes Care*, 2010

ADA research shows that the DASH (Dietary Approaches to Stop Hypertension) eating plan benefits individuals with type 2 diabetes. DASH emphasizes keeping calories in check and eating low-glycemic foods that convert into glucose more slowly for a reduced insulin production. The DASH diet stresses whole grains and natural, unprocessed foods--not the processed or sugary, high-glycemic kinds.

For 8 weeks, diabetic patients were assigned to the DASH diet or a control diet. Diabetics following the DASH diet reduced their weight, waist circumference, blood pressure, fasting blood glucose level, and A1c level.

Diabetes Care, 2010

A person with type 2 diabetes who carefully eats DASH diet-recommended foods can reduce hemoglobin A1c; lose weight; lower blood pressure; lower cholesterol; and reduce the risk of kidney disease. If the person adds daily exercise, type 2 diabetes will improve and may even reverse itself.

2. Hypertension

Hypertension, the second leading cause of CKD, is also impacted by diet. As we age, we are more likely to have high blood pressure. According to the American Heart Association (AHA), over 70 percent of U.S. adults ages 65 and up are hypertensive, and nearly all people with kidney disease (even in early stages) suffer from it.

> **The USRDS reports between 63 and 94% of CKD patients-- depending upon age and CKD stage--suffer hypertension, compared to 29% of the general population.**

Despite the high incidence of hypertension, the AHA reports that only 20 percent of CKD patients and less than half of non-CKD individuals control their blood pressure. Uncontrolled blood pressure leads to heart disease, stroke, and further kidney damage.

The AHA stresses that eating a heart-healthy diet may prevent and will help manage high blood pressure. That diet should emphasize fruits, vegetables, whole grains, beans, fish, lean meats, and low-fat dairy products. The AHA recommends the DASH eating plan.

Studies show that the DASH diet has the same effect as taking blood-pressure-lowering medication. The DASH plan is rich in fruits and vegetables (eight to ten servings a day for someone on a 2000-calorie diet), grains (six to eight servings daily of mostly whole grains), and low-fat protein sources. It's also low in saturated fats and added sugars.

People following the DASH diet reduce blood pressure, regardless of age, gender, ethnicity, or initial blood pressure readings. In the DASH study, researchers followed people on three different diets. One diet was the typical American diet-- low in fruits, vegetables, and dairy and high in fat and cholesterol. A second was rich in fruits and vegetables, and the third was the DASH plan.

DASH dieters experienced a significant reduction in blood pressure compared to people who followed the other two diets. The sodium was about the same high amount (3000 mg.) in all three diets, so the blood pressure effect was attributable to other components of the diet: the calcium from the dairy, the magnesium from the nuts and grains, and the potassium from the fruits and vege- tables. For hypertensive individuals with blood pressures ranging from 140/90 to 160/99 mmHg, the DASH diet's effectiveness in reducing blood pressure was similar to the effectiveness resulting from antihypertensive medication.

> The Joint National Committee on Prevention, Detection, Evaluation, and Treatment of High Blood Pressure has adopted the DASH diet, with sodium restrictions, in its JNC 7 Guidelines.

3. Cardiovascular Disease

Cardiovascular disease (CVD), another disease related to diet, is closely linked to kidney disease. As explained in Chapter 7, the existence of even a microscopic amount of protein in the urine (microalbuminuria) escalates the risk of CVD. Add the impact of excess weight, diabetes, and hyper- tension, and it becomes understandable that most kidney patients develop CVD and then die from it.

The risk of CVD events (e.g., heart attacks, heart failure, strokes) increases as kidney function declines. The NKF classifies kidney patients as "high risk" for coronary artery disease. The NKF notes that up to 20 percent of individuals with Stage 3 CKD (when the person may not even know about the kidney disease) have had a prior heart attack or stroke, compared to less than 10 percent of the general population. In dialysis patients, the risk of CVD events is 20 times greater than in the general population.

Accordingly, heart and blood vessel protection must be a goal for kidney patients and for people with diabetes and/or hypertension, the leading causes of kidney disease. Nutrition is a key to protection from CVD.

The AHA recommends the DASH eating plan to avoid cardiovascular disease. In a 2010 study published in the AHA's Journal, researchers found that DASH lowered the 10-year risk of heart attacks by nearly 20 percent. While both whites and African-Americans benefited from the DASH diet in this study, African-Americans had the greatest benefit.

> **The higher your waist measurement relative to your hip measurement, the greater your heart attack and stroke risk, even if you are not overweight.**
> **Avoid abdominal fat.**
> *Neuroepidemiology, 2010*

The AHA notes that DASH emphasizes non-meat sources of protein. Red meat is particularly heart-damaging.

RECENT RESEARCH → Researchers followed 84,136 healthy women ages 30 to 55, assessing their diets every 4 years during the 26-year study. Higher intakes of poultry, nuts, and fish reduced heart disease risk by 30% compared to red meat intake.
Circulation, 2010

Processed meats (bacon, sausage, salami, luncheon meats, hot dogs) are especially threatening to the heart and are associated with an increased risk of diabetes. In a study that included 1.2 million people, those eating just 50 grams (equal to one hot dog or two slices of salami) of processed meat daily had a 42 percent greater risk of heart disease and a 19 percent

> **Processed meats have 4 times more sodium and 50% more cancer-inducing nitrate preservatives than natural meats.**
> *Circulation, 2010*

increased risk of diabetes. The researchers of this study advised eating no more than one serving of processed meat per week and placing greater emphasis on health-protective foods.

C. Other Troublesome "Foods"

1. Shake the Salt

Too much salt in the diet is linked to many serious diseases. In a recent study, researchers concluded that cutting sodium consumption to 1500 mg. per day would slash strokes and deaths by up to 92,000 annually. Likewise, the DASH diet

> **Reducing salt by as little as 1/2 teaspoon per day could prevent nearly 100,000 heart attacks and 92,000 deaths each year, reports the AHA.**

was shown to reduce blood pressure even more effectively if sodium intake in the diet is restricted to less than 1500 mg. per day. Even people with resistant hypertension-- blood pressure that does not drop even with multiple anti-hypertensive drugs--saw a decrease in pressure when they ate no more than 1150 mg. of sodium each day.

Reducing sodium to the 1500 mg. daily limit recommended by the AHA is difficult for people who eat fast foods and prepared convenience foods. Eating a single meal at a typical fast-food restaurant may throw you over the sodium limit for the entire day.

RECENT STUDY → New York City Health Department researchers reviewed the cash receipts for 6,580 lunches bought at 11 different fast-food chains by ordinary customers, adding up the sodium content of the meals. The average lunch contained 1,751 mg. of sodium. Researchers noted: "Fast food is not only a high-calorie but also a high-sodium food."

Archives of Internal Medicine, April 2010

Natural salt in food accounts for only about 10 percent of total intake. Salting at the table or while cooking is another 5 to 10 percent. The rest of our salt intake (75 percent) comes from salt added to processed foods by manufacturers and cooks at restaurants. Packaged foods include canned foods, processed meats such as bacon and hot dogs, frozen dinners, canned and boxed soups, and prepared snacks such as chips and crackers. Much of the food served in restaurants is this pre-packaged, high-sodium food.

Who would guess these common foods are salt demons?

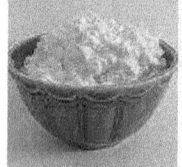 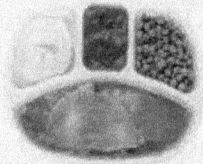 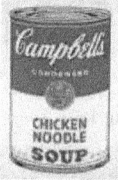 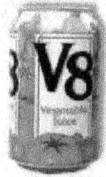 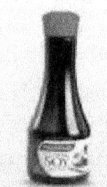

| 1 cup cottage cheese 820 mg. | 1 Banquet frozen turkey dinner 1060 mg. | 1 can chicken noodle soup 980 mg. | 1 12-oz can V-8 Juice 690 mg. | 1 Tbs. soy sauce 1000 mg. |

The Food and Drug Administration has set the following guidelines for labeling of low-salt foods:

Label	Sodium Content
Sodium / Salt-free	Less than 5 mg. per serving
Very Low Sodium / Salt	35 mg. or less per serving
Low Sodium / Salt	Less than 140 mg. per serving
Unsalted/No Salt Added	No salt added
Light in Sodium / Salt	50 percent less than original
Reduced Sodium / Salt	Sodium level reduced by 25 %

Monitoring sodium intake requires careful review of nutritional food labels on packaged foods and keeping sodium ingestion to no more than 500 mg. per meal. If your diet relies primarily on manufactured and fast-food restaurant products, the sodium limit can be challenging.

Salt is particularly troublesome for kidney patients. Researchers have found that diets high in salt are associated with decreased GFR (*i.e.,* lower kidney function).

One out of three American adults has high blood pressure, and 25% of CKD cases are caused by high blood pressure.

Patients with CKD demonstrate salt-sensitive hypertension; that is, their bodies respond to salt by increasing blood pressure. The CKD patient's impaired kidneys are unable to excrete sodium effectively, resulting in excess bloodstream sodium levels. This attracts excess fluid and prompts a blood pressure increase. The hypertensive response, in turn, damages the cardiovascular system and further increases kidney damage.

Scientists conclude that nearly all CKD patients exhibit some degree of salt sensitivity. The sensitivity is particularly troublesome in African-Americans. When compared to hypertensive individuals of European descent, hypertensive individuals of African descent excrete sodium less efficiently, especially during the daytime. This results in a higher blood pressure response to excess sodium.

Similarly, the kidneys of obese people who also have metabolic syndrome show impaired sodium excretion.

The American Society of Hypertension issued a position paper recommending less than 1500 mg. of salt daily, in addition to a DASH-style diet, to lower blood pressure.
Journal of Clinical Hypertension, 2009

Obese blacks are unusually vulnerable to high blood pressure and resulting kidney damage from excess sodium. A study of 397 African-Americans reported a 94 percent prevalence of high blood pressure in metabolic syndrome subjects compared to 37 percent in subjects without metabolic syndrome.

The bottom line: excess salt raises blood pressure and is particularly harmful in people who have kidney disease; are obese; have metabolic syndrome; or are black. Salt restriction generally lowers most individuals' blood pressure.

The NKF recommends people with kidney disease follow a reduced-sodium DASH-style diet (with modifications as necessary to control excess potassium and phosphorus) to help control blood pressure.

2. Sugar -- Not Sweet for Health

Fructose is a sugar used in corn syrup and accounts for one-half of the sugar molecules in table sugar. High-fructose corn syrup (HFCS) is often used in packaged sweetened products because of its low cost and long shelf life. The consumption of fructose has increased nearly 2000 percent over the past three decades. This increase coincides with the epidemics of obesity, metabolic syndrome, diabetes, hypertension, and CKD. The USDA estimates that each American consumes about 63 pounds of HFCS each year, 70 percent of this from soft drinks and fruit-flavored drinks.

Data from recent health studies link regular sugar-laden cola to elevated uric acid and creatinine levels and a corresponding increased risk for hypertension and kidney disease. For example:

RECENT STUDY → Researchers analyzed data from 15,745 patients who completed dietary question-naires and who had their levels of uric acid and creatinine measured for kidney function. Consumption of more than 1 soda per day increased the odds of high uric acid levels by 31 percent and was associated with up to a 159 percent increased risk of kidney disease.
Kidney International, 2010

Similarly, a study presented at the American Heart Association's (AHA) 2009 High Blood Pressure Research Conference showed that men consuming a HFCS diet for just two weeks experienced an increased incidence of high blood pressure and metabolic syndrome and an associated increased risk of CKD.

Is the danger only in the name?
Because of current media attention on the dangers of HFCS, the Corn Refiners Association has petitioned the FDA to change the name to "corn sugar."

Added sugars, particularly HFCS, also appear to harm heart health. The decades-long, 88,000-woman Nurses' Health Study found that drinking one 12-ounce can of regular soda daily boosts a woman's risk of having a heart attack by 24 percent. Two or more servings raise the risk by 35 percent.

Likewise, sugar consumption is linked to unhealthy cholesterol levels:

RECENT RESEARCH ➔
> Using data from 1999 through 2006, researchers divided 6113 NHANES study participants into five groups based on percentage of total calories from sugars. Groups ranged from sugar intake of less than 5 percent (about 3 t. sugar/day) to 25 percent (46 t./day). As sugar consumption increased, HDL cholesterol decreased and LDLs and triglycerides increased. The highest sugar consumers were more than three times as likely to have unhealthy levels of all blood lipids.
>
> *Journal of the American Medical Association,* 2010

Defenders of HFCS suggest it is not the soda, but instead the lifestyle behaviors (eating too many calories, obtaining little physical activity, and choosing high-salt diets) so often associated with soda drinking that cause kidney disease, diabetes, and high blood pressure. That is the position of the USDA in the *2010 Dietary Guidelines*. Leading authorities agree that Americans consume too much sugar, including too much HFCS, and the excess harms health.

The AHA recommends that women consume no more than 100 calories of added sugar (*i.e.,* 25 grams, about 6 teaspoons) per day, and men take in no more than 150 calories of sugar per day (37.5 grams, 9 teaspoons). The AHA also encourages the DASH diet for heart health because DASH limits sugar intake. To keep sugar in check, the AHA suggests:

- Check food labels for terms indicating added sugar: brown sugar, corn sweetener, corn syrup, fruit juice concentrates, high-fructose corn syrup, honey, invert sugar, malt sugar, syrup, sugar molecules ending in "-ose."

- Buy sugar-free.

- Buy fresh fruits; fruits canned in water; or fruits canned in 100% natural juice.

- Add fresh or dried fruit to cereal instead of sugar.

- Substitute spices for sugar.

A regular soft drink contains
8 teaspoons of sugar

3. High-Protein Diets and CKD

Many people purposely choose high-protein diets (limiting their intake of fruits, vegetables, and grains) in an attempt to lose weight. Other individuals unknowingly eat high-protein diets by selecting large quantities of meat, cheese, and eggs, while again limiting important foods. Either way, kidney function is jeopardized.

Red meat and animal protein may be particularly harmful to kidney function. Several studies suggest that CKD advances more quickly in red meat eaters:

RECENT RESEARCH → A study of 3,348 women participating in the Nurses' Health Study showed that just 2 servings of red meat per week was associated with increased microalbuminuria, an early sign of kidney damage.

Clinical Journal of the American Society of Nephrology,
2010

In a similar 2010 study, researchers examined the impact of dietary fat on kidney function. They found that higher saturated fat intake (from red meat and processed meat products, such as hot dogs, sausage, luncheon meats) was significantly associated with the prevalence of high albuminuria. Other types of dietary fat had no negative impact on kidney function.

A 4-oz piece of chicken contains 28 grams of protein. One cup of milk has 8 grams.

The NKF in its K/DOQI Clinical Guidelines states that even modest limitations in dietary protein slow progression of CKD, particularly in diabetics. Consequently, the NKF recommends that individuals in Stages I through IV of CKD limit dietary protein to that recommended for all adults, which is 0.8g/kg of body weight per day (about 54 grams of protein per day for a 150-pound person). This protein limitation "should stabilize or reduce albuminuria, slow the decrease in GFR, and may prevent CKD Stage V," states the NKF.

Studies referenced in the NKF's Guidelines suggest that vegetable or soy protein sources may spare kidney function in comparison to red-meat sources, particularly in diabetes and CKD. The NKF recommends that individuals with CKD follow a DASH-like diet that emphasizes sources of protein other than red meat, *e.g.,* lean poultry, fish, grains, beans, and vegetables.

Some authors discussing CKD suggest extreme protein-restricted diets to delay the progression of kidney disease. Certainly, the available research suggests that individuals with CKD should avoid *over*eating protein and should limit red and processed meats. However, protein is critical for growth, tissue repair, a strong immune system, and building muscle. We need sufficient protein for good health. It is important to consult with your nephrologist and a dietitian trained in kidney disease to create a proper diet. Excessively limiting protein can result in muscle loss, wasting, and even death.

4. Alcohol--a Little is Okay

Excessive alcohol consumption (more than two drinks per day for men and one drink for women) leads to sustained elevated blood pressure. Studies indicate that alcohol interferes with blood flow by moving nutrient-rich blood away from the heart. Alcohol also reduces the effectiveness of anti-hypertensive drugs. Binge drinking--having at least four drinks consecutively--can cause a significant and rapid increase in blood pressure.

What is a "drink"?
- **12 oz beer**
- **½ oz vodka/gin**
- **1½ oz 80% whiskey**
- **5 oz wine**

We regularly enjoy a glass of red wine. Moderate red wine consumption is shown to have cardiovascular benefits and may be kidney-protective. In a small study, participants with type 2 diabetic nephropathy were asked to drink 4 ounces of either red or white wine daily for six months. The serum creatinine of the red wine imbibers (but not the white wine drinkers) significantly decreased during the study period.

18.

FOOD – HOW MUCH AND WHAT KIND?

Achieving and sustaining appropriate body weight and doing so by consuming nutrient-dense foods, are vital to maintaining good health and avoiding (perhaps reversing) heart disease, type 2 diabetes, hypertension, and kidney disease. Calorie control is key to weight management. Controlling calories requires an understanding of your particular calorie needs and the appropriate food sources for those calories.

A. Weight and Calorie Needs

Food provides the body with energy to support basic involuntary functions (*e.g.,* breathing, heartbeat, maintaining body temperature). The minimum energy needed for these involuntary bodily functions is determined by your **basal metabolic rate** (BMR), which is your baseline rate of metabolism measured when your body is at rest. You also expend energy through the activities you perform, whether sedentary or vigorous. All of your body's energy needs are met by the foods you consume and from your body's energy stores.

The energy you obtain from food is measured in **calories.**[*] The higher your BMR, the more calories you need. Men generally have higher BMR's than women because of greater percentage of muscle mass. Older adults generally have lower BMR's and require fewer calories. Also, the more active a person is, the higher the BMR and the associated calorie need. Eating more calories than you require for your metabolic needs results in weight gain.

---

[*] One calorie represents a tiny amount of energy, and kilocalories (1,000 calories = one kilocalorie) are used in nutritional analysis. However, the term "calories" has come to be used as a shorthand reference to kilocalories. Each type of nutrient generates a specific amount of energy. Three ounces of protein generates 400 calories. Three ounces of carbohydrate generates 400 calories. Three ounces of fat generates 900 calories.

1. Identify Your Weight Status

The terms "overweight" and "obese" describe ranges of weight that are unhealthy for a given height. People often don't know if their weight is healthy or if they have crept into the overweight category or, worse, the obese category. Either category means a greater risk of disease. You may assess your weight (and associated health risks) a couple of ways:

A. BMI

Body mass index (BMI) is a tool used to estimate your weight status. BMI is a measurement of body fat based on height and weight. For example, a 5-foot, 4-inch person who weighs 130 pounds has a BMI of 22.3 and has a healthy weight. The BMI of a 175-pound male who is 5 feet, 8 inches is 26.6, and he is overweight.

Overweight..........or Obese?

Category	BMI
Healthy Weight	$18.5 - 24.9 \text{ kg/m}^2$
Overweight	$25.0 - 29.9 \text{ kg/m}^2$
Obese	$30.0 - \text{ kg/m}^2$ or higher

Calculate your BMI at: http://www.nhlbisupport.com/bmi/ or link to a BMI calculator at KidneySteps.com.

B. WAIST CIRCUMFERENCE

Your body weight distribution can indicate your health risk if you are overweight or obese. If more of your fat is around your waist than at your hips, you are at a higher risk for disease, particularly diabetes, heart disease, and high blood pressure. Measure your waist, placing the tape measure just above the hip bones. The risk goes up if your waist measurement is above 35 inches (for a woman) or 40 inches (for a man).

Once you know your body weight status, you are ready to determine your daily calorie needs.

2. Determining Calorie Needs

While most U.S. adults need (and are trying) to lose weight, few have any idea how many calories they should consume. According to the 2010 Food & Health Survey

> **To figure your calorie goal,** see www.mypyramid.gov/ mypyramid/index.aspx **or link to it at KidneySteps.com.**

Council, 65 percent of respondents chose food with losing weight in mind. Only 17 percent of respondents, though, accurately estimated how many calories they actually needed.

A person's calorie needs are based on age, height, weight, sex, and activity level. Here are examples of the number of daily calories adults need to maintain their current weight, depending on activity level:

Estimated Daily Calorie Needs

Gender	Age	Physical Activity Level		
		Sedentary	Moderately Active	Active
Female	19-30	1800-2000	2000-2200	2400
	31-50	1800	2000	2200
	51+	1600	1800	2000-2200
Male	19-30	2400-2600	2600-2800	3000
	31-50	2200-2400	2400-2600	2800-3000
	51+	2000-2200	2200-2400	2400-2800

Knowing your daily calorie needs is a useful reference. However, the best way to assess whether you are eating the appropriate number of calories is to monitor your body weight by weighing yourself regularly and then adjusting the number of calories you consume based on changes in your weight over time.

The USDA states that the usual calorie intake of most Americans exceeds daily needs. The top 6 sources of these excess calories are:

1. Grain-based desserts (e.g., cakes, cookies, donuts)

2. Yeast breads (e.g., white bread, rolls, bagels)

271

3.   Chicken and chicken mixed dishes (*e.g.*, chicken nuggets, fingers, patties)

4.   Soda/energy/sports drinks

5.   Pizza

6.   Pasta (*e.g.*, macaroni cheese, spaghetti, noodles)

Health authorities such as the USDA encourage Americans to limit these sources of calories and increase the intake of fruits, vegetables, whole grains, nuts, and low-fat dairy.

3. What is the Most Effective Diet?

Excess weight is about calories. Which diet you choose does not matter, so long as you receive a wide range of heart-healthy, low-in-saturated-fat foods. These include plenty of fruits, vege-tables, whole grains, low-fat

> **For every 2 lbs. of excess body weight a person carries, his/her risk of diabetes increases 4.5%.**

dairy, nuts, and legumes, as well as a reasonable amount of protein. However, as stated in Chapter 17, if you have diabetes or CKD, avoid high-protein diets.

Interview, Sue: *I have CKD and am obese. I try to diet all the time. I joined an advertised diet program recently. I like the convenience of eating what I am told. At my last doctor's appointment, my nephrologist mentioned that I should watch my protein intake. So I called my diet coach, and she told me my diet was high-protein. I had no idea that eggs for breakfast, meat and cottage cheese for lunch, and meat for dinner meant the diet was high-protein. I thought I would need to be eating protein bars and drinking protein powders for the diet to be high-protein.*

Recently, scientists at Harvard University and Louisiana State University studied more than 800 adults in mid-life who were overweight or obese. The volunteers were randomly placed into one of four different heart-healthy diets. Two of the diets were higher in carbohydrates, and two were higher in protein but varied in fat amount.

272

The results showed no substantial difference in weight loss among the four diets. The important factor was how many calories the volunteers took in and whether they stayed with the diets. The volunteers in all four groups lost an average of 19 pounds in the first six months and kept off an average of eight pounds after two years. All of the diets provided the same food satisfaction to the volunteers, and the weight loss included improved lipid levels and fasting insulin levels.

To lose weight, individuals must either reduce calories to below the number needed to maintain current weight, or increase activity level. Studies have shown that reducing calories is the most effective way to reduce weight. The USDA recommends a reduction of 500 calories per day as a common initial goal for weight loss for adults.

B. Sources of Calories/Nutrients

Carbohydrates, protein, and fat are the main sources of calories and nutrients in our food. Most foods contain combinations of these nutrients in varying amounts. We need all three nutrient groups to live and function properly. Our bodies' cells utilize the nutrients to create energy for numerous body processes: heartbeat, digestion, respiration, kidney function, brain processes, etc.

1. Carbohydrates

Carbohydrates are the primary energy source to fuel bodily activities. Carbohydrates also help in processing fat and in building body tissues. We obtain carbohydrates from grains, breads, pasta, fruits, vegetables, legumes, and dairy products. Each carbohydrate gram provides 4 calories.

Of the 7.5 ounces of grains consumed per person each day in the U.S., less than 1 ounce is whole grain. The rest are refined grains.

Carbohydrates are classified as simple or complex, depending upon their structure. When digested, simple carbohydrates quickly break down into simple sugars (*e.g.,* glucose, fructose). This rapid release of simple sugars into the blood causes an immediate release of insulin. When manufacturers refine whole grains to create white bread, white rice, and snack foods, they convert a complex carbohydrate to a simple carbohydrate largely devoid of nutrients.

Complex carbohydrates include starches and fibers found in beans and whole grains. They occur naturally in nearly all plant foods and are high in nutritional value. They also contain vitamins, minerals, phytochemicals, and protein. Complex carbohydrates are digested more slowly, resulting in a steady--rather than abrupt--release of insulin. Most of your carbohydrates should come from these whole foods.

Glycemic Index

The glycemic index (GI) classifies foods according to how fast they release glucose (sugar) into the bloodstream. High-GI foods release glucose quickly, causing a rapid rise in blood glucose levels. The body reacts to high blood glucose levels by releasing insulin, which stimulates fat storage. Low-GI foods, in contract, release glucose steadily over several hours, so less insulin is released.

So long as your carbohydrates consist of fruits, vegetables, and whole (not refined) grains, you need not worry about the GI, according to the USDA.

Complex carbohydrates that contain fiber are critical for digestive health. The two types of dietary fiber are **soluble** (dissolves in water) and **insoluble** (does not dissolve in water). Soluble fiber slows the breakdown of complex carbohydrates into simple sugars, thereby slowing absorption of sugar and reducing

> **Required Daily Fiber:**
>
> **20 to 40 grams**

levels in the blood. During digestion, soluble fiber forms a gel-like mass that binds cholesterol to the stool. If eaten in sufficient amounts, soluble fiber can help reduce the levels of cholesterol in the blood. Good sources of soluble fiber include grains (oats, barley, rye), vegetables, citrus fruits, and beans.

274

Fiber in Food

Food	Serving Size	Fiber Content (grams)
Oatmeal, dry	½ cup	8.4
Kidney beans	1 cup	6.4
Lima beans, boiled	1 cup	13.5
Lentils, boiled	1 cup	7.9
Whole wheat bread	1 slice	1.6

Insoluble fiber occurs naturally in brown rice, whole wheat bread, cereals, seeds, legumes, and fruit and vegetable skins. It is neither digested nor absorbed by the body, but insoluble fiber helps keep the intestinal tract clean and promotes regular bowel movements. It does this by drawing water into the stools, making them larger, softer, and easier to pass.

> The ideal bowel movement is S-shaped, medium brown, the consistency of toothpaste, about 6 to 8 inches long, and enters the water smoothly--without making a "plop" sound.

Studies show that high-fiber diets help prevent diabetes, heart disease, and obesity; and, they reduce the risk of colorectal cancer. Most people consume too little fiber and too much added sugar and refined grains.

2. Protein

Protein is used for energy and is important in building and maintaining tissues, muscles, and organs. We need protein to make most enzymes and hormones and for a healthy immune system. Protein provides 4 calories per gram.

The body breaks protein down into amino acids (the components of protein), which are absorbed into the bloodstream. This pool of amino acids provides the elements needed to build new proteins in the body. To obtain a full range of essential amino acids, we require a variety of protein foods.

Studies show that people who eat less red meat and eat more protein from plants have a lower risk of developing cardiovascular disease, certain cancers, and CKD; they may also live longer.

RECENT STUDY → Researchers analyzed data on over one-half million volunteers in the National Institutes of Health-AARP Diet and Health Study. Participants were ranked by meat consumption. The one-fifth who ate the most red meat (the equivalent of a quarter-pound hamburger daily) were more likely to die during the 10-year analysis than the quintile eating the least red meat (1-2 servings per week).

Archives of Internal Medicine, 2009

Plant sources of protein include beans and peas, nuts, seeds, and soy products. Most leading health authorities recommend obtaining protein from plant sources and limiting meat intake. Meat and meat products contain fat, particularly saturated fat. The worst offenders are sausage, hot dogs, bacon, chicken skin, and marbled beef steaks. Sausage and hot dogs, for example, are about 80 percent fat. These products are also very high in sodium. Better meat choices are fish, shellfish, and skinless white poultry.

3. The Skinny on Fats

Besides providing energy, fats form a major part of all the body's cell membranes. Fats are necessary for absorption of fat-soluble vitamins from foods. Fat cushions the body's organs to

> **Fats (the good ones) don't make you fat. Excess weight results from eating too many calories from *any* food source.**

prevent injury and also acts as skin insulation to maintain body temperature. About one-third of your daily calories should be fat calories. Each gram of fat provides 9 calories.

A. LIPIDS/LIPOPROTEINS.

Lipids are a group of fats that include triglycerides, waxes, and sterols. Cholesterol is a well-known sterol.

> **The National Heart, Lung and Blood Institute says the optimal blood level of HDL is at least 60 mg/dL.**
> **You can raise HDLs with omega-3s from fatty fish and with exercise.**

Cholesterol is a major component of every body cell and helps in the manufacture of vitamin D. Your body makes its own cholesterol, and you do not require much from your diet.

Cholesterol circulates in the blood attached to compounds known as lipoproteins. Low-density lipoproteins (LDLs), which carry cholesterol to tissues and organs, are often called "bad" cholesterol, because high levels in the blood are associated with increased risk of cardiovascular disease.

High-density lipoproteins (HDLs) carry cholesterol away from the tissues and back to the liver. HDLs are known as "good" cholesterol, because high levels decrease the risk of cardiovascular disease and cancer.

RECENT STUDY → Researchers examined data from 24 studies covering a five-year period and found that cancer risk dropped 36 percent for every 10 mg/dL higher increment of HDL cholesterol in the blood. The higher the HDL level, the better, concluded the researchers.

Journal of the American College of Cardiology, 2010

B. SATURATED, TRANS, AND NON-SATURATED FATS.

Fats are referred to as "good" or "bad," depending upon whether their chemical bonds are **saturated** with hydrogen or are **unsaturated**. The body uses saturated fats for numerous cell functions, but it makes enough to meet those needs. People therefore have no dietary need for saturated fat. Yet, we consume excessive amounts from animal and dairy products, including red meat, whole milk, butter, cheese, cream, and ice cream. Tropical plant oils (coconut, palm) also contain saturated fats. Excessive intake of saturated fat increases the risk of cardiovascular disease by raising unhealthy LDL levels. The USDA recommends consuming less than 10 percent of daily calories from saturated fat and replacing it with unsaturated fat.

Trans fatty acids are found naturally in some foods and are formed during food processing. The body does not need them, and they are associated with cardiovascular disease. Therefore, Americans should avoid trans fats.

Unsaturated fat is classified as **mono-** or **polyunsaturates,** which differ in nutritional make-up. A diet high in monounsaturated fats (found in olive oil, nuts, and avocados, for example) helps lower blood levels of LDLs and triglycerides, reducing the risk of heart disease and stroke.

> **You may link to the USDA's food composition site through KidneySteps.com to determine nutrients in various foods.**

Polyunsaturated fats consist of two major groups: omega-3 fatty acids found in fish oils, and omega-6 fatty acids found in vegetable oils (such as canola, sunflower, and corn). Omega-3's are linked to a wide range of health benefits. Omega-6's are more controversial, and some studies suggest they have inflammatory effects if not balanced with omega-3's. We require both omega-3 and omega-6 fatty acids for good health.

4. How Much of Each?

The United States' National Academy of Sciences' Institute of Medicine issued the *Dietary Reference Intakes* (DRIs) to guide us as to specific amounts of each nutrient we need daily to maintain good health and to prevent chronic disease. The DRIs include intake ranges for carbohydrates, fats, and protein (as well as fiber, vitamins, minerals, and water). Consuming these nutrient types in these ranges ensures you meet both your calorie and nutrient needs, and you reduce risk of chronic disease, particularly cardiovascular disease, obesity, diabetes, high blood pressure, and kidney disease.

DRIs

Nutrient	Daily
Carbohydrates	45 to 65 % of calories
Protein	10 to 35 % of calories
Fats	20 to 35 % of calories
Fiber	20 to 40 grams

Let's say you wish to eat 2000 calories per day. Applying the DRI guide, you would eat the following proportions of carbohydrates, protein, and fat:

Nutrient	Daily Calories	Grams
Carbohydrates	1,100 calories (55% of total)	275
Protein	300 calories (15% of total)	75
Fats	600 calories (30% of total)	60

In the next chapter, we provide the DASH eating plan, which includes the serving size of each food category to eat in a day. By following the serving sizes and food choices recommended in the plan, you avoid the need to calculate grams or specific calories for each meal.

If you follow a different diet, you will find food labels helpful in determining the quantity of each nutrient you eat/drink.

5. Food Labels are Useful

Nutrition Facts

Serving Size 1 cup (85g) (3 oz.)

Servings per container 2.5

Amount per serving

Calories 45   Calories from Fat 0

	% Daily Value*
Total Fat 0g	0%
Saturated Fat 0g	0%
Cholesterol 0mg	0%
Sodium 55 mg	2%
Total Carbohydrate 10g	3%
Dietary Fiber 3g	12%
Sugars 5g	
Protein 1g	

Vitamin A 360% • Vitamin C 8% • Calcium 2% • Iron 0%

*Percent Daily Values are based on a 2,000 calorie diet. Your daily value may be higher or lower depending on your calorie needs.

		Calories:	2,000	2,500
Total Fat	Less than		65g	80g
Sat. Fat	Less than		20g	25g
Cholesterol	Less than		300mg	300mg
Sodium	Less than		2,400mg	2,400mg
Total Carbohydrate	Less than		300mg	375mg
Dietary Fiber	Less than		25g	30g

Calories per gram: Fat 9 • Carbohydrate 4 • Protein 4

Ingredients: Carrots

The Nutrition Facts food label and the ingredients list on packages of foods are useful in evaluating and comparing the nutritional content and ingredients in different foods. The label shows the number of calories per serving of a particular food, as well as the number of grams of fats, protein, carbohydrates, and fiber in the food item. The label also provides information on certain nutrients that should be limited in the diet, including saturated fat, trans fat, cholesterol, sodium, and sugar.

The labels may show some vitamins or minerals in the product, particularly if the product supplies a significant amount of the DRI. Because most foods contain a combination of carbohydrates, protein, and fat, we require a daily intake of a range of nutritious, non-processed foods.

C. Components of a Good Eating Plan

In the next chapter, we offer food selections based on a DASH-like diet because of its proven health benefits. Any sound eating plan will focus on the following components.

1. Whole Grains

Foods from the grain group (bread, cereal, rice, and pasta) are excellent sources of carbohydrates and are the basis of a good diet. Choose *whole* rather than refined grains. Whole grains improve cholesterol levels and lower risk of cardiovascular disease because they are low in saturated fat and high in fiber, vitamins (especially vitamin B), minerals, and antioxidants.

RECENT STUDY →

An analysis of data from 31,684 men finds that men who ate the most whole grains (52 grams per day) were 19 percent less likely to develop hypertension than men eating the least.

American Journal of Clinical Nutrition, 2009

Refined grains (white rice, white flour, processed foods such as potato chips, corn chips) raise blood sugar levels and can contribute to diabetes and cardiovascular disease.

Eat Whole Grains

A whole grain is an unprocessed grain. It contains the bran, germ, and endosperm inside an inedible hull. About 90 percent of the nutrients are in the bran and germ. The bran is an excellent source of fiber. The germ is the embryo of a new plant and provides protein, vitamins, and minerals and contains polyunsaturated fats. The endosperm supplies carbohydrates.

When grains are processed, the hull, bran, and germ are removed, leaving a product--such as white flour-- that is deficient in protein, vitamins, and fiber.

---

2. Vegetables

Vegetables are excellent sources of vitamins (particularly vitamins C and A), antioxidants, folate, potassium, and fiber. Experts emphasize spreading vegetable selections across all varieties: dark green and orange vegetables, beans and peas, starchy vegetables, and the red, yellow, white, and purple varieties.

Studies show that diets high in vegetables reduce the instance of cardiovascular disease. The fiber in vegetables helps keep the intestinal tract in good working order and may reduce the risk of colon cancer. Yet, only 6 percent of men and 4 percent of women (ages 40 to 59) eat the recommended 5 servings per day.

3. Fruits

Fruits are naturally sweet, high in vitamins and fiber, and low in calories and fat. Fruits are rich in vitamin C and phytochemicals, including antioxidants. Antioxidants destroy harmful substances in the body, called free radicals, which build up and can cause cancer.

The AHA, the National Cancer Institute, and the American Cancer Society recommend eating 5 servings of fruits and vegetables a day. Yet, less than 39 percent of American adults currently do so.

> The AHA cautions against getting too much of your fruit from juice. Juice generally offers quick calories but zero fiber.

According to the NHANES study, the risk of cardiovascular disease is reduced in people who eat more than three servings of fruits and vegetables a day. Mounting evidence suggests that eating at least five servings daily halves the risk of developing many types of cancer. In addition, eating plenty of fruits and vegetables can help with weight control because they are higher in fiber, which creates a feeling of fullness.

4. Dairy

Milk and other dairy products are excellent sources of protein, vitamins, and minerals--particularly calcium for healthy bones and teeth. You may choose cow, goat, sheep, rice, or soy milk. Choose low-fat or fat-free dairy products to limit ingested saturated fat.

RECENT STUDY → Researchers examined the effects of calcium from diet (not supplements) for 23,266 men over 10 years. Men who consumed an average of 1957 mg. of dietary calcium per day (versus 990 mg. daily for the lowest calcium measures) had a lower rate of death from all causes.
Journal of Epidemiology, 2010

Calcium is important throughout life for bone health. Studies suggest that calcium from dairy food is utilized by your body better than calcium in pill form.

5. Meat, Poultry, Fish, Legumes, Nuts, Seeds, Eggs

Animal sources of protein include meat, poultry, fish and shellfish, as well as eggs. Protein is also prominent in grains and many vegetables. Health authorities regard fish as the healthiest source of animal protein, particularly oily fish such as salmon, herring, tuna, and sardines, which are rich in omega-3 fatty acids and help reduce the risk of developing cardiovascular disease. Prominent health authorities recommend that people eat less red meat and eat more protein from plants (grains, nuts, seeds, legumes, beans) to lower their risk of developing cardiovascular disease and certain cancers.

6. Fats, Oils / Sweets

The AHA and DASH recommend 2 to 3 daily servings of fats and oils, such as 1 tablespoon low-fat mayonnaise, 2 tablespoons light or 1 tablespoon regular salad dressing, or 1 teaspoon vegetable oil. Food experts concur on the importance of limiting saturated fats and eliminating trans fats. Choose mono- and polyunsaturated fats that offer health benefits. These include olive oil, canola oil, and nut oils.

You can calculate your own daily fat limits online at www.americanheart.org/myfattranslator

Food experts also agree on the need to limit intake of sugar-sweetened beverages and sweets. Only the occasional dessert is recommended. The AHA and DASH recommend limiting sweets to 5 servings per week.

D. A Special Word About Dialysis

A patient in Stage IV or V (on dialysis) of CKD is concerned about sufficient protein, excess fluid, and a balance of sodium, potassium, and phosphorus.

Protein and Calories. Malnutrition from an inadequate intake of nutrients is a common problem for dialysis patients. Over one-third of hemodialysis patients and over one-half of peritoneal dialysis patients exhibit malnutrition. Contributing factors include acidosis (refer to chapter 15); protein and mineral losses into dialysate; anorexia; alterations in the capacity to taste; and, concurrent illnesses that interfere with ability to eat.

Dialysis patients may lose several grams of protein during dialysis. Thus, the NKF recommends a dialysis patient increase his or her protein intake to 1.2 to 1.3 grams of protein per kilogram of body weight per day (70 to 77 grams of protein for a 154-pound person). This quantity helps prevent muscle wasting.

> **The American Association of Kidney Patients offers a nutritional reference for kidney patients that lists hundreds of foods and their associated amounts of sodium, phosphorus, protein, potassium, and calories. You may obtain it at: www.aakp.org/brochures/nutrition-counter.**

The NKF also recommends that dialysis patients take in sufficient calories to help prevent malnutrition. The recommended calories are 30 to 35 calories per kilogram of body weight (about 2,450 calories for a 154-pound person).

Sodium. Healthy kidneys maintain sodium balance by excreting excess sodium. However, damaged kidneys lose that ability. During CKD Stages I through IV, the undamaged nephrons adapt to kidney damage by excreting a higher percentage of sodium to maintain the internal balance. When GFR falls below 10 mL/min, too few functioning nephrons remain to excrete excess sodium. The excess raises blood pressure and creates thirst, which is a problem for hemodialysis patients who must control fluid intake to prevent edema and heart issues. Thus, sodium restriction may become necessary to help control blood pressure, edema, and risk of congestive heart failure. Restricting sodium to 1500 milligrams per day may be sufficient to prevent an excess sodium problem.

Potassium. If the kidneys fail to maintain the proper levels of potassium, the excess potassium causes irregular heartbeat and can even result in death. Too much potassium retained in the blood can also lead to calcium deposits in the eye, heart, and joints. Dietary potassium restriction for hemodialysis patients is necessary to avoid heart rhythm abnormalities, heart failure, and muscle weakness. Potassium accumulates in the body between dialysis treatments if the patient no longer has sufficient urine output.

The NKF recommends 2000 to 3000 milligrams per day of potassium for hemodialysis patients. Peritoneal dialysis patients don't usually require a potassium restriction. CKD patients in their earlier stages may also require potassium restriction based on their individual disease, metabolism, and blood test results.

Phosphorus. In the earlier states of CKD, the kidneys adapt to excrete excess phosphorus from the blood. When GFR falls to less than 20 mL/min (late Stage IV), excess blood phosphorus levels usually become evident.

The NKF recommends dietary phosphorus restriction sufficient to maintain normal blood serum levels. Phosphorus binding medications are frequently required. The phosphate binders bind to the phosphorus consumed or ingested and prevent its absorption in the gastrointestinal tract.

19.

Now, Let's Eat

Managing body weight requires a focus on total calorie intake. Excess weight usually results from overeating calories. Controlling weight requires limiting calories, and achieving good health requires making deliberate food choices so the limited calories consumed come from nutrient-dense foods. Processed, sugared, and fatty foods are generally low in nutrient density but high in calories. Consuming such foods encourages disease. Each food taken in throughout the day should meet a nutrient need.

While we have selected a DASH-like eating plan for Kidney Steps, you may prefer another diet. So long as the foods you eat and drink are varied and nutrient-rich and your calorie intake is appropriate, enjoy the diet. Any eating pattern you select should reflect the 10 elements set out below.

A. 10 Good-Eating Elements

1. **Monitor calorie intake**. People most successful at maintaining a healthy weight consume only enough calories from food and drink to meet their needs. If you are overweight, reduce your calorie intake.

2. **Make every calorie count**. Americans consume too many calories from refined grains, added sugar, and saturated fats. Those replace the nutrient-dense foods necessary for good health and a healthy weight. Emphasize whole grains, vegetables, fruits, low-fat dairy, and fish and seafood.

3. **Avoid sugar-sweetened beverages**. Sugar-sweetened drinks (colas, sodas, fruit-flavored juices) provide excess calories and few nutrients, and they lead to obesity and other diseases.

4. **Increase intake of whole grains**. Individuals who eat whole grains control weight more successfully and exhibit better health compared to adults who indulge in refined grains (donuts, packaged sweets, white bread).

5. **Vary your vegetables/fruits**. A health-promoting diet reflects a variety of vegetables and fruits, not just a few favorites. Throughout the week, consume dark green, yellow, red, purple, blue, and orange vegetables and fruits for a mix of nutrients.

6. **Limit eating out**. Most restaurant food contains excessive fat, sodium, and sugar. Cook and eat more meals at home. When eating out, select small portions and choose lower-calorie options.

7. **Cut back on sodium**. Reduce sodium intake to 1500 mg. a day. The best way to do so is to eat more fresh foods and fewer packaged and processed foods. Go easy on sodium-laden condiments such as soy sauce, bottled salad dressings, and ketchup. Read food labels to check for sodium content.

8. **Limit solid fats and added sugars**. Saturated fats are found in meats and dairy products. Trans fats are in fried and baked goods, particularly packaged foods. Added sugars also are in most packaged baked items. Avoid trans fats and limit saturated fats to no more than 7 percent of dairy calories.

9. **Drink only moderately**. While moderate alcohol consumption can be beneficial, heavy drinking is harmful to health. Heavy drinking is defined as more than 3 drinks on any day or more than 7 per week for women, and more than 4 drinks on any day or more than 14 drinks per week for men.

10. **Increase physical activity**. You prevent and/or reduce overweight and obesity through improved eating and physical activity. Limit time spent in sedentary behavior (watching television, sitting at a computer, etc.). See KidneyStep 5 for exercise tips.

B. DASH -- for Good Health

The *Dietary Approaches to Stop Hypertension* (DASH) eating plan is recommended by multiple health authorities, including the National Heart, Lung and Blood Institute; the American Heart Association; and, the American Society of Hypertension. DASH is similar to, and forms the basis for, the USDA's revised *2010 Dietary Guidelines*. The American Diabetes Association supports DASH, and the National Kidney Foundation endorses a DASH-like diet in its K/DOQI clinical guidelines for people in Stages I through IV of CKD.

As discussed in the two previous chapters, DASH lowers blood pressure and improves response to medication in people with more severe hypertension. DASH helps lower cholesterol, reduces insulin resistance, and encourages weight loss. Following a DASH-like diet is shown to reduce risks of diabetes, stroke, heart disease, kidney stones, and kidney disease.

For these reasons, DASH is the basis of the eating plan presented here, with additional modifications to reduce total sodium to less than 1500 milligrams per day (for enhanced blood pressure benefit) and to limit total protein to a modest level (to aid in kidney health).

1. The DASH Eating Plan

This version of the actual DASH reflects DASH serving recommendations for a person requiring 2000 calories per day.

Food Group	Average Daily Servings	Serving Sizes	Best Options/ Recommendations
Bread, pasta, cereals, and whole grains	6-8	1 slice whole grain bread 1 oz dry cereal 1/2 cup cooked whole grain, rice, or pasta	To get the most fiber and nutrients, look for whole-grain or whole-wheat products, such as whole-grain bread, brown rice and whole-wheat pasta.
Vegetables	4-5	1 cup raw leafy vegetables ½ cup raw or cooked vegetables ½ cup vegetable juice	Tomatoes, carrots, broccoli, sweet potatoes, greens and other vegetables are full of fiber, vitamins, and minerals.
Fruits	4-5	½ cup no-sugar, 100% juice 1 medium fruit ½ cup fresh, frozen, or canned fruit ¼ cup dried fruit	Fruits such as apples, bananas, oranges, mangoes, melons, peaches and berries are packed with vitamins and minerals. Certain citrus fruits and juices (grapefruit) can interact with certain blood pressure medications.

Food Group	Average Daily Servings	Serving Sizes	Best Options/ Recommendations
Low-fat and fat-free dairy	2-3	1 cup skim milk or yogurt 1 ½ oz cheese	Milk, yogurt, cheese and other dairy products are major sources of calcium, vitamin D and protein. Choose low-fat or fat-free. Also, go easy on cheese—it's typically high in sodium.
Meats, poultry, and fish	6 or fewer	1 oz cooked meat, poultry, or fish 1 egg (limit yolks to no more than 4/week)	Meat is a good source of protein, B vitamins, iron and zinc. Yet, even lean varieties contain fat and cholesterol, so try cutting back your usual portions. Eat more fish and seafood. Also, trim away skin and fat from meat, and skip frying in favor of broiling, grilling, or roasting.
Nuts, seeds, and dry beans	4-5 per week	1/3 cup nuts 2 T. peanut butter 2 T. seeds ½ cup cooked beans, peas	Almonds, sunflower seeds, kidney beans, peas, lentils, and other foods in this family are good sources of magnesium, potassium, and protein. They're also full of fiber and plant compounds (phytochemicals). Calories count, so keep serving sizes small.
Fats and oils	2-3	1 tsp vegetable oil 1 tsp margarine (soft) 1 T. salad dressing 1 T. mayonnaise	Choose unsaturated fats (e.g., olive oil), and limit saturated fat (found in meat, butter, cheese and high-fat dairy products). Avoid trans fats (commonly found in processed foods that are baked or fried).
Sweets and added sugars	5 or less per week	1 T. sugar 1 T. jelly, jam ½ cup sorbet, gelatin dessert 1 cup lemonade	When you eat sweets, opt for fat-free or low-fat, such as sorbets, fruit ices, jelly beans, hard candy, or graham crackers.

The DASH diet places special emphasis on fruits, vegetables, and whole grains (to increase potassium and magnesium in the diet) and low-fat dairy (for extra calcium). Calcium, potassium, and magnesium are shown to counter the blood pressure effects of excess sodium intake. DASH also limits meats and encourages nuts to supply magnesium.

Saturated fat is reduced to less than seven percent of total calories. Red meats, sugars, and sweets are discouraged.

2. CKD Patients

Recent research has shown that the typical "Western" diet of most Americans is associated with a greater likelihood of the development of microalbuminuria and rapid decrease in kidney function when compared to a more healthful diet. A 2011 study included 3071 participants of the Nurses' Health Study. The researchers compared the kidney function of individuals who followed the Western diet (high in red meat, processed meats, saturated fats, and sweets) or one of two other diets, including a DASH-style diet. Individuals following the Western diet over the 16-year study period experienced a loss of kidney function and an increase in urine albumin. Following a DASH-like diet, though, was associated with a preservation of kidney function.

Cutting back on salt and fighting high blood pressure with a DASH-like diet has additional benefits for people with CKD. An Australian study found that the low-sodium DASH diet also reduced acidosis and the excretion of calcium in urine, indicating a beneficial effect on bone health.

The National Kidney Foundation in its Clinical Practice Guidelines recommends that patients with CKD follow a DASH-like diet. However, patients on dialysis or who have imbalances in blood levels of potassium and phosphorus will require dietary modifications. Failing kidneys often have difficulty in maintaining the balance of potassium and phosphorus, and the DASH food components (dairy, nuts, vegetables, and fruits) are high in those minerals. If you are on dialysis or if your blood tests show a rise in levels of these minerals, consult with your dietitian for an appropriate modification of the DASH diet.

C. Eat Breakfast

You've heard it before, but breakfast really is the most important meal of the day. Eating a proper breakfast helps you reach your daily quota of vitamins, minerals, anti-oxidants, and other important nutrients. It can also help you control cholesterol, improve insulin sensitivity and maintain a healthy weight. According to the National Weight Control Registry--a database of Americans who have lost weight and kept it off--80 percent of its successful weight-loss members eat breakfast daily.

> **An ABC News poll found that 40% of U.S. adults don't eat breakfast.**

Breakfast jump-starts the brain, which relies on glucose as an immediate fuel source. Glucose is also an immediate source of energy for the rest of the body's cells. Because blood glucose is depleted overnight, eating in the morning replenishes the glucose supply for improved overall function. Regular breakfast eaters have lower rates of type 2 diabetes, lower risk of heart failure, and may even live longer.

RECENT RESEARCH →

In a recent study, scientists investigated certain health effects associated with eating breakfast. They found that study participants who ate breakfast had lower BMIs and waist circumferences than non-breakfast-eaters. Participants who ate cereal for breakfast had higher intakes of several vitamins and minerals than both non-breakfast-eaters and consumers of other breakfast choices.

American Journal of Lifestyle Medicine, 2009

Components of a Good Breakfast

Protein - Look for lean sources like eggs, beans, low-fat dairy such as yogurt or milk.
Carbohydrates - Select complex ones for the nutrients and fiber--whole grains, fruits, and vegetables.
Healthy Fats - Including olive or canola oil, nuts, seeds, fatty fish.

For breakfast to provide its benefits, it must be nutritious. Forgo the donuts, white bread products, fast-food offerings, and bacon or sausage. Such items are largely stripped of nutrition and often loaded with sugar, salt, saturated fat, and trans fatty acids. Stick with the more traditional fare: whole grain cereals, eggs, low-fat milk products (including yogurt), and fruit.

Following are easy-to-prepare and nutritious choices for breakfast. Each breakfast serves one person and is around 400 calories (some even less). Vary your breakfast choices to obtain a variety of nutrients throughout the week.

10 Quick Breakfasts

Nutritious Smoothie

Blend until smooth:
1 cup fruit (½ med. banana, fresh pineapple, mango, kiwi, peach, papaya, or melon)
1 c. fat-free, plain Greek yogurt
½ c. non-fat milk or calcium-fortified juice
½ c. frozen blueberries or other berries
1 T wheat germ
1 T almonds, walnuts, pecans, or ground flaxseed

Total Calories: 388

Egg Salad

Mix: 2 chopped, hard-boiled eggs with 2 T. light mayonnaise
Spread on:
1 slice whole-wheat toast
Top with:
1 slice (1oz) swiss cheese
Tomato slices and lettuce
Enjoy with ½ c. 100% pomegranate juice combined with ½ c. carbonated water over ice.

Total Calories: 374

Yogurt Sundae

Top 1 c. non-fat plain Greek yogurt
With: ¾ c. fresh berries
2 T chopped nuts or seeds

Total Calories: 401

Omelet

Prepare a 2-egg omelet, topped with
½ c. chopped asparagus
½ c. chopped tomato
2 T. grated Parmesan cheese
Serve with:
1 slice multi-grain toast
1 c. non-fat milk

Total Calories: 379

Pocket Scramble

Sauté in ½ T extra-virgin olive oil over medium heat:
1-2 T chopped onion
6 cherry tomato halves
3 sliced mushrooms
When soft, add and scramble together:
1 c. baby spinach
2 med. eggs
Fill ½ of a whole-wheat pita pocket.
Enjoy with: 1 c. fresh fruit and hot unsweetened green or black tea

Total Calories: 340

Whole Wheat Bagel

Smear ½ small (3-in) whole-wheat bagel with:
2 T low-fat ricotta cheese
Top with:
2 oz. smoked salmon
Black pepper, herbs, sliced onion, and a squirt of lemon, if desired
Serve with:
1 c. calcium-fortified 100% orange juice and hot unsweetened green tea

Total Calories: 275

Cereal to Sip

Blend until smooth:
1 c. non-fat milk
½ c. cooked barley (or brown rice, or quinoa)
1 c. frozen blueberries
¼ t. cinnamon, cardamom, or nutmeg

Total Calories: 285

Oatmeal

Stir into 1 c. boiling water:
½ c. oatmeal
¼ t. cinnamon
1 T. wheat germ
Serve with:
1 c. non-fat milk
1 c. mango cubes

Total Calories: 374

Whole-Grain Cereal

1 c. whole-grain cereal (with more than 5 g fiber and less than 7 g sugar per serving)
Top with:
1 c. sliced strawberries
1 c. non-fat milk
Enjoy with:
1 orange (or grapefruit)

Total Calories: 305

PB and Toast

Spread 1 T all-natural peanut or almond butter on
1 slice toasted whole-wheat plain or raisin bread.
Top with:
banana (or apple) slices.
Enjoy with:
1 cup non-fat milk

Total Calories: 394

D. Replenish Nutrients at Lunch

Regular meals, including eating a midday meal, help you maintain stable blood glucose and lipid levels and replenish energy. Studies show that irregular meal frequency (skipping meals) disturbs energy metabolism, increases insulin resistance, and raises fasting blood lipid levels in both lean and obese people. The components of a good lunch include some protein, carbohydrates, a little good fat (nuts, seeds, olive oil), and fiber.

Limit fast foods, which are loaded with saturated and trans fats, salt, and sugar. Eating the typical offerings of common fast-food restaurants is proven to lead to poor health. A McDonald's Quarter Pounder with cheese and a small milk-shake contain 38 grams of fat and nearly 1200 milligrams of sodium. Add fries for another 30 grams of fat, and that's more fat than is recommended for the entire day.

> **A statin would not cancel the ill effects of the excess sodium and calories and the lack of nutrients in fast food.**

Because of the insult on health imposed by most fast-food choices, British researchers recently suggested that fast-food restaurants offer customers a statin (*e.g.,* Lipitor) to go with their meals, one that could be found alongside the salt and pepper. The researchers argued (in the 2010 issue of *American Journal of Cardiology*) that one statin pill would offset the ill effects of the unhealthy fast-food meal, thereby reducing the risk of heart disease brought on by the meal. However, fast-food fare threatens more than just the heart, and eating for good health is about proper food selection and moderation in intake. We cannot expect a pill to cancel the health assault from poor eating.

Here are 10 healthful lunch choices that provide needed nutrients and reduce risk of chronic diseases--not add to the risk as do most fast-food restaurant choices. Each of these 10 lunches contains 450 calories or less and is low in saturated fat and sodium. Again, vary your lunch choices from day to day so you obtain a variety of nutrients from different foods throughout the week.

10 Easy Lunches

Pocket Sandwich

Saute until softened, 1½ c. sliced vegetables
(*e.g.*, mushrooms, carrots, onions, cabbage, celery) in 1 T extra virgin olive oil
Stuff into a whole wheat pita
Enjoy with 1 med. apple and unsweetened iced tea

Total Calories: 413

Tuna Salad

Combine:
1 can (3 oz) albacore tuna (in water, drained)
¼ c. salsa (regular or pineapple)
Serve on a salad of:
3 c. mixed organic baby greens
1 c. sliced cucumbers,
1 c. sliced red bell peppers
Enjoy with: 1 c. non-fat milk and 3 Triscuits

Total Calories: 408

Seafood Roll

Combine:
1 c. cooked, chopped lobster
1 T each chopped celery and onion
2 T light mayonnaise
1 t. lemon juice
1 t. tarragon
Black pepper
Place into: whole-wheat hot dog bun
Top with:
¹/₂ c. chopped cabbage, mixed with 1 t. light mayonnaise
4 cherry tomatoes
½ c. sliced cucumbers
½ c. red pepper slices
Enjoy with unsweetened iced tea and 1 orange.

Total Calories: 350

Chopped Salad

Combine:
3 c. chopped romaine lettuce
½ c. white beans or chickpeas (low-sodium, drained and rinsed)
Add:
¼ c. each chopped tomato, cucumber, radishes, red bell pepper, celery
1 sliced green onion
Chopped fresh parsley
Dress with:
1 T red wine vinegar
½ T extra-virgin olive oil
Black pepper
2 T dried cranberries
Enjoy with 5 multi-grain crackers and 1 c. non-fat milk.

Total Calories: 371

Gazpacho

Puree until smooth:
4 chopped plum tomatoes
2 c. low-sodium tomato juice
1 chopped red bell pepper
1 c. chopped cucumber
½ c. chopped onion
½ jalapeño pepper
   (seeded, deveined)
1 clove garlic
¼ c. basil leaves
¼ c. cilantro
Makes 3 2-cup servings.
Top each with ⅓ chopped
   avocado.
Enjoy with: 15 baked blue
   corn chips and 1 med. apple
Total Calories: 405

Veggies 'n' Dip

Blend:
1 can garbanzo beans,
   rinsed and drained
1 clove garlic
1 T extra-virgin olive oil
¼ c. water
¼ c. tahini
2 T lemon juice
Serve ½ cup with a mix of
   raw vegetables
   (broccoli, celery, carrot or
   zucchini sticks, radishes,
   bell pepper).
Enjoy with: ½ c. 100%
   pomegranate juice mixed
   with ¾ c. carbonated or
   sparkling water
Total Calories: 425

Bruschetta

Combine:
⅓ c. chopped Haas avocado
½ c. chopped tomato
1 T lemon juice
1 T chopped onion
1 T chopped cilantro
Black pepper
Spread over:
2 slices whole-wheat toast
Enjoy with:
10 sweet, raw cherries and
   unsweetened iced tea
Total Calories: 428

Summer Salad

Combine:
3 c. organic baby spinach
½ c chopped mango
½ c. sliced strawberries
¼ c. each chopped red bell
   pepper, carrots, red onion,
   celery, and cucumber
Sprinkle salad with:
2 T walnuts
1 T extra-virgin olive oil
1 T vinegar
2 T feta cheese
Total Calories: 450

Soup / Salad

Enjoy:
 1 ½ c. lentil soup
 1 small whole wheat roll
With:
 2 c. torn Romaine lettuce
 topped with 1 med. toma-
 to, ¼ avocado, and 1 T
 light vinaigrette dressing.

Total Calories: 427

Quinoa (keen-wah)

Mix:
 ½ c. cooked quinoa
 1 c. combination of diced
 carrots, onion, cucumber,
 and celery
Add:
 1 T sunflower seeds
 2 T low-fat feta cheese
Dress with:
 1 T each red wine vinegar
 and extra-virgin olive oil
Enjoy with unsweetened iced
 tea.

Total Calories: 423

E. Dinner

Sitting down for family dinners has several advantages over eating in front of a television or in the car. Studies indicate that families who eat together have better overall nutrition and, in turn, lower risks of disease and of being overweight.

RECENT RESEARCH → Researchers collected data from students in sixth, seventh, and eighth grades regarding meals. The students who reported frequent family dinners had a higher quality diet than students who ate few family dinners. Likewise, skipping breakfast and lunch was negatively associated with diet quality.

Other Benefits of Family Dinners:
- **Children less likely to take drugs.**
- **Children do better in school.**
- **Parents have better rapport with children.**

Following are dinner menus that are nutrient-dense and varied. Again, select a different dinner each night for a full spectrum of important nutrients. Each dinner has 500 or fewer calories. If you ate meat for lunch, select a meatless dinner to help control your daily protein intake.

10 Delicious Dinners

Pesto Pasta

Toss: 1 ½ c. whole wheat penne pasta with 2 T pesto (Blend 1 c. spinach, basil, or arugula with 2 t. extra-virgin olive oil and black pepper)

Top with:
A mix of sliced mushrooms, onions, and broccoli sautéed in 1 T. extra-virgin olive oil
2 T. Parmesan or Romano cheese

Have 1 c. sliced fresh fruit for dessert.

Total Calories: 495

Simple Salmon

Grill: 3 oz. piece of salmon

Enjoy with:
1 c. steamed broccoli
½ c. brown rice, cooked with ¼ c. diced onions
2 small whole-wheat roll

Have: 1 c. fresh strawberries for dessert.

Total Calories: 500

Salad/Shrimp Night

Toss together:
3 c. mix of organic baby spinach and arugula

Top with
¼ c. thinly-sliced red onion
6 grape tomatoes
$1/3$ c. sliced avocado
½ c. blueberries

Add:
4 large grilled shrimp

Enjoy with: 1 slice crusty whole-wheat bread and a 4 oz. glass red wine.

Total Calories: 462

Tomato-Basil Cod

Grill: 3 oz. cod filet

Top with a mix of:
1 diced tomato
2 T choped basil
½ t. minced garlic
1 t. extra-virgin olive oil

Serve with:
8 grilled or steamed asparagus spears
½ c. barley (cooked with chopped onion, garlic, and herbs of your choice).

Total Calories: 505

Veggie Pizza for 1

Break open:
A 4-inch multigrain pita
Brush with:
1 t. extra-virgin olive oil
Top with:
¼ c. marinara sauce
¾ c. mix of sautéed
mushrooms, diced onions,
chopped garlic, chopped
green pepper
Add: 2 T low-fat mozzarella
cheese
Broil until cheese melts.
Serve with:
2 c. chopped, organic
Romaine lettuce topped with
chopped tomato and
2 T light Italian dressing.

Total Calories: 426

Baked Potato Night

Bake: 1 medium organic
potato (eat the skin, too!)
Top with your choice of:

1 c. cooked broccoli
2 T. parmigiano-reggiano
cheese

$1/_2$ c. shredded chicken breast
1 T. sliced green onion
1 T. barbecue sauce

¼ c. low-fat ricotta cheese
2 T. sliced green onion

½ c. tomato salsa (see
Vegetable recipes, Sec. G)

Enjoy with: 2 c. spinach
topped with 2 T lemon juice
1 ½ t. extra-virgin olive oil.
Small whole-wheat dinner roll

Total Calories: 471 (varies
with topping)

Vegetarian Delight

Choose:
1 c. each of 3 different-
colored vegetables from
the list of Vegetables in
Section G, below
Add:
$1/_3$ c. cooked brown rice
Enjoy with a small whole-
wheat roll

Total Calories: 400
(depending on vegetable
choices)

Tuna Tonight

Grill:
3 oz. tuna steak, as you like
Top with:
½ onion thinly sliced and
3 sliced mushrooms,
sautéed in 2 t. extra-virgin
olive oil
Add: 1 t. sesame seeds
Enjoy with 1 c. sweet potato
French fries (see Vegetables
in Section G).
2 c. cooked spinach

Total Calories: 438

Italian Night

Cook:
  Whole-wheat ziti per
  package directions
Sauté in 1 T extra virgin
  olive oil:
  ½ c. chopped onion
  2 cloves chopped garlic
  ½ c. chopped flat-leaf
    parsley
  ½ c. chopped basil
Steam:
  4 c. broccoli florets
Toss pasta with other
  ingredients.
  (1 serving = 2 cups)
Enjoy with 4 oz. red wine.

Total Calories: 452

Mexican Salad

Top 3 c. organic mixed baby
  greens with:
  ½ black beans, rinsed and
  drained
  ¼ c. corn kernels (thawed from
  frozen)
  ¼ c. thinly-sliced sweet onion
  ¼ c. diced red pepper
  ½ c tomato salsa (see Sec. E
  for recipe
  $^1/_3$ c. sliced avocado
Enjoy with lime juice
  combined with carbonated
  water over ice and a cup of
  diced mango for dessert.

Total Calories: 433

F. Snacks/Desserts

Healthful snacks fill the gap between meals to keep blood
sugar levels even and provide additional calories for energy.
Desserts are pleasant and should supply nutrients, not just
calories. Each snack and dessert presented here contains
200 calories or less. Add 2 snacks during the day if you have
a 1600 calories-per-day goal. Add additional 200 calorie-
snacks for 1800, 2000, or 2200 calories per day.

Satisfying Snacks/Desserts

½ c. whole-grain cereal
½ c. non-fat milk

1 c. low-fat (sodium-free)
cottage cheese
1 c. strawberry halves

1 c. salsa (combine ¾ c. diced
tomato, ½ c. diced red pepper, ¼ c. chopped onion,
1 clove minced garlic,
2 T. chopped cilantro
2 T lime juice, 1 T olive oil)
12 baked blue corn chips

1 red bell pepper, sliced into
strips
1 carrot, cut into strips
1/3 c. hummus

1 ½ c. cooked edamame
(green soybeans) in their
pods. Top with lime juice
and black pepper.

Spread 4 RyKrisp crackers
each with:
1 T low-fat ricotta cheese and
top with strawberry slices.

Blend and drink:
½ c. unsalted tomato juice
½ c. carrot juice
½ c. baby spinach
1 T. ground flaxseed
½ small ripe avocado
2 T. lemon juice
2 T. fresh parsley

1 c. lentil soup

1 c. blueberries
2 T walnuts or almonds

1 c. non-fat yogurt
1 c. raspberries

Heat together:
1 ½ c. non-fat milk
1 t. extra dark cocoa
½ t. honey
½ t. cinnamon
1 t. vanilla

1 cup strawberries topped
with
2 T. dark chocolate sauce

1 cup fat-free sorbet
(under 180 calories)

1 small baked apple, topped
with cinnamon
and
2 T chopped walnuts

1 frozen banana, rolled in
2 T. chopped pecans

30 dark-chocolate-covered
raisins

4 pineapple slices (1/4 inch
each)
grilled with a sprinkle of
brown sugar

½ c. red grapes

2 sticks low-fat mozzarella
string cheese

G. Eat More Vegetables

We love vegetables. We can enjoy large portions of most vegetables without worrying about excess calories, and we receive a nutritional bonus with each bite. Vegetables are high in vitamins, minerals, phytochemicals, antioxidants--all important in preventing many diseases. Vegetables also provide carbohydrate and some protein energy, without much fat.

Diets high in vegetables are known to help reduce risks of hypertension, cancer, heart disease, and diabetes. Yet, less than a quarter of U.S. adults consume the recommended 5 servings of vegetables per day. This inadequate consumption could account for the epidemic rates of several diet-related diseases.

We list our favorite vegetables, with a recipe for each. You can enjoy a serving of one of the vegetables as a snack anytime during the day.

Our Favorite Vegetables (Fast and Delicious)

Asparagus	**Drizzle** clean asparagus with 1 T extra-virgin olive oil and fresh ground black pepper. **Spread** asparagus in single layer on a baking pan, and roast at 425° for about 10 min.
Beans (Green)	**Steam** green beans covered over simmering water, 4 to 5 minutes. **Drizzle** with 1 T extra-virgin olive oil, sautéed garlic, grated ginger, toasted almonds.
Beets	**Roast** fresh beets in a covered baking dish in 1 inch of water at 450° for 40 minutes. Cool and rub off skins. **Slice** beets and combine with sliced red onion, 2 T sunflower seeds, 1 t. dill, 2 T red wine vinegar, 2 t. extra-virgin olive oil. **Chill** before eating.
Broccoli	**Arrange** organic florets in a steamer basket and steam, covered over simmering water for about 5 minutes, until tender. **Serve with** 1 T light Italian dressing.

Brussels sprouts	**Sauté** ½ c. chopped onion and 2 sliced cloves of garlic in 1 T extra-virgin olive oil for about 4 minutes. **Stir in** ¾ lb. Brussels sprouts, halved and thinly sliced, sauté 2 minutes. **Add** ½ c. water and cook 5 minutes to absorb liquid, stirring frequently. **Sprinkle** with 4 t. chopped walnuts.
Cabbage	**Toss together:** 1 small head thinly sliced red cabbage 1 thinly sliced unpeeled apple 1 thinly sliced onion ¼ c. fresh lemon juice ⅓ c. chopped fresh parsley ¼ c. low-fat mayonnaise ¼ c. non-fat, plain yogurt Fresh-ground black pepper 2 oz. crumbled bleu cheese **Refrigerate** 2 to 3 hours.
Carrots	**Place** in a small saucepan: 1 t. butter 1 t. extra-virgin olive oil 3 organic carrots, cut into 1-inch pieces ½ t. cinnamon **Cook** over medium heat, about 10 minutes until carrots are tender.
Cauliflower	**Steam** separated florets from 1 head of cauliflower 5 to 6 minutes until tender; drain. **Heat** together just until warm: 2 T extra-virgin olive oil 1 clove minced garlic 3 T chopped fresh parsley 1 T balsamic vinegar **Pour** sauce over steamed cauliflower.
Swiss Chard, Collards, or Kale	**Cook** over medium heat, until wilted, about 5 min.: 1 lb. greens, stems removed 2 T extra-virgin olive oil **Add** 3 cloves minced garlic **Cook** 1 minute more. **Serve** with your choice of ¼ c. crumbled feta cheese, toasted pine nuts, or raisins.

Corn	**Soak** unhusked corn in cold water to cover for 30 min. **Roast** corn in a 400° oven or on a barbecue grill; turn once. **Serve** hot.
Cucumbers	**Slice** 2 fresh cucumbers. **Mix** with ½ sliced small red onion, 2 T apple cider vinegar, ½ t. dill. **Refrigerate**.
Eggplant	**Prick** 1 large eggplant with a fork, and roast in a shallow dish for 450° for about 1 hour. Cool. **Halve** eggplant and scoop out flesh. **Blend** together with flesh: 3 T extra-virgin olive oil ½ small onion 2 cloves garlic 3 T fresh parsley 2 T lemon juice Dash hot pepper sauce **Chill** and serve as a vegetable or pita dip.
Garlic	**Cut** ¼-inch slice from top of 4 heads of garlic. **Drizzle** heads with extra-virgin olive oil. **Bake**, uncovered, in baking dish for 30 minutes at 300° **Cover** dish with foil and continue baking another 1 to 1½ hours, until garlic is creamy. **Squeeze** garlic from heads onto crusty whole grain bread and serve.
Parsnips	**Toss** 2 lbs. parsnips, peeled and cut into 3-inch pieces, with 1 T extra-virgin olive oil and fresh ground black pepper. **Roast** at 400° until tender, about 45 minutes.

Potatoes	**Best Ever "French Fries":** **Cut** 2 cleaned, unpeeled organic potatoes (sweet or white) into French fry slices. **Toss** potatoes with 1½ t. extra-virgin olive oil and fresh ground pepper. **Spread** potatoes in a single layer onto a parchment-paper-lined baking sheet. **Bake** at 450° for 20 to 25 minutes, until golden brown. **Serve** immediately.
Spinach	**Add** 2 t. extra-virgin olive oil to saucepan and sauté ¼ c. thinly sliced onion until tender. **Add** washed organic spinach, tossing from time to time, until spinach collapses, about 2 minutes.
Squash	**Bake** large winter squash (such as butternut) at 375° for 45 minutes until tender. Cool and remove flesh. **Blend** squash flesh together with: ¼ c. non-fat milk 2 t. cinnamon 1/8 t. each nutmeg, ground cloves, and ginger ¼ c. dark brown sugar. **Bake** in non-stick spray-coated dish for 20 minutes at 350°.
Tomato Salsa:	**Combine** in a small bowl: 2 medium chopped tomatoes 1 jalapeño pepper (seeded and minced) ½ medium red onion (minced) 2 bunches green onion (thinly sliced, white and green parts) 1 clove garlic, minced ½ c. fresh chopped cilantro ¼ c. fresh lime juice 2 T extra-virgin olive oil Fresh ground black pepper. **Chill** salsa several hours.

Zucchini	**Cut** 2 or 3 zucchini into ¼-inch slices.
	Drizzle lightly with extra-virgin olive oil and fresh ground black pepper.
	Grill about 10 minutes, turning once.

For more on DASH, visit the National Heart, Lung, and Blood Institute at www.nhlbi.nih.gov. Also, the KidneySteps.com website provides delicious menu choices, as well as nutrition tips.

KIDNEYSTEP 5

EXERCISE FOR THE KIDNEY

Deciding to exercise is one of the best lifestyle choices you can make to improve your health, better your kidney function, and improve your odds of longer survival. A sedentary lifestyle is dangerous, substantially increasing your risks of obesity, diabetes, metabolic syndrome, high blood pressure, CKD, cardiovascular disease, cancer, and cognitive decline. Sedentary adults die years earlier and in poorer physical condition than physically active individuals.

KidneyStep 5 illustrates:

- How exercise aids kidney health.

- The impact of exercise in preventing, delaying, or improving chronic diseases common in people at risk of or with CKD.

- The principles of a sound physical activity program.

- Exercises for people who are sedentary and want to begin activity.

- How to advance a beginner's exercise program.

20.

STAYING ACTIVE MEANS STAYING ALIVE

For individuals with chronic kidney disease (CKD), staying active may mean staying alive. Many people with CKD die prematurely from conditions that develop concurrent with the kidney disease, including particularly cardiovascular disease. Nearly all individuals with CKD have hypertension, and many have diabetes, are overweight, and develop bone disease. Research shows that if kidney patients get off the couch, they increase their odds of survival, lessen the likelihood of developing other diseases, and may even improve kidney function.

> **Even though CKD patients have the ability to exercise, they are over twice as likely as the general population to be inactive.**

A. Exercise--Medicine for the Kidneys

If you think physical activity is unimportant to kidney health, think again. Exercise significantly increases long-term survival in people with kidney disease, and the ability to exercise is the single most powerful predictor of their longevity. This study illustrates the need to be active:

RECENT STUDY → Researchers analyzed data collected from 15,368 adult participants of the U.S. National Health and Nutrition Examination Survey, III (NHANES) health study. Of those, 5.9% had CKD, and 28% of the CKD participants were inactive compared to 13.5% of participants without kidney disease. Researchers found that the participants with kidney disease who were active were 56% less likely to die during the 9 year study compared to the inactive CKD participants. Increasing physical activity has a survival benefit in the CKD population, researchers concluded.

Clinical Journal of the American Society of Nephrology
October 2009

Not only can people with CKD increase the chances of a lengthier, healthier life simply by exercising, they can also improve kidney function with exercise. Physical activity is shown to lower proteinuria/albuminuria, the key sign of CKD and the best known predictor of cardiovascular disease.

CURRENT STUDY → Researchers examined 3,587 participants with a mean age of 58.6 years in the NHANES health study. Participants who exercised (walking) the most reduced their albuminuria levels.

American Journal of Epidemiology, March 2010

The reduction in albuminuria from exercise is most obvious in individuals with CKD caused by diabetes, but also occurs in exercisers with other causes of kidney disease.

Research likewise emphasizes the positive effect of exercise on kidney function in overweight individuals. Excess weight is linked with diabetes and the development of microalbuminuria, an early sign of CKD. Losing weight may preserve kidney function in overweight people. Researchers at the Cleveland Clinic analyzed 13 studies that looked at the effects of weight loss intervention in obese CKD patients. The analysis showed that weight loss from diet and exercise decreased proteinuria and could even prevent additional decline in kidney function.

Most individuals with CKD also have hypertension, which threatens kidney function in all individuals. The *Seventh Report of the Joint National Committee on Prevention, Detection, Evaluation, and Treatment of High Blood Pressure* recommends that all patients with hypertension engage in regular aerobic physical activity, such as brisk walking, for at

A meta-analysis of 54 trials showed that previously sedentary adults decreased their blood pressure with regular aerobic exercise

least 30 minutes per day on most days of the week. This recommendation is based on considerable evidence from clinical studies of hypertensive patients assigned to regular exercise. Regular exercise lowers blood pressure.

Exercise also helps protect aging kidneys. While kidney function naturally declines with age, high levels of physical activity seem to slow the rate of decline. Preserving kidney function is particularly important for the aging CKD patient:

RECENT STUDY ➜ A 7-year study consisting of 4,011 people ages 65 or older showed that those who exercised most had a 28 percent lower risk of renal function decline.

Archives of Internal Medicine, 2009

Typically, patients with CKD are physically inactive and report reduced physical function. As in the general population, reduced physical function and inactivity are associated with increased mortality and poor quality of life. Cardiovascular exercise increases both physical functioning and life quality in kidney patients:

RECENT RESEARCH ➜ Researchers reviewed prior studies on the effects of exercise in reducing the physical and psychological limitations encountered by CKD patients. Exercising CKD patients showed improvements in physical fitness, physical function, manual dexterity, reaction time, and lower extremity muscle strength. All of these factors helped to improve quality of life for CKD patients.

Medscape Journal of Medicine, 2008

Even if the CKD patient is on dialysis, physical activity has important health benefits. When a patient has ESRD, the patient often has several co-existing medical conditions that can interfere with the physical and psychological aspects of life. One common problem is muscle wasting. In an interesting study, dialysis patients were asked to lift hand weights during dialysis. The results showed that the weightlifting counteracted muscle wasting and improved health for these fragile patients.

THE STUDY ➜ Researchers gave 49 dialysis patients 12 weeks of high-intensity, progressive resistance training administered during hemodialysis treatment. Each patient performed two sets of 10 exercises at high-intensity using hand weights three times a week for 12 weeks. The patients showed significant improvements in muscle strength, mid-thigh and muscle circumference, and C-reactive protein.

Journal of the American Society of Nephrology, 2007

313

Because of the obvious and overwhelming benefits of physical activity for individuals with kidney disease, the National Kidney Foundation (NKF) revised its K/DOQI Guidelines to recommend that nephrologists counsel patients to increase physical activity. Yet, researchers report that few nephrologists are doing so. Recently released recommendations aim at encouraging practitioners to counsel patients:

> **KidneySteps.com provides regularly updated tips to help you meet your health and fitness goals. Tips include exercises you can do in your home, healthful recipes, and more.**

- In 2010, the National Coalition for Promoting Physical Activity released the *National Physical Activity Plan* to encourage the U.S. to meet the minimum physical activity guidelines. The planning strategies include a recommendation to healthcare providers to counsel patients about the health benefits of exercise.

- The American College of Sports Medicine (ACSM) and the American Medical Association have developed the *Exercise is Medicine Health Care Provider Action Guide* to encourage health practitioners to counsel with patients about exercise benefits.

- Every 10 years the U.S. Department of Health and Human Services (HHS) releases national health objectives to encourage improvement in addressing major health concerns. These objectives reflect recent scientific findings, current data, and trends about major health risks in our population. One important goal in *Healthy People 2020* is for physicians to provide counseling/education on exercise to all patients with chronic diseases.

B. Exercise--Medicine for the Whole Body

In the 2009 results of the American Time Use Survey of the Bureau of Labor Statistics, only 21% of men and 16% of women engaged in sports, exercise, or recreation on any given day.

The CDC estimates that over one-third of Americans are sedentary. They avoid even the minimum walk of 30 minutes per day recommended by most health and fitness authorities.

We sit commuting to and from work; we continue to sit while at work; then we sit at home watching television, at the computer, or reading a book. The American Heart Association (AHA) reports that every hour spent in front of a television daily is associated with:

- An 11 percent increased risk of death from all causes;

- A 9 percent increased risk of cancer death; and

- An 18 percent increased risk of a cardiovascular disease-related death.

People who watch TV more than 4 hours daily (compared to less than 2 hours) have a 46 percent higher risk of death from all causes and an 80 percent increased risk of cardiovascular disease-related death. All in all, this inactivity is making America fat, diabetic, disabled from many chronic diseases, and is shortening lifespans.

Watching TV and riding in a car for more than 23 hours in a week (compared to less than 14 hrs/wk) increase risk of cardiovascular death by 82%.
Exercise and Sports Science Review, 2010

1. Wide Sweeping Benefits

Few lifestyle choices have as large an effect on mortality as physical activity. The HHS lists the following benefits of physical activity in adults:

Exercise lowers risk of:	Exercise can also:
• Early death • Coronary heart disease • Stroke • High blood pressure • Adverse blood lipid profile • Type 2 diabetes • Metabolic syndrome • Cancer, including colon, breast, prostate	• Result in weight loss, particularly when combined with reduced calorie intake • Improve cardiorespiratory and muscular fitness • Prevent likelihood of falls • Reduce depression and anxiety • Preserve cognitive function

CKD patients often have a host of co-existing chronic diseases (e.g., diabetes, hypertension, cardiovascular disease) for which exercise is beneficial. Cardiovascular disease alone accounts for half of the deaths of CKD patients. Besides improving kidney function and heart health, physical activity reduces the risk for these other chronic illnesses, wards off cognitive decline and disability, and slows the process of aging.

A growing and convincing body of scientific evidence illustrates that regular exercise as simple as a brisk 30-minute walk five days a week improves the body's ability to avoid diseases of all kinds. This is true across all age groups, ethnic groups, and among the disabled. Regular physical activity:

Strengthens the Heart

The cardiovascular benefits of exercise, both aerobic and strength exercises, are substantial. Studies show that exercise:

- Reduces the incidence of high blood pressure by 40 percent, according to the ACSM

- Reduces coronary heart disease in women by up to 40 percent

- Reduces risk of any cardiovascular event by 60 percent

316

Improves Overall Health

A 2010 study of 13,535 Nurses' Health Study participants ages 70 or older showed that higher levels of physical activity in midlife are associated with exceptional health status in older years.

Prevents Cancer

Numerous studies connect exercise with a lowered risk of cancer. According to the ACSM, exercise can:

- Reduce mortality and the risk of recurrent breast cancer by about 50 percent.
- Lower the risk of colon cancer by over 60 percent.
- Reduce the risk of prostate cancer by 35 percent.

Contributes to Healthier Weight Loss

During a 10-year American Cancer Society study, 44,000 women in their 40's or early 50's lost, rather than gained, weight over that period by exercising at least 4 hours per week.

Builds Bone

High impact activities such as running, jumping, and playing basketball, volleyball, or soccer, increase and prevent loss of bone mineral density, studies show. In a 2010 study, researchers found that women who exercised more than 180 minutes per week retained greater bone density than non-exercisers.

Prevents Diabetes

In the Finnish Diabetes Research Study, 522 overweight, middle-aged people were divided into an exercise/diet group and a control group. At a 3-year follow-up, the people in the lifestyle group who exercised at least 30 minutes per day reduced their risk of diabetes by 58 percent, compared to the control group of non-exercisers.

Improves Blood Cholesterol Levels

In a study of 8700 middle-aged people over 12 years, those who increased their activity by one hour of mild or 30 minutes of moderate activity per week, decreased their triglycerides and raised their good HDLs. Women also reduced their bad LDLs.

317

Adds Longevity

Even a little extra exercise may add years to your life. Researchers divided 4,384 middle-aged and older Americans into five groups based on fitness and followed them for nine years. The least fit group was four times more likely to die during the study than the fittest group. While 25 percent of the least fit group died during the study, only 13 percent of the next-fittest participants did. Better still, only 6 percent of the fittest group died.

Improves Memory

The ACSM reports that exercise can reduce the risk of developing Alzheimer's disease by nearly 40 percent. Also, in a study reported in 2010, researchers followed 3903 participants, ages 55 and older, for two years. The most active participants (exercising more than 3 times per week) had reduced incidence of cognitive impairment compared to the non-active participants.

Decreases Depression

Numerous studies evidence that depression is decreased by exercise. For example, in a 2010 study of obese women asked to exercise, those spending the most minutes exercising saw a decrease in depression and anxiety, as well as a reduction in waist circumference.

Reduces Stroke Risk

A new analysis of data on 39,315 women ages 45 and up over 12 years found the more the women walked, the lower their stroke risk. Two-hours per week of moderate walking led to an 18 percent reduction in stroke risk, and a faster-paced walk reduced stroke risk by up to 37 percent.

In a separate study of 3,298 people over age 69, men who engaged in intense physical activity were 63 percent less likely to suffer a stroke than the couch potatoes.

Remain Independent

Researchers from Indiana University at Indianapolis reviewed 121 trials involving 6700 people over age 60 who strength trained two days each week. Training significantly improved muscle strength and the ability to perform simple daily activities, such as getting out of a chair or climbing stairs.

2. Never Too Old to Exercise

Age is no excuse for avoiding exercise. You are never too old to begin a physical activity program. In fact, becoming active even late in life increases life expectancy and helps you remain independent.

An Israeli study of people over age 70 found that those elderly people lived longer and better if they were physically active at least four hours each week. The physically active seniors were up to 58 percent less likely to die during the 18-year study than their sedentary peers, and up to 92 percent more likely to remain independent while performing the activities of daily living:

THE STUDY →

> Researchers followed 18,021 people for 18 years, from ages 70 to 88.
> - Between ages 70 and 78: a quarter of the sedentary group died compared to 15 percent of the active group.
> - From ages 78 to 85: nearly 41 percent of the sedentary participants died compared to one-fourth of the active seniors.
> - From ages 85 to 88: over 24 percent of the sedentary seniors died versus just 6.8 percent of their physically active peers.
>
> *Archives of Internal Medicine,* 2009

If you are out of shape, resuming exercise can restore your fitness. In a famous study originally done in 1966 (Dallas Bed Rest and Training Study), scientists put five healthy men, all age 20, to bed for 3 weeks and measured their physical deterioration, which was significant. The researchers then assigned the men to 8 weeks of training to see if they could bring them back to their baseline fitness level, which worked.

People who regularly exercise briskly, at an intensity that makes them perspire and breathe a little heavily, live an average of 3 years longer than sedentary people.

Thirty years later, the researchers tracked down the five men, who were now out of shape and a little flabby, and put them on a six-month training program. By the end, they were as aerobically fit as they had been at age 20, although still heavier.

No restrictions to physical activity apply to the older exerciser. The physical activity recommendations for older adults over age 50 are the same as for other adults, but with an additional focus on flexibility and balance. If older adults have physically limiting chronic conditions, the ACSM and the AHA recommend that they be as physically active as their abilities and conditions allow.

C. Physical Activity Basics

Physical activity is nothing more than body movement that expends calories. Activities such as gardening, walking a dog, or performing housework are physical activity. **Exercise** is structured activity like running, aerobics, weight-lifting, or kick-boxing. We use the terms "exercise" and "physical activity" interchangeably. All movement counts.

1. Components of Fitness

According to all leading fitness authorities, a good physical fitness plan to improve health and physical condition includes three separate components: cardio-vascular, strength, and flexibility.

A. CARDIOVASCULAR.

Patient Interview: Nicole has CKD, and she exercises to avoid the development of heart disease. "I joined the YMCA for its cardio classes. I like having an instructor tell me what to do in a class environment. I really like the cardio mix class. We do a variety of activities that keep my heart rate up," Nicole tells us.

Your heart, just like your body, puts on fat and weakens with disuse. If you don't make your heart pump hard on a regular basis, it becomes surrounded by a fatty layer and sluggish. Cardiorespiratory (or aerobic) exercise gets you breathing hard and your heart pumping. Aerobic means "with oxygen" and is a continous activity that most benefits your cardiovascular system (heart, blood, and blood vessels). During aerobic exercise, your heart beats faster and delivers more oxygen-carrying blood to your tissues. The more fit you become, the more efficiently your heart pumps.

Research suggests that people who are physically active for approximately 7 hours a week have a 40% lower risk of dying early than those who are active less than 30 minutes a week.

Choose aerobic activities you enjoy, perhaps brisk walking, running, workout classes or DVDs, bicycling, skating, etc. To benefit sufficiently from the cardio activities you choose, the ACSM and the AHA recommend that you:

- Perform a cardio activity at least four days each week. You will see better health benefits if you perform a cardio activity five to seven days each week.
- Spend at least 20 minutes performing the cardio activity, but 30 to 45 minutes are even better.
- Exercise at an intensity level that ranges between 65 percent and 85 percent of your **maximum heart rate**. This percentage is your **target heart rate** and the intensity range recommended by the ACSM and the AHA.

You may break the cardio down into two or more 10-minute sessions, if you are a beginner.

Here's how to estimate your maximum heart rate and target heart rate:

 Target Heart Rate Calculator

Step 1: Calculate your Maximum Heart Rate (MHR) = 220 – your age
Step 2: Calculate your Target Heart Rate below ↓

Intensity	Target Heart Rate
For a low-intensity workout	**50% to 60% of your MHR (beginners)** This rate is sufficient to reach some cardiovascular benefit. You can easily carry on a conversation in this heart rate zone.
For a moderate-intensity workout	**65% to 70% of your MHR** You burn calories from fat in this zone and strengthen the heart. Talking requires some effort in this zone.
For a high-intensity workout	**75% to 85% of your MHR** Talking is out of the question if your heart rate is in this zone.

Example: For a 50-year-old working at a moderate intensity, the target heart rate equals 220-50 = 170 x 65% =110.5 beats per minute.

The best way to monitor your heart rate is with a heart-rate monitor. Monitors are easy to use and are a fun and accurate way to assure you stay in your workout zone. Exercising at an intensity above the high intensity heart rate zone is hard to maintain and may be harmful for beginners. Let your heart be the indicator of your workout intensity.

The easier and cheaper way to monitor your heart rate and the method recommended by the CDC is with the *Borg Rate of Perceived Exertion*, or RPE. Some experts call the RPE the "talking test." You determine how hard you are working based on your perception of your own exertion. The Swedish scientist Gunnar Borg created his RPE scale using numbers 1 through 20. We prefer the modified scale that includes only 10 exertion ratings. It is more convenient to use.

Modified RPE Scale

1	**No exertion at all** sitting at rest
2	**Very, very light** walking slowly on flat surface
3	**Very light** walking slowly, on a slight grade, talking is easy
4	**Light** moving faster but can still talk effortlessly
5	**Fairly light** not completely comfortable but still can talk easily
6	**Somewhat hard** can talk in full sentences but slightly breathless
7	**Hard** can speak only a few words at a time
8	**Very hard** can't talk except in single words
9	**Very, very hard** talking is not possible
10	**Maximum exertion** probably too high

- If you can talk easily, you are in a low-intensity zone (around level 3 to 4).
- If you are breathing heavily and talking takes some effort, you have hit the moderate intensity zone (level 5 to 6).
- If you are sweating, breathing heavily, can barely talk, and your heart is beating rapidly, you are in the vigorous-intensity zone (level 7 or 8). Never go to the point that you are gasping for breath.

323

As your heart gets fitter, it may take longer to reach your target heart rate, and your pulse returns to normal faster after your workout is over. Also, your resting heart rate-- your heart rate when you are not exercising--might become lower as your heart becomes stronger and healthier. A recent George Washington University School of Medicine study found that individuals with the highest resting heart rates (above 76 beats per minute) were 26 percent more likely to have a heart attack than those with the lowest (62 beats per minute or less).

B. STRENTH TRAINING

Even if you are not interested in bigger biceps, strength training benefits your overall health in ways that extend beyond your resulting improved looks. Experts believe that strength training may be the key to preventing disability as you age. Declining muscle mass contributes to heart disease, type 2 diabetes, and other chronic diseases by slowing the body's metabolic rate, which allows fat to accumulate. Strength training halts the decline in muscle mass, and has a host of other benefits not obtained by cardio workouts alone. Consequently, a good fitness plan will include strength exercises at least twice a week.

> **Between the ages of 50 and 70, strength can drop by 15% per decade.**

You can increase your strength with dumbbells, barbells, or resistance bands. Each time you workout for strength, you will perform repetitions and sets.

Repetitions - Repetitions or "reps" are the number of times you perform the particular strength exercise. The CDC and the AHA recommend that you try to perform 8 to 12 reps per weight activity (8 bicep curls or 12 abdominal crunches). If you are older than 50, you are to attempt up to 15 reps for each exercise.

Sets - A set is the completed number of repetitions. If you are lifting the weight 8 times, you have performed a set after all 8 lifts. Beginners might choose to start with 1 set of reps for each exercise; over time, increasing the number of sets.

Strength train 2 to 3 days each week, but not on consecutive days. You will perform 8 to 10 strength exercises, working each of the major muscle groups (arms, shoulders, back, chest, hips, legs, abdomen).

C. FLEXIBILITY

As we age (or if we have not exercised recently), our muscles shorten and our joints stiffen. In other words, we are not flexible and our body is not fit. Flexibility is important for full-range motion and to keep the spine upright and elongated to stand straighter and taller. It is important for balance and to avoid falls and resulting injuries. One in three people age 65 and up will fall each year doing the normal activities of daily living, but falls are preventable with stretching and balance programs.

Research also suggests that low-intensity exercises like yoga or tai chi can help reduce blood pressure. Researchers at the Stanford Prevention Research Center had 39 sedentary seniors perform 60 minutes of tai chi three times a week for 12 weeks. On average, the group lowered resting systolic blood pressure by 13 percent and resting diastolic blood pressure by 10 percent. These results were similar to results obtained from medication use.

A person's flexibility may indicate their heart health:

RECENT STUDY ➔ Researchers studied 526 healthy, non-smoking adults, 20 to 83 years old, with a normal BMI. The participants performed a "sit and reach" test for flexibility. Participants with less flexibility had stiffer arteries measured by blood pressure and pulse rate. The researchers speculated that improving flexibility might improve the health of arteries.

American Journal of Physiology Heart Circulation Physiology, 2009

Your authors enjoy the de-stressing aspect of stretching, as well as the muscle toning and joint flexibility. We each attend yoga classes that challenge our balance and strength and improve joint movement. Pilates classes also increase our flexibility, in addition to developing core strength (strength in the back and abdominals).

2. How Much of Each?

The *2008 Physical Activity Guidelines for Americans* were the first-ever guidelines released by the Department of Health and Human Services for exercise. The guidelines resulted from extensive analysis of scientific information on physical activity and health.

While any physical activity is better than little or no activity, a certain amount of minimum activity is directly tied to improved health. The *2008 Guidelines* suggest the following amounts of exercise as a minimum for all adults:

Fitness Component	Guideline Amount
CARDIO	**Moderate-intensity** At least 150 min. per week (2 hours and 30 min.) **or** **Vigorous-intensity** 1 hour and 15 min. a week
STRENGTH	**8 to 10 exercises, 8 to 15 reps each** (2 or 3 non-consecutive days per week) • **Moderate to vigorous intensity** • **Involve all major muscle groups**
FLEXIBILITY (for older adults)	**At least 10 minutes of stretches** (2 or more days per week) • **Use a static stretch, holding each stretch to a level of mild discomfort 10 to 30 seconds** • **Repeat each stretch 3 or 4 times, breathing normally** • **Practice balance exercises, also**

The *2008 Guidelines* set out the minimum exercise necessary for health benefits. Yet, 77 percent of Americans fail to meet the *2008 Guideline* minimums.

21.

LEARNING TO MOVE IT

If you are new to exercise or have not exercised in some time, this chapter is for you. Start slowly and progress gradually. Regular exercise decreases the risk of heart disease, stroke, high blood pressure, type 2 diabetes, obesity, some cancers, and osteoporosis. Regular exercise also improves mood, decreases anxiety and depression, aids in stress management, helps control weight, and maintains healthy bones, muscles, and joints. With regular exercise, you may enjoy these benefits, too.

A. Exercising with CKD/Diabetes

Because exercise is so important in helping to prevent diabetes, high blood pressure, heart disease, cancer, osteoporosis, and other chronic diseases; and, because it improves blood pressure, liver profiles, kidney function, and overall feelings of well-being for kidney patients, the National Kidney Foundation (NKF) encourages patients to be physically active. The NKF also makes the following recommendations regarding exercise for individuals with more advanced CKD:

- Talk with a nephrologist before starting an exercise program.

- Start with low impact exercise (walking, cycling, water exercise) that involves the large muscles.

> **The ACSM has listed very high blood pressure as a contraindication to exercise:**
> - **Systolic blood pressure greater than 200 mmHg;**
> - **Diastolic pressure greater than 115 mmHg.**

- Start with shorter sessions, 10 to15 minutes each, and gradually build up to 30 to 60 minutes most days of the week.

The above-listed recommendations are aimed at patients who have not exercised recently and who are in the later stages of CKD. No specific precautions apply to all other people with CKD who already are physically active. Your author with CKD regularly exercised, at vigorous intensity through all stages of CKD.

For individuals who have not exercised recently, gradual progression is essential to health improvement. If you are on dialysis, you should exercise (*e.g.*, lift hand weights) during those dialysis treatments, recommends the American Association of Kidney Patients. Improving your exercise ability can be the difference between living independently or becoming disabled and unable to continue working.

The CDC reports that diabetes in the U.S. increased 25%. between 2005 and 2008.

If you have CKD and are concerned about whether an activity is safe for you, talk with your nephrologist. If you are on dialysis, your nephrologist can refer you to a rehabilitation specialist to get you started. If you don't need this level of care, you may exercise on your own at home or at a fitness center.

For people with diabetes, the American Diabetes Association (ADA) cautions that beginning exercisers check with their physicians before starting vigorous activity. If diabetes is uncontrolled, avoid strenuous exercise so that you do not injure blood vessels in the feet or legs, but do not avoid exercise entirely.

In late 2010, the ADA and the ACSM issued new exercise guidelines for diabetics, recommending the same 150 minutes/week of vigorous activity expressed in the *2008 Physical Activity Guidelines*. People with diabetes are to spread out the aerobic exercise over at least 3 days per week, with no more than 2 consecutive days between bouts of aerobic activity. The ADA states that this amount of physical activity could prevent or delay type 2 diabetes by 57 percent.

Some fitness centers, such as the YMCA, have programs for people with chronic diseases and disabilities. Consult a fitness expert at a fitness center to design a program appropriate for you at your physical level.

B. Make Exercise a Habit

People living in "healthier" neighborhoods (access to walking paths, exercise facilities, and fresh produce) are 38% less likely to develop diabetes.
Archives of Internal Medicine, 2009

You soon will see and feel the results of regular exercise, perhaps in just one month. Your biceps muscles may show some definition as you flex your arms. Your blood tests might indicate improved lipid levels, higher HDL's (the good lipids), and lower blood glucose levels. You will notice more energy and better sleep. If you are over-weight, you may reduce your clothing size, begin looking healthier, and move more easily.

For these changes to occur, physical activity must become a priority and part of your daily routine. Your survival and health depend on making a habit of exercise. Select a time of day that works best, and activities that you enjoy. Studies show that morning exercisers tend to be more consistent exercisers. One of your authors exercises mornings at 5:30 a.m. The rest of the day, she is more energetic and free to focus on her job and other activities. Your other author fits in exercise at different times, depending on the day. But, it is one of the "must-do" items on her daily check list. Her body feels something is missing if she fails to exercise.

Too many of us start an exercise program--perhaps even join a gym--with good intentions of losing weight and getting fit. After a while, the novelty wears off, and we find ourselves back on the couch. Consider the couch dangerous:

RECENT RESEARCH ➔ In a 2010 study of 53,440 men and 69,000 women over 14 years, those who sat more than six hours per day increased their risk of early death by 40 percent (for females) and 20 percent (for males). The participants who sat the rest of the day (watching TV or reading, for example) increased their death rates over the study period by 94 percent in the least active females and 48 percent in the least active males.

American Journal of Epidemiology, 2010

It helps to find activities you like that also increase heart rate for at least 20 minutes, because you'll be more likely to exercise consistently. For example:

Claire: *"I'm a busy lawyer with little motivation to go out and jog or swim. I joined Arthur Murray Dance Studio on a lark and fell in love with dancing. I now go to a line-dancing place once each week and to the dance studio twice a week. The dancing really gets my heart pumping and my body sweating."*

Ed: *"I've never been a jock or an exerciser. I joined a gentle yoga class a few years ago and found it helped relieve my joint pain and really increased my flexibility. After a few months, I tried a vinyana yoga class, which is very aerobic, and I am hooked. This form of yoga is great for my heart, muscle strength, and overall flexibility. I get all the components of exercise at one time, and I look good and feel fantastic."*

You may wish to try a variety of physical activities until you find the one activity (or combination of activities) that is right for you.

C. Cardio--Just Begin

Walking is an easy way to begin a fitness program and is the cardiovascular exercise of choice for beginning exercisers. However, even advanced exercisers often maintain their heart and vessel fitness by moderate to vigorous walking. We love walking and routinely walk 45 minutes or so daily. Walking only requires a good pair of shoes and a safe route.

> **Volunteers who spent 20 minutes on cardio exercise had better moods than non-exercisers for up to 12 hours.**
> *ACSM, 2009*

Start by doing what you can. You might only walk 5 to 10 minutes in the beginning, but even that is better than no activity, according to the *2008 Physical Activity Guidelines for Americans*. If 10 minutes is your limit, then walk that long four or five days the first week or two. Add two minutes each week after that. In time, you will cover two miles in about 30 minutes on a daily basis, which is the goal for beginning exercisers.

Here is a sample walking schedule for those new to exercise and unable to begin with a full 30-minute-per-walk schedule:

The Beginner Begins

Week	1	2	3	4	5	6
Walk slowly	5 min.	5 min.	5 min.	5 min.	5 min.	5 min.
Walk briskly	5 min.	7 min.	9 min.	11 min.	13 min.	15 min.
Total Time	10 min.	12 min.	14 min.	16 min.	18 min.	20 min.
Week	7	8	9	10	11	12
Walk slowly	5 min.	5 min.	5 min.	5 min.	5 min.	5 min.
Walk briskly	18 min.	20 min.	23 min.	26 min.	28 min.	30 min.
Total Time	23 min.	25 min.	28 min.	31 min.	33 min.	35 min.

If you can only walk 5 minutes at a time, try doing it three times each day, increasing the minutes per walk as you progress. Once you are able to walk two miles daily, time yourself to make sure you eventually cover each mile in 15 minutes. When you reach that goal, you are ready to modify your walking program with heart-strengthening variations by moving into the next chapter for more advanced exercisers.

If you prefer, you can increase the benefits of your walk by covering more than two miles each day. An easy

Research shows pedometer users take nearly 2500 more steps a day-- enough to lose 10 pounds in a year-- than non-users.

way to motivate yourself to walk farther each day is to wear a pedometer. Pedometers are streamlined devices that clip to your waist, sit in your pocket, or hang around your neck as they count every step you take. The American Heart

Association (AHA) encourages walkers to take 10,000 steps (about five miles) each day, realizing that every step counts, even when you walk from a chair to the kitchen.

Diana: *Diana has CKD and is obese. She tells me, "I love wearing a pedometer. I just clip it on the waist of my pants each morning, and off I go. I know I walk more now than when I didn't use the pedometer. I log about 8,000 to 9,000 steps on average. This is much better than the 1,500 or so steps I walked when I first started a couple of months ago. My daughter and I compete. She wins, taking about 12,000 steps each day, but soon I will catch her!"*

Dialysis patients who used pedometers increased the steps they walked by up to 50%.
Journal of Nephrology 2010.

For those needing a little encouragement to keep moving, enroll in START! The AHA START! program is free; just log on at www.startwalkingnow.org. Because a brisk walk is one of the best steps you can take for a healthier heart, the AHA instituted this national movement to encourage everyone to walk more, eat well, and make other healthy habits part of everyday life. When you enroll in START!, you receive a monthly e-newsletter; connect with others across the U.S. who share your goals; have the ability to record your walk time and distance on the online tracker; develop a personalized walking plan; and locate online walking paths in your area.

Another walking motivator is befriending a pooch. A recent study at the University of Missouri found that walking a dog, even a neighbor's dog, leads to weight loss and adherence to a walking schedule. Participants in the study walked a "loaner" dog for 20 minutes, five days a week for 26 or 50 weeks. The 50-week group lost an average of 14.4 pounds, and 72 percent stuck with the walking schedule because the dogs "need us to walk them," they reported.

D. Beginning Strength and Flexibility

It is difficult to overstate the importance of muscle strength. Your 640 or so skeletal muscles (muscles you can control) comprise up to 50 percent of your body weight and power every move you make. Additional internal muscles often never rest--your continuously beating heart and the muscles controlling the lungs and intestines, for example.

Beginning at age 40, we lose about 5% of muscle mass per decade. By age 70, we might have lost 25% of muscle mass.

Your more obvious skeletal muscles surround and move your bones and impact how you look and how easily you perform daily activities. Skeletal muscles can have defined shape, giving your body attractive contours, or can waste away from disuse or disease.

Unfortunately, as we grow older, we lose muscle, replacing it with fat. This loss of muscle mass makes us more vulnerable to cardiovascular disease, type 2 diabetes, and obesity. Decreased muscle strength also threatens our ability to remain independent, avoid falls, or otherwise enjoy an active lifestyle. Studies show that exercising prevents muscular wasting and even preserves bone strength, in addition to muscle strength.

The U.S. government's *2008 Physical Activity Guidelines for Americans* recommend that you choose at least eight strength training exercises that work your major muscle groups--those in your abdomen, arms, chest, legs, shoulders, and upper and lower back. According to the CDC, beginners only need 10 to 12 repetitions of each exercise, though you will see extra benefits if you do a second set.

The CDC reports that one-third of adults over 65 fall each year, and 30% of these falls results in injury.

A well-rounded fitness plan also includes flexibility and balance exercises to counter the tendency of our muscles to shorten and stiffen as we age. Adding a balance exercise reduces the risk of future falls and promotes body stability.

333

If you enjoy stretching, try a yoga or tai chi class. Studies suggest that both yoga and tai chi have numerous benefits for good health. In a 2009 study, researchers found that the heart rate variations involved in a yoga practice improved the health of the heart.

There are numerous exercises you can perform for each muscle group. The combined strength, stretch and balance exercises presented in this Chapter are specifically for beginners. As you perform these moves, follow these steps:

1) **Warm up** your muscles before you work them. Spend five minutes walking or jumping to avoid muscle injury.

2) **Perform the exercises slowly.** Slower movement helps stimulate muscle growth.

3) **Perform hardest first.** Some exercises may be easier to perform than others. To address your weaknesses, perform the harder exercises first in your workout. Strive to improve the movements most difficult for you.

> **Women who drank 2 glasses of milk after weight lifting gained more muscle and lost more fat compared to women who drank sugar-based energy drinks.**
> *Medicine and Science in Sport and Exercise,* 2010

4) **Breathe.** Exhale during the lifting or pushing phase, and inhale doing the lowering phase. Continuous breathing helps keep blood pressure stable.

5) **Rest between exercises.** Unless you want the aerobic edge from a quick-paced workout, rest a minute or two between exercises.

6) **Twice a week is enough.** Rest a day or two between strength-training days. This allows your muscles to rebuild and helps you avoid muscle injury.

7) **Maintain good posture** by keeping your spine straight and your shoulders dropped (this takes practice and focus!). Use your legs, not your back, when picking weights up from the floor.

E. Beginning Exercises

These exercises are designed by Daniel Hubbard, exercise physiologist and certified physical trainer, for presentation here. Author and kidney donor Jennifer demonstrates the exercises. Repeat each exercise four or more times.

1. Supine Hip Bridges

This exercise strengthens thighs, hips, and lower back. Hold your abdominal muscles in as you perform the bridges to increase your core strength.

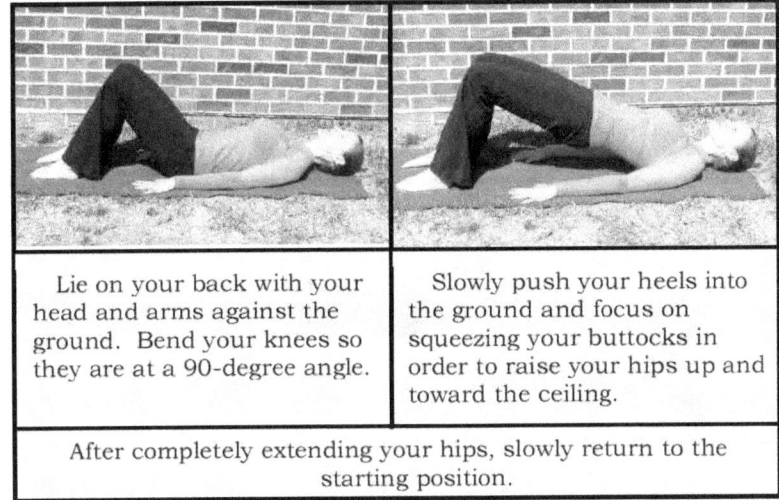

Lie on your back with your head and arms against the ground. Bend your knees so they are at a 90-degree angle.	Slowly push your heels into the ground and focus on squeezing your buttocks in order to raise your hips up and toward the ceiling.
After completely extending your hips, slowly return to the starting position.	

2. Side Bridges (on knees)

The side bridge strengthens your core, lower back, and shoulders.

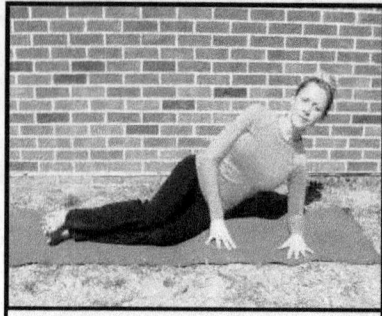 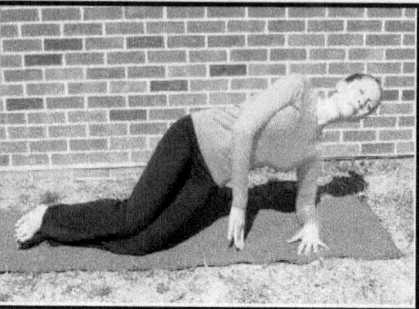

Start by positioning your body on its side, with your knees and elbow closest to the floor at 90 degrees.	With your knee, lower leg, and forearm in contact with the ground, lift your hips up until your torso is in a straight line.

Hold your torso up in the straight position for at least five seconds, then lower your hips to the ground. Switch sides.

3. Quadriped Reaching

This exercise is another core move that strengthens the abdomen and lower back. It also challenges your balance.

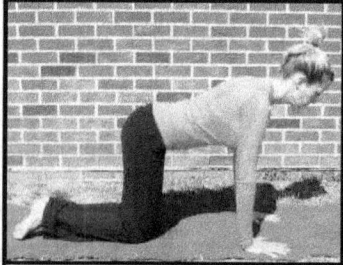 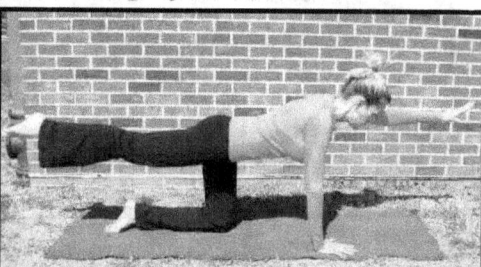

Start by positioning your body on all fours. Maintaining your back straight and hips in line with shoulders, brace your torso muscles.	Slowly lift your arm up and forward and your opposite leg up and back. Hold your abdomen in tightly as you maintain your leg, torso, and arm in the straight position for at least five seconds.

Return to the starting position on all fours.
Repeat, alternating the arms and legs.

4. Prone Bridges / Down Dog

The bridge is a shoulder and core strengthening move.
The down dog works your back, hips, shoulders, and hamstrings.

Start on your hands and feet, in a push-up position, maintaining a horizontal back.

Begin the movement by pushing your hips back and shrugging your shoulder blades up toward your ears.

Keep your back flat as you continue to elevate your hips. The height of your hips will depend on the flexibility of your legs.

After your hips reach their maximum height, return to the starting position by slowly lowering your hips down to the starting position.

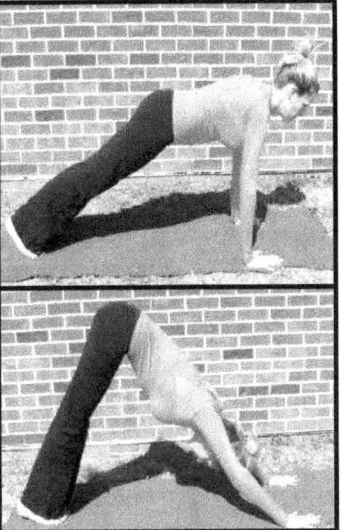

5. Split-Stance Stabilization and Reach

This exercise is another core move that strengthens the abdomen and lower back. It also challenges your balance.

While standing with both feet hip width, lift one foot, draw it back, and keep the toe of that foot in contact with the ground.

Slowly hinge at your hip, leaning forward, and slide the foot, with only the toe in contact with the ground, back.

Hold your abdomen in tightly as you maintain your leg, torso, and arm in the straight position for at least five seconds.

Return to the starting position by extending your hip.

Alternate legs as you continue repeating the exercise.

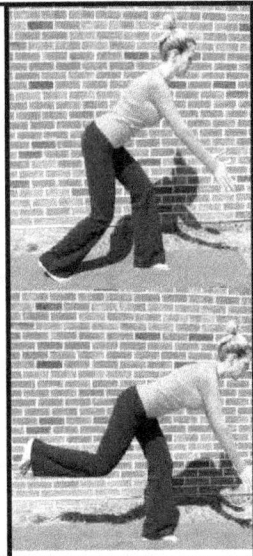

6. Back Squeeze

This move strengthens your upper back.

Stand straight, abs pulled in, with your arms extended in front of your chest.

Squeeze your shoulder blades back and down, and draw your elbows back, trying to keep your elbows high.

Hold the position for at least two seconds, and return to the starting position

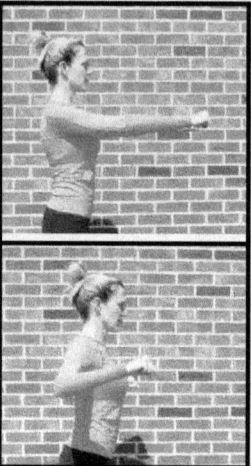

7. Floor Slides

This move looks easier than it is. Keep your elbows and back of hands on the floor as you perform the arm movements.
You will feel this in your shoulders and arm muscles.

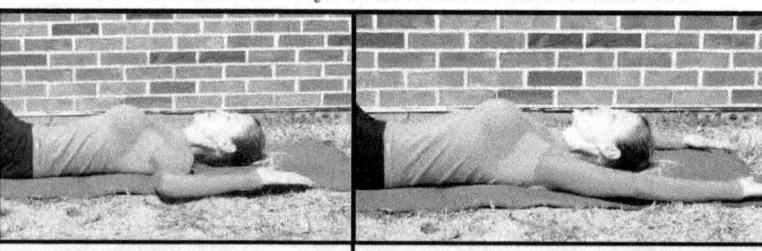

Lie on the ground with your feet drawn towards your hips, your elbows bent at a 90-degree angle, and forearms resting against the ground.	Shrug your shoulder blades up towards your ears as you slowly slide your hands above your head as far as you comfortably can. Shrug your shoulder blades down, away from your ears, as you slide your forearms toward your hips. (As in previous photo.)

Repeat sliding your hands up and down, while trying to keep your forearms in contact (or as close as you can) with the ground.

8. Step Over

The step-over is a hip, quadriceps,
and balance exercise.

Stand with your feet at hip
width.

Slowly lift one foot 4-6 inches
off the ground and move it out
and over an imaginary hurdle. As
it reaches the other side of the
imaginary hurdle, shift your
weight onto that leg.

After your first leg steps over
the imaginary hurdle, step the
second leg over in a slow, controlled manner.

Repeat the steps in the
opposite direction, stepping back
and forth with each repetition.

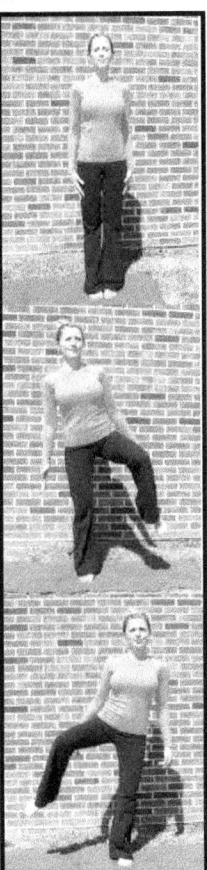

22.

KICK IT UP A NOTCH

The *2008 Physical Activity Guidelines for Americans* emphasize that people who are physically active can "gain additional and more extensive health and fitness benefits" by becoming even more active. Performing greater amounts of moderate-intensity activity (turning your 30-minute walk into a 60-minute walk), or more vigorous activity (making that 30-minute walk a jog, instead), further reduces your risk for chronic illness and helps you control weight.

> **Lose twice as much weight in a year by walking faster.**
> *Circulation,* 2009

A tried-and-true method to give your exercise routine a boost is interval training--a mix of moderate and vigorous exercise intensity. You add short spurts of higher intensity exercise to increase the effectiveness of activities you already perform. Rather than turning your 30-minute walk into a 30-minute run, you vary how fast you walk, such as alternating between a moderate and fast pace every two or so minutes. Or switch from walking on a level surface to walking up a hill. Your heart will feel the difference. If you swim, intersperse a vigorous crawl with your more leisurely backstroke. If you bike, alternate between fast and moderate pedaling.

Want other ways to increase the effectiveness of your workouts for added health benefits?

- When you strength train, add a cardio aspect by jumping rope, performing jumping jacks, or running in place for one minute between strength sets. (This is the ultimate time-saver: combining muscle training with cardio).

- Try a vigorous form of yoga for simultaneous flexibility, cardio, and strength training benefits.

- Join a fitness facility, such as the YMCA, for group classes that are fun; provide exercise variety; and often combine cardio, strength, and stretching into one-hour classes.

341

- Buy or rent DVD's for multilevel workouts at home.

- Take a Pilates class to combine core strengthening with flexibility moves. Strong core muscles (abdominal and lower back muscles) provide a solid foundation for all physical activities.

- Add a new activity to your schedule, such as dance classes, kickboxing, or karate.

- Try a rowing machine, boating, kayaking, swimming, or cross-country skiing. These activities recruit muscles throughout the body, making your heart work harder in the process.

- Be active throughout the day to burn more calories and become healthier. If you have a job, get up and walk, run an errand, or wear a pedometer to measure your activity outside of your normal exercise time.

Varying your exercise routine is called **cross-training**, and it has the advantage of working different muscle groups to enhance your overall fitness. For example, if you routinely perform yoga, intersperse an occasional Pilates class. If you use hand weights to strength train, try resistance bands or barbells periodically. You may enjoy the variety, and you will strengthen your muscles in a different way.

A. Revving up Your Cardio

It is easy to turn a moderate intensity walk into a vigorous intensity one, simply by increasing your walking speed to a 7- to 8-level on the PRE scale--the point when talking is difficult and your heart rate is in your 75 to 85 percent target heart rate zone (revisit Chapter 20). You can also achieve this level of intensity by switching your walk to a jog (between a fast walk and a run) and, as you advance, a run. When a slow run becomes comfortable, intersperse that comfortable run with some 30-second intervals of sprints every two minutes.

1. The Benefits of Interval Training

Studies suggest that performing **intervals** (alternating between moderate- and vigorous-paced cardio) during a walk or run is unrivaled for preventing heart disease and diabetes, losing weight, and efficiently improving fitness. When you combine short bursts of high intensity exercise with slightly longer periods of active recovery, you continuously raise and lower your heart rate. This improves vascular function, burns calories, and makes the body better able to eliminate fats and sugar from the blood.

Interval aerobic training is so effective in improving heart health that it is used in cardiac rehabilitation. Interval training improves cardiovascular function more effectively than moderate continuous training in patients after coronary artery bypass surgery and with heart failure, as well as in people with metabolic syndrome, obesity, or diabetes, and in healthy subjects. As an example:

RELEVANT RESEARCH → Researchers divided 32 people with metabolic syndrome into three groups. One group walked, a second group interval trained, and the third group was given no specific exercise instructions. After 16 weeks of exercising three times per week, both exercise groups lost weight. However, only the interval training group also lowered blood lipid levels. Nearly half (40%) of the interval group no longer met the criteria for metabolic syndrome.

Circulation, 2008

Here is an example of an interval walk schedule for people wanting to begin interval training:

Interval Walk

Amount of Time	5 min	21 min	5 min
Speed	Warm-up	Alternate 1 min moderate & 30 sec fast for a total of 14 times	Cooldown
Perceived Intensity	3-5	Moderate: 5-6 Fast: 7-8	3-4

With this schedule, you still exercise 30 minutes, but the exercise is more vigorous for increased health results, as compared to a steady, moderate-intensity walk.

2. Exercise to Maintain Weight Loss

You will probably not lose large amounts of excess weight by exercise alone, unless you are a long distance runner or extreme exerciser. Reducing your calories is what counts in weight loss, but exercise does increase your metabolism to assist you in weight loss. Once you have lost weight, regular exercise is indispensable for maintaining that loss. The CDC reports that the only way to maintain weight loss is to be engaged in regular physical activity, and the ACSM agrees.

In March 2010, the ACSM announced an update to its earlier 2001 recommendation for weight loss to reflect that long-term maintenance of weight loss requires 250 to 300 minutes per week of physical activity--that is 50 to 60 minutes of exercise 5 days each week. The revised recommendations are based on substantial research, similar to the following:

RECENT STUDY ➔ In The Womens' Health Study, researchers analyzed data of 34,079 healthy women, average age 54. Over the 13-year study period, the women gained an average of nearly six pounds. The 13.3% of women who managed to gain less weight were of normal weight and averaged 60 minutes daily of moderate physical activity (such as brisk walking). If the women were overweight (BMI of 25 and up), diet was required to keep off pounds. *JAMA*, 2010

The bottom line: to maintain your body weight, you need about 60 minutes of moderate-to-vigorous intensity activity on most days of the week, while avoiding excess calories. If weight loss is your goal, increase the moderate-to-vigorous physical activity to at least 60 to 90 minutes daily, and cut calories from your diet.

B. Strength/Stretch Exercises

Kidney transplant donor/author Jennifer demonstrates a slightly more difficult set of exercises than the ones presented in Chapter 21. These are combination exercises that strengthen multiple muscle groups simultaneously and provide balance and muscle toning. Perform each exercise at least four times.

1. Split Squats

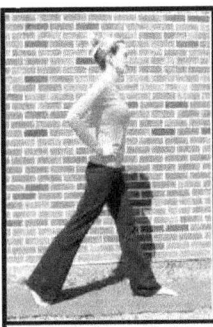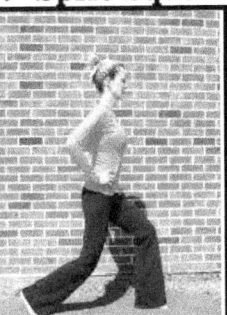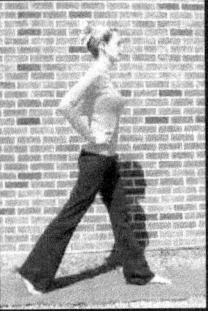

Assume a split-stance position by moving one foot forward and one foot back, and hip width apart.	Keeping your torso vertical, slowly lower your hips by equally bending both legs. Lower until your back knee is within 2 to 4 inches of the ground.
Raise back up to the starting position by extending both legs, keeping the torso vertical and back straight.	

2. Push-ups (on knees) and Down Dog

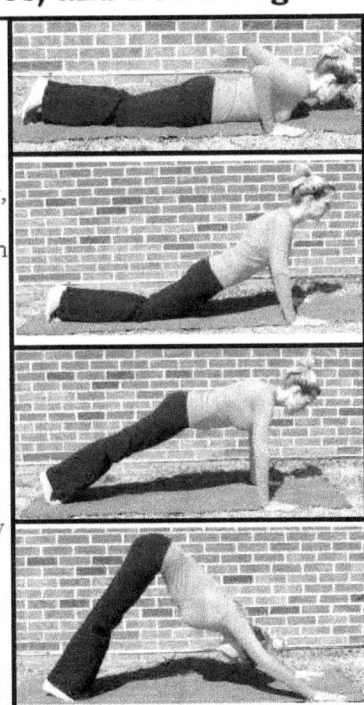

Lie face-down on the ground, knees slightly bent, and hand slightly lower and wider than your shoulders.

Push your body up from the floor, keeping your torso straight, and your knees and toes in contact with the ground.

Lift your knees up from the ground and straighten them. You will be on your hands and feet

Push your hips back and up while your knees and back remain straight so hips are higher than your shoulders.

Return to the starting position by lowering hips and knees to the ground.

3. Side Bridges (legs straight)

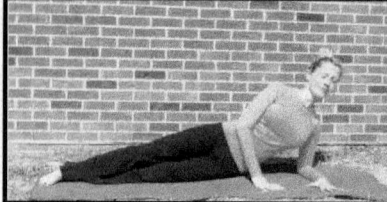 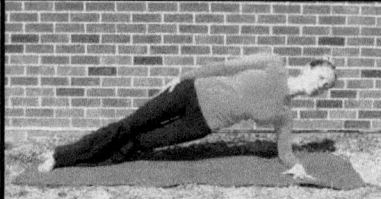

Lie on your side with your legs straight and stacked one on top of the other. Position your lower arm with the elbow bent 90 degrees, directly under your shoulder.	Lift your hips and torso off the ground so your body makes a straight line from heel to shoulder. Lower your hips to the ground.

Repeat this sequence on your right side as you gradually crawl forward, maintaining a horizontal back and straight legs.

4. Bear Crawl

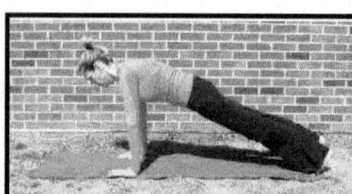 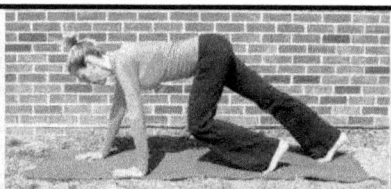

Assume a push-up position on your hands and feet with your back horizontal to the ground.	Keep your knees straight as you take a small step with your left foot, following with a small step with your left hand.

5. Back Squeeze

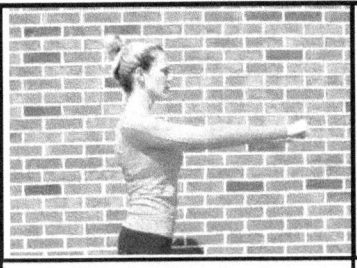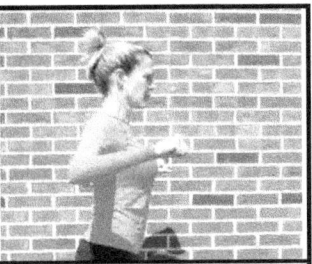

Stand straight, abs pulled in, with your arms extended in front of your chest.	Squeeze your shoulder blades back and down, and draw your elbows back, trying to keep your elbows high.

Hold the position for at least two seconds, and return to the starting position.

6. Single-Leg Deadlift and Reach

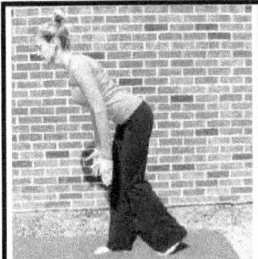

Standing with both feet at hip width, lift one foot off the ground and stabilize the hips with the other foot. Reach arms out and in front of your body for balance as you slowly hinge forward.	The leg that is off the ground should go back as the torso leans forward. Hinge until your torso makes a 45-degree angle, then smoothly return to the starting position. Move slowly and controlled in a manner that allows you to keep the leg you are standing on stable.

7. Alternating Floor Slides

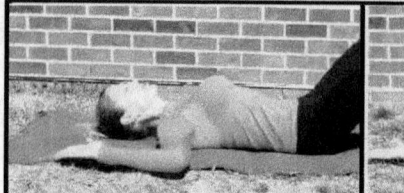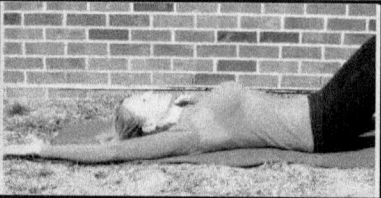

Lie on your back on the ground, your feet drawn close to your hips and elbows out to the side at a 90-degree angle.	Trying to keep your elbows and back of your hands against the floor, slide one of your shoulder blades and hands up over your head. At the same time, slide the other shoulder blade and arm toward your hips, in the opposite direction of the other hand.

Once you reach as far as you can comfortably go above your head, reverse the directions of each arm and, again, move as far as you can comfortably.

C. Vary How You Exercise

The strength exercises presented thus far use body weight alone. As you advance, you may try different exercises using dumbbells, kettleballs, barbells, resistance bands, a Swiss ball, sand bags, medicine balls, or the equipment at a fitness center. They each work your muscles differently, and that variety increases strength and prevents boredom. Jennifer demonstrates several exercises using dumbbells.

1. Biceps Curls

Biceps curls work your biceps muscles
in the front of your upper arms.

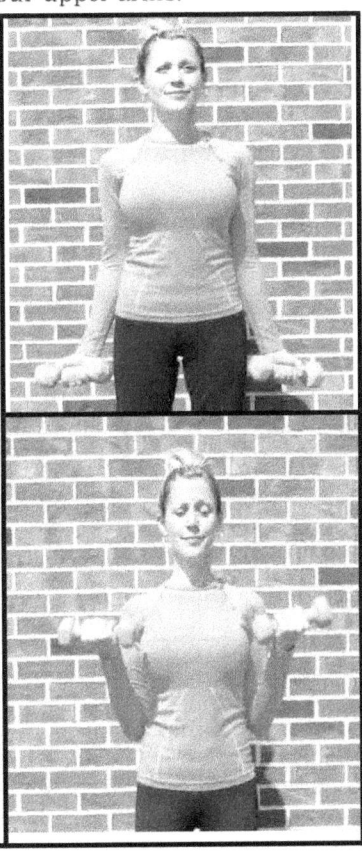

Start with feet shoulder-width apart and arms at sides. Hold a dumbbell in each hand, palms facing forward.

Exhale as you keep your elbows locked against ribcage and curl both arms up toward your shoulders three-quarters of the way.

Hold for a beat as you squeeze your biceps but not your hands.

Inhale as you slowly lower arms to starting position.

Repeat 8 reps for 1 set.

2. Overhead Press

The overhead press focuses on shoulder muscles.

Stand tall with feet hip width apart and abs pulled in. Hold a dumbbell in each hand, arms bent at shoulder level. Your upper arms should be parallel to the ground.

Exhale as you press both arms up over your head so the weights slightly touch. Straighten your arms doing this move.

Hold for a beat, and inhale as you lower your arms to starting position.

Repeat 8 reps for 1 set.

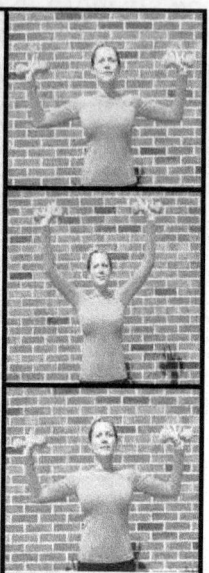

3. Dumbbell Row

This exercise targets the upper and middle back.

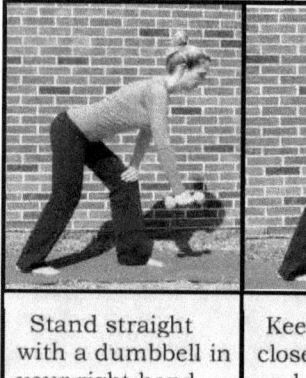 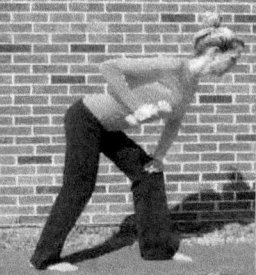 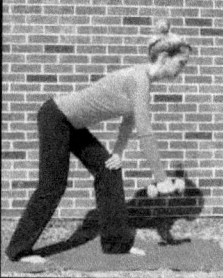

Stand straight with a dumbbell in your right hand. Bend forward at the waist until your torso is almost parallel with the ground. Your arm is hanging down with your palm facing in.	Keeping your arm close to your torso, and your back as flat as possible, exhale and pull the dumbbell up until it touches the side of your chest. Squeeze your shoulder blade toward your spine.	Slowly lower the weight back toward the ground as you inhale. Repeat 8 reps for 1 set, then switch arms.

4. Lunge

Targets the glutes, quads, hamstrings and calves.

Stand in a wide stride with one leg in front of the other. Your back is straight and abs pulled in tightly.

As you inhale, bend both knees until your back thigh is parallel to the ground. Your front knee never travels past your toes, and your spine is straight up and down.

Exhale as you lift back to starting position.

Repeat 8 reps for 1 set, then switch legs.

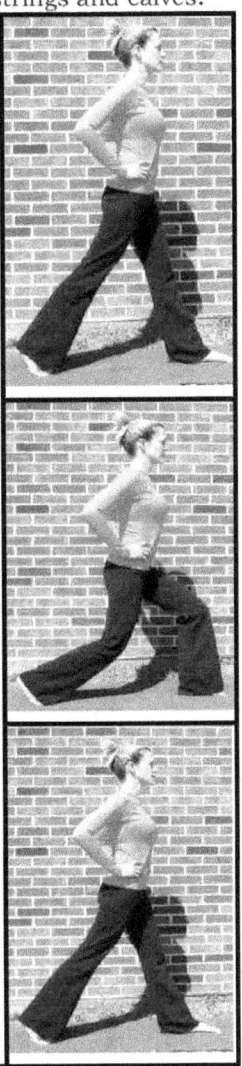

5. Squat

The squat strengthens the glutes, quads, and hamstrings.

Stand tall with feet hip width apart, your weight on your heels and abs tight.

Lower yourself back and down as if you are sitting in a chair. Keep your chest high and back straight. Lower until your thighs are parallel to the ground.

Exhale and raise to starting position.

Perform 8 reps for 1 set.

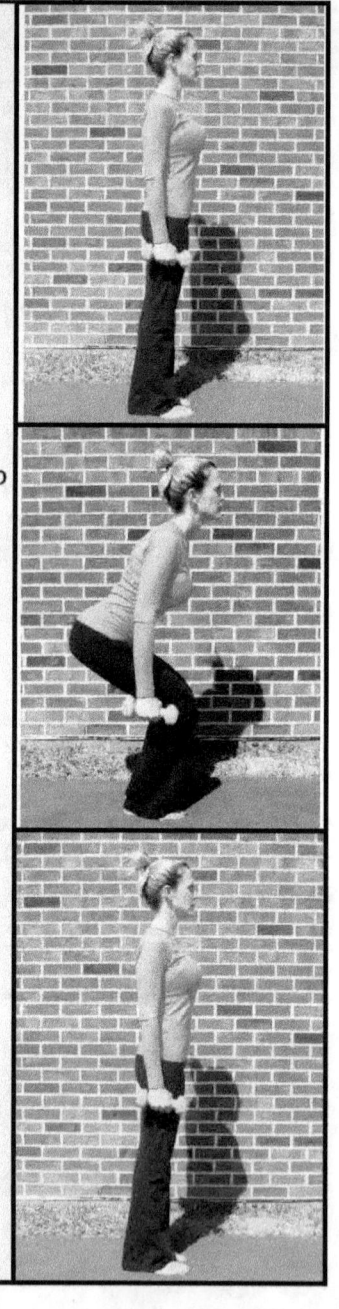

6. Push-Up

The push-up is a must-do! It targets the chest, shoulders, triceps, and abs. This version is easier than the full push-up.

Place your hands on the floor directly under your shoulders. Put your knees back far enough so that your head, back and butt are in a straight line.

Inhale as you slowly lower your chest to the ground. Keep your eyes focused on the ground in front of you and your abs tight.

Exhale as you raise back up to starting position.

Perform 8 reps for 1 set.

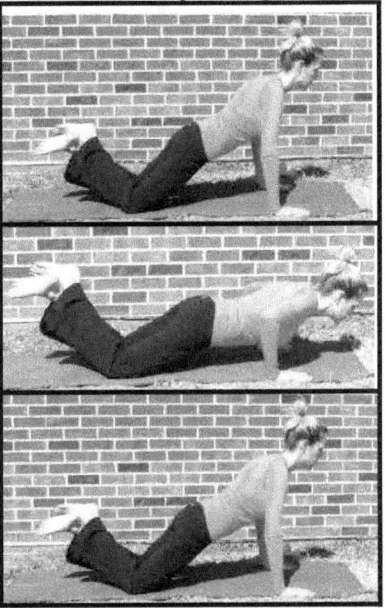

7. Triceps Extension

This exercise targets the triceps, muscles in the back of your upper arms.

Lie on the ground, knees bent, holding a dumbbell in your right hand, palm facing in and arm straight up. You may place your left hand lightly on the back of your right arm to stabilize the arm.

Inhaling, bend your right arm, lowering the dumbbell behind your head. Your elbow is pointed straight up and your arm is close to your head.

Exhale and raise the weight back to starting position. Your upper arm (the part you are holding with your left hand) never moves during the exercise.

Perform 8 reps, switch arms and repeat the exercise.

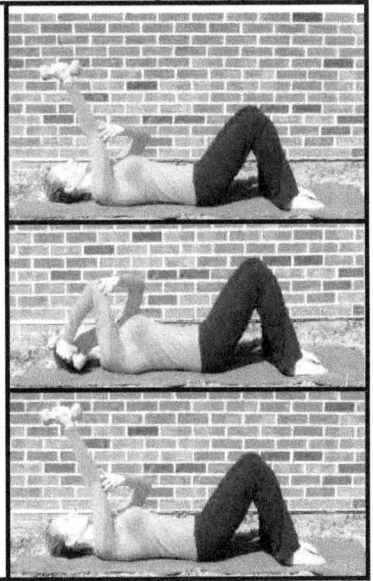

8. Plank

The plank is an excellent overall exercise that particularly tones the abs, lower back, chest, and shoulders.

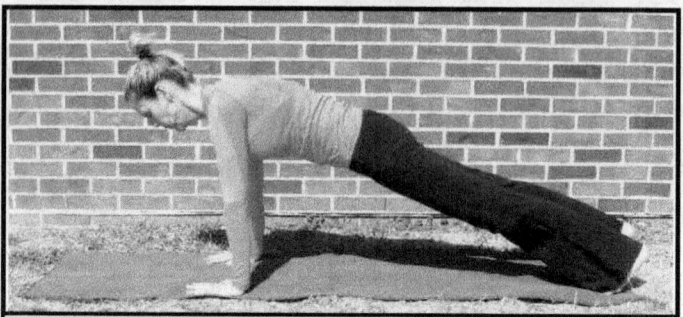

Start in push-up position with your hands on the ground directly under your shoulders. Keep your legs straight behind you, feet together, butt level (not up in the air). Pull your abs in tightly. Hold the position as long as you can, working up to 2 minutes.

9. Bicycle

The bicycle is an overall ab-toning exercise.

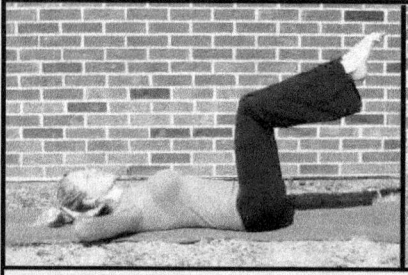 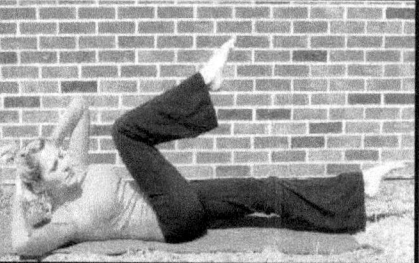

Lie on your back with your hands loosely behind your head and your elbows back so you cannot see them. Your knees are lifted. Keeping your elbows back, lift your head as you tightly pull in your abs. At the same time bring your right armpit toward your left knee.

Your right leg straightens.

Switch armpits and knees. Slowly move back and forth from one side to the other as if you are riding a bicycle.

Continue (with abs tight) until you have done 8 lifts on each side for 1 set.

Balance/Stretches

1. Balance

Balance exercises are important
to lessen the odds of falls.

Stand tall with your feet hip distance apart and your abs pulled in tight.

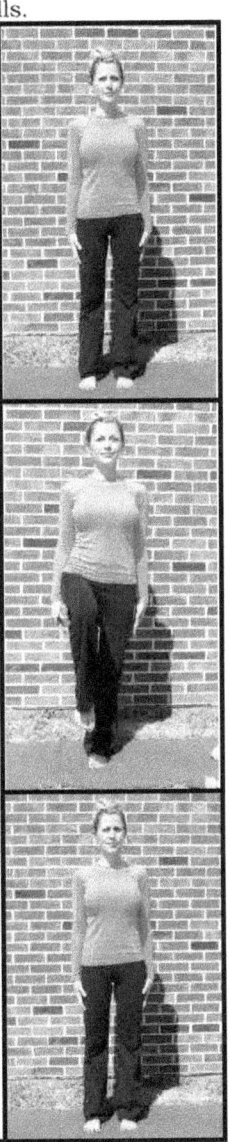

Slowly lift one knee until your thigh is parallel to the ground. Hold for at least 10 seconds and slowly lower the foot to the ground. The taller you stand and the tighter you keep your abs, the easier it is to balance.

Repeat with the opposite leg.

2. Oblique Stretch

Stand tall with feet hip distance apart, abs pulled in and back straight.

Raise arms straight up over your head, keeping them fully extended. Touch palms together.

Exhale as you bend to the right. Keep arms straight and shoulders in line. Do not bend the upper shoulder forward. Hold stretch as you complete your slow exhale.

Inhale as you slowly raise back to start.

Repeat on the opposite side.

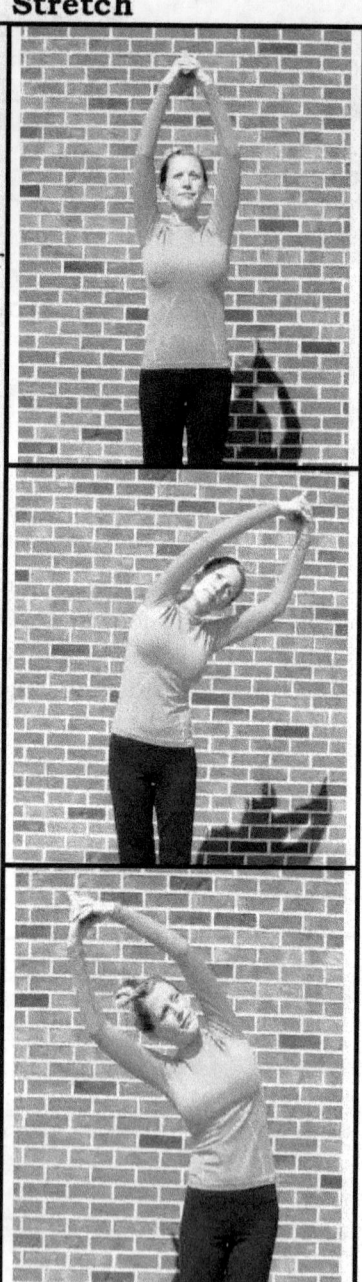

3. Spinal Twist

Sit tall on the ground with your legs bent in front of you.

Your back should be straight and you are sitting tall.

Bring your right hand behind you and rest it on the floor. Keep your back very straight.

Turn the body to the right as you bring your left hand over your right knee.

Exhale as you twist (back straight) to the right, looking over your right shoulder.

Repeat on the opposite side.

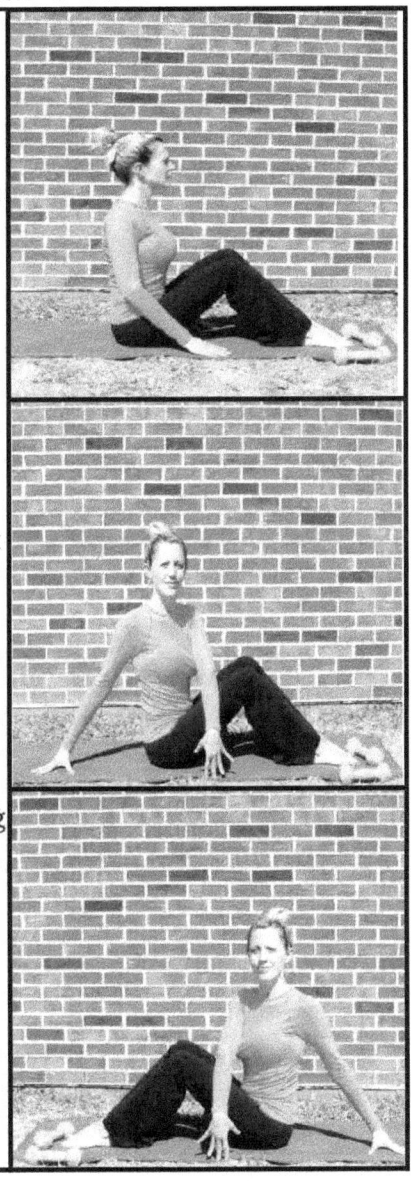

357

REFERENCES

Chapter 6. The Amazing Kidney

Abercrombie D. *Professional Guide to Diseases*, Lippincott Williams & Wilkins, 9th Ed. 2009; pp. 372-374 (location of kidneys, drops as move, internal structure, description, 1-3 million nephrons, box information – total bladder capacity; homeostasis, renin system, EPO, calcitriol).

Clifford RL, Knox AJ. Vitamin D-a new treatment for airway remodeling in asthma? *B J Pharmacol.* 2009; 158(6):1426-8.

Holick MF. Vitamin D deficiency. *N Engl J Med.* 2007; 347:266-81 (calcitriol and effects).

Marieb EN. *Essentials of Human Anatomy & Physiology*, Pearson Benjamin Cummings, 2009; pp. 518-533 (bean-shaped, color, location, size, structures, functions, blood pressure, summary of functions, filtering capaci, ureters, bladder, urethra, urea and description, glomeruli filtering, urine components, homeostasis and water balance, renin).

Marieb EN, Mitchell, SJ. *Human Anatomy & Physiology Laboratory Manual*, Pearson Benjamin Cummings, 8th Ed., 2008; pp. 609-615 (organs of urinary system, right kidney lower, internal structures and descriptions, glomeruli function and pressure, box info (25% of blood), box info (bladder capacity), urochrome, darker urine, homeostasis).

Millis RM. Epigenetics and hypertension. *Curr Hypertens Rep.* 2011; 13(1):21-8 (renin gene affected by mother's environment).

Murphree DD, Thelen SM. Chronic kidney disease in primary care: interventions to slow the progression of kidney disease. *J Am Board Fam Med.* 2010; 23(4):542-550 (effects of malfunctioning kidneys).

Publication No. 09-3195 of the National Kidney and Urologic Disease Information Clearinghouse, a service of the National Institutes of Health, National Institute of Diabetes and Digestion and Kidney Diseases, Bethesda, MD, February, 2009 (single kidney).

Roberts A. *The Complete Human Body*. DK Publishing, 2010, pp. 366-369 (1 million nephrons, components of nephrons, filtering capacity, anatomy, urine contents, bladder capacity).

Saladin KS, *Anatomy & Physiology: The Unity of Form and Function*, The McGraw Hill Companies, Inc., 4th Ed., 2007; pp. 899-935 (kidney weight, box information, internal structures and descriptions, nephron, tubules, glomeruli, blood pressure in glomeruli, vulnerable to hypertension, functions, urine quantity, nitrogen wastes, BUN, urine components, renin system, tubule reabsorption).

United States Renal Data System: USRDS 2010 Annual Data Report: Atlas of Chronic Kidney Disease and End-Stage Renal Disease in the United States, National Institutes of Health, National Institute of Diabetes and Digestive and Kidney Diseases, Bethesda, Md. 2010; Vol 1, Ch. 1 and 2 (blood pressure medication statistics).

www.usatoday.com/community/utils/dmap/28396893.story (accessed October 1, 2010)(Meng brothers drinking urine).

Chapter 7. What is Kidney Disease?

A. Acute Kidney Injury

Abercrombie D, *et al. Professional Guide to Diseases*, Lippincott Williams & Wilkins, 9th Ed. 2009, pp. 383-395; 422-424 (AKI and causes, kidney stones).

Anglani F, Mezzabotta F, Ceol M, *et al.* The regenerative potential of the kidney: What can we learn from developmental biology? *Stem Cell Rev* 2010 Aug; www.ncbi.nim.nih.gov/pubmed/20714827 (accessed Sept. 3, 2010)(Kidney repair after acute kidney injury; regeneration).

Bellomo R, Ronco C, Kellum JA, *et al.* Acute renal failure—definition, outcome measures, animal models, fluid therapy, and information technology needs: The Second International Consensus Conference of the Acute Dialysis Quality Initiative (ADQI) Group. Critical Care, 2004;8(4):R204-R212.

Coca, SG. Long-term outcomes of acute kidney injury. *Curr Opin Nephrol Hypertens* 2010 May; 19(3):266-72.

Herzog CA. Kidney disease in cardiology. *Nephrol Dial Transplant.* 2010; 25(2):356-360 (AKI and cardiac surgery).

Himmelfarb J, Ikizler TA. Acute kidney injury: Changing lexicography, definitions, and epidemiology. *Kidney Int.* 2007; 71(10):971-976.

Kheterpal S, Tremper KK, Heung M, *et al.* Development and validation of an acute kidney injury risk index for patients undergoing general surgery: results from a national data set. *Anesthesiology.* 2009; 110(3):505-15.

Negishi K, Niori E, Doi K, *et al.* Monitoring of urinary L-type fatty acid-binding protein predicts histological severity of acute kidney injury. *Am J Pathol.* 2009 Apr; 174(4):1154-9 (using protein in urine to identify AKI early).

Ricci Z, Ronco C. Kidney Diseases beyond nephrology: intensive care. *Nephrol Dial Transplant.* 2009; 24(2):391-395.

Saladin KS. *Anatomy & Physiology: The Unity of Form and Function*, The McGraw Hill Companies, Inc., 4th Ed., 2007, p. 921 (kidney stones, lower back injury for AKI).

Taylor EH, Fung TT, Curan GC. DASH-style diet associates with reduced risk for kidney stones. *J Am Soc Nephrol.* 2009 Oct; 20(10):2253-9.

United States Renal Data System: USRDS 2010 Annual Data Report. Atlas of Chronic Kidney Disease and End-Stage Renal Disease in the United States, National Institutes of Health, National Institute of Diabetes and Digestive and Kidney Diseases, Bethesda, Md. 2010; Vol. 1, Ch 8:121-132 (box information and all statistics regarding AKI).

Vaidya VS, Ford GM, Walkar SS, *et al.* A rapid urine test for early detection of kidney injury. *Kidney Int.* 2009; 76(1):106-14.

Waikar SS, Winkelmayer WC. Chronic on acute renal failure: long-term implications of severe acute kidney injury. *JAMA.* 2009; 302(11):1227-9.

Wald R, Quinn RR, Luo J, *et al.* Chronic dialysis and death among survivors of acute kidney injury requiring dialysis. *JAMA.* 2009; 302(11):1179-1185 (70% die if AKI while hospitalized).

U.S. Department of Health and Human Services, Centers for Medicare and Medicaid Services. End-Stage Renal Disease (ESRD) payment regulations and notices. CMS-14.
www.cms.gov/ESRDPayment/01_overview.asp# (accessed September 2010).

B. Chronic Kidney Disease

Collins AJ, Foley RN, Herzog C, *et al.* Excerpts from the U.S. Renal Data System 2009 Annual Data Report. *Am J Kidney Dis.* 2010 Jan; 55(1Suppl):S1-420, A6-7.

Coresh J, Selvin F, Stevens LA, *et al.* Prevalence of chronic kidney disease in the United States. *JAMA.* 2007; 298(17):2038-47 (10-year increase in CKD related to increase in hypertension and diabetes).

Flessner MF, Wyatt SB, Akylbekova EL, *et al.* Prevalence and awareness of CKD among African-Americans; the Jackson Health Study. *Am J Kid Dis.* 2009; 53(2):238-47 (CKD more common in African-Americans; 17% of population with CKD).

Heron M, Hoyert DL, Murphy SL, *et al.* Deaths: final data for 2006. *Natl Vital Stat Rep.* 2009; 57(14):1-134 (CDC reports kidney disease is 9th leading cause of death in US).

Hossain M, Goyder EW, Rigby JR, *et al.* CKD and poverty: a growing global challenge. *Am J Kidney Dis.* 2009; 53(1):166-74 (poverty and social deprivation risk factors for CKD).

Levey A, Eckardt K, Tsukamoto Y, *et al.* Definition and classification of chronic kidney disease: a position statement from Kidney Disease: Improving Global Outcomes (KDIGO). *Kidney Int.* 2005; 67:2089-100.

Meyer TW, Hostetter TH. Uremia. N Engl J Med. 2007; 357(13):1316-25.

Murphee DD, Thelen SM. Chronic kidney disease in primary care. *J Am Board Fam Med.* 2010; 23(4):542-50 (definition of CKD; risk factors; interventions).

National Kidney Foundation Fact Sheet at http://www.kidney.org/news/newsroom/fs_new/KDaGrowing Problem.cfm (last accessed 2/1/11)(CKD numbers).

Plantinga LC, Boulware LE, Coresh J. Patient awareness of chronic kidney disease: trends and predictors. *Arch Intern Med.* 2008; 168(20):2269-75.

Plantinga LC, Crews DC, Coresh J, *et al.* Prevalence of Chronic Kidney Disease in U.S. adults with undiagnosed diabetes or prediabetes. *Clin J Am Soc Nephrol.* 2010; 5(4):673-82 (18 million in U.S. with undiagnosed CKD).

Saran R, Hedgeman E, Plantinga L, Burrows NR, *et al.* Establishing a national chronic kidney disease surveillance system for the United States. *Clin J Am Soc Nephrol.* 2010 Jan; 5(1):152-61 (CDC established CKD surveillance system).

Snyder J, Foley R, Collings A, *et al.* Prevalence of CKD in the United States: a sensitivity analysis using the National Health and Nutrition Examination Survey (NHANES) 1999-2004. *Am J Kidney Dis.* 2009; 53(2):218-28.

Szczech L, Harmon W, Hostetter TH, *et al.* World Kidney Day 2009: problems and challenges in the emerging epidemic of kidney disease. *J Am Soc Nephrol.* 2009 Mar; 20(3):453-5.

United States Renal Data System: USRDS 2010 Annual Data Report: Atlas of Chronic Disease and End-Stage Renal Disease in the United States, National Institutes of Health, National Institute of Diabetes and Digestive and Kidney Diseases, Bethesda, Md. 2010; Introd: 12-39; Vol. 1, Ch 1:40-52, (CKD statistics); Vol II, Intro: 212 (ESRD statistics).

C. CKD and Being Older

Ahmed AK, Brown SH, Abdelhafiz AH. Chronic kidney disease in older people: disease or dilemma? *Saudi J Kidney Dis.* 2010; 21(5):835-41 (elderly and CKD).

Choudhury D, Levi M. Renal function and disease in the aging kidney. In Schrier RW (ed): *Diseases of the Kidney,* 6th ed. Philadelphia, Lippincott Williams & Wilkins, 2007; pp. 2088-2120.

Hemmelgarn BR, Zhang J, Manns BJ, *et al.* Progression of kidney dysfunction in the community-dwelling elderly. *Kidney Int.* 2006; 69(12):2155-61.

United States Renal Data System: USRDS 2010 Annual Data Report: Atlas of Chronic Kidney Disease and End-Stage Renal Disease in the United States, National Institutes of Health, National Institute of Diabetes and Digestive and Kidney Diseases, Bethesda, Md 2010; Vol 1, Ch 1:40-52 and Ch 2:54-64 (statistics, metabolic abnormalities at stage III, 5-stage CKD staging).

D. CKD and Its Sister: Cardiovascular Disease

Breiethardt T, Mebazaa A, Mueller CE. Predicting progression in nondiabetic kidney disease: the importance of cardiorenal interactions. *Kidney Int.* 2009; 75(3):253-5 (20 million at risk of CKD; interplay between CKD and CVD; cardiorenal syndrome).

Herzog C. Can we prevent sudden cardiac death in dialysis patients? *Clin J Am Soc Nephrol.* 2007; 2(3):410-2.

Herzog CA. Kidney disease in cardiology. *Nephrol Dial Transplant.* 2010; 25(2):356-360.

Nitsch D, Lawlor DA, Patel R, *et al.* The association of renal impairment with all-cause and cardiovascular disease mortality. *Nephrol Dial Transplant.* 2010; 25(4):1191-9.

Stevens LA, Viswanathan G, Weiner DE, *et al.* Chronic kidney disease and end-stage renal disease in the elderly population: current prevalence, future projections and clinical significance. *Adv Chronic Kidney Dis.* 2010 Jul; 17(4):293-301 (high prevalence of CKD in elderly and associated cardiovascular diseases).

United States Renal Data System: USRDS 2010 Annual Data Report: Atlas of Chronic Kidney Disease and End-Stage Renal Disease in the United States, National Institutes of Health, National Institute of Diabetes and Digestive and Kidney Diseases, Bethesda, Md 2010; Vol 1, Ch 1:40-52 and Ch 5:87-98 (CVD with CKD).

Chapter 8.   Detecting Kidney Disease

A.   Outward Signs

Abercrombie D, *et al. Professional Guide to Diseases*, Lippincott Williams & Wilkins, 9th Ed. 2009; p. 375.

Marieb EN. *Essentials of Human Anatomy & Physiology*, Pearson Benjamin Cummings, 2009; p. 526 (CKD occurs silently; CKD symptoms).

Publication No. 09-3195 of the National Kidney and Urologic Disease Information Clearinghouse, a service of the National Institutes of Health, National Institute of Diabetes and Digestive and Kidney Diseases, Bethesda, MD, February, 2009.

B.   Internal Signs

Alanock RJ. Estimated glomerular filtration rate: time for a performance review. *Kidney Int.* 2009; 75(10):1001-3.

American Diabetic Association: Standards of medical care in diabetes--2008. *Diabetes Care* 2008; 31(Suppl1):S12-54.

Brito-Ashurat I, Varagunam M, Raftery MJ. Bicarbonate supplementation slows progression of CKD and improves nutritional status. *J Am Soc Nephrol.* 2009; 20:2075-2084.

Chobanian AV, Bakris GL, Black HR, *et al.* Seventh report of the Joint National Committee on Prevention, Detection, Evaluation and Treatment of High Blood Pressure. *Hypertension* 2003; 42:1206-52.

D'Apolito M, Du X, Zong H, *et al.* Urea-induced ROS generation causes insulin resistance in men with chronic renal failure. *J Clin Invest.* 2010; 120:203-13 (high urea levels may cause insulin resistance).

Dzielinska Z, Januszewicz A, Wiecek A, *it al.* Reduced kidney function estimated by cystatin C and clinical outcomes in hypertensive patients with coronary artery disease: association with homocystic and other cardiovascular risk factors. *Kidney Blood Pressure Res.* 2010; 33(2):2117-22.

Eknoyan G, *et al.* Proteinuria and other markers of chronic kidney disease: a position statement of the National Kidney Foundation (NKF) and the National Institutes of Diabetes and Digestive and Kidney Diseases (NIDDK). *Am J Kidney Dis.* 2003; 42(4):617-622.

Fassett RG, Owen JE, Fairley J, *et al.* Urinary red-cell morphology during exercise. *Brit Med J.* 1982; 285(6353):1455-1457.

Fogazzi GB, Cameron JS. Urinary microscopy from the seventeenth century to the present day. *Kidney Int.* 1996; 50(3):1058-1068 (urinalysis by nephrologist).

Fogazzi GB, Verdesca S, Carigali G. Urinalysis: core curriculum 2008. *Am J Kidney Dis.* 2008; 51(6):1052-1067.

Gaspari F, Perico N, Remuzzi G. Timed urine collections are not needed to measure urine protein excretion in clinical practice. *Am J Kidney Dis.* 2006; 47(1):1-7.

Glanook RJ. Estimated glomerular filtration rate: time for a performance review. *Kidney Int.* 2009; 75(10):1001-3.

Go AS, Chertow GM, Fan D, *et al.* Chronic kidney disease and the risks of death, cardiovascular events, and hospitalization. *N Engl J Med.* 2004; 351(13):1269-1305.

Grossfeld GD, Wolf JS, Litwin MS, *et al.* Evaluation of asymptomatic microscopic haematuria in adults: The American Urological Association best practice policy. *Urology* 2001; 57(4):604-610.

Haick H, Hakim M, Patrascu M, *et al.* Sniffing chronic renal failure in rat model by an array of random networks of single-walled carbon nanotubes. *ACS Nano* 2009; 3(5):1258-66.

Hallan SI, Ritz E, Lydersen S, *et al.* Combining GFR and albuminuria to classify CKD improves prediction of ESRD. *J Am Soc Nephrol.* 2009; 20(5):1069-77.

Henry JB, Fuller CE, Threatte GA. Basic examination of the urine. In Henry JB (ed): Clinical Diagnosis and Management by Laboratory Methods, 20th ed. Philadelphia, WB Saunders, 2001: 367-402.

Ju W, Eichinger F, Bitzer M, *et al.* Renal gene and protein expression: signatures for prediction of kidney disease progression. *Am J Pathol.* 2009; 174(6):2073-2085. (identify early markers of CKD)

Jurkovitz C, *et al.* Family members of patients treated for ESRD have high risks of undetected kidney disease. *Am J Kidney Dis.* 2002; 40(6):1173-1178.

Kanal E, Barkovich AJ, Bell C, *et al.* ACR guidance document for safe MR practices: 2007. *AJR Am J Roentgenol.* 2007; 188(6):1447-74.

Levey AS, Coresh J, Balk E, *et al.* National Kidney Foundation practice guidelines for chronic kidney disease: evaluation, classification, and stratification. *Ann Intern Med.* 2003; 139(2):137-47.

Levey AS, Coresh J, Greene T, *et al.* Expressing the Modification of Diet in Renal Disease Study equation for estimating glomerular filtration rate with standardized serum creatinine values. *Clin Chem.* 2007; 53(4):766-72 (estimating GFR).

Levey AS, Schoolwerth AC, Burrows NK, *et al.* Comprehensive public health strategies for preventing the development, progression, and complications of CKD: report of an expert panel convened by the Centers of Disease Control and Prevention. *Am J Kidney Dis.* 2009; 53(3):522-35.

Li HX, Xu GB, Wang XJ, *et al.* Diagnostic accuracy of various glomerular filtration rates estimating equations in patients with chronic kidney disease and diabetes. *Clin Med J.(Engl).* 2010; 123(6):745-51.

Lorenz EC, Vrtiska TJ, Lieske JC, *et al.* Prevalence of renal artery kidney abnormalities by computed tomography among healthy adults. *Clin J Am Soc Nephrol.* 2010; 5(3):431-438.

Madero M, Sarnak M, Stevens L. Serum cystatin C as a marker of glomerulus filtration rate. *Curr Opin Neph Hyper.* 2006; 15:610-6.

360

Marieb EN, Mitchell SJ. *Human Anatomy & Physiology Laboratory Manual*, Pearson Benjamin Cummings, 8th Ed 2008; p. 62 (color of urine).

National Kidney Foundation. K/DOQI Clinical Practice Guidelines for Chronic Kidney Disease: Evaluation, Classification, and Stratification. *Am J Kidney Dis*. 2002; 39(2 Suppl 1):S1-266 (GFR, chart).

National Kidney Foundation. Modification of Diet in Renal Disease study calculator. Available at www.kidney.org/professional/tools. (accessed September 2010).

National Kidney Foundation: Clinical Practice Guidelines for Chronic Kidney Disease: Evaluation Classification and Stratification. Part 4: Definition and classification of stages of chronic kidney disease. *Am J Kidney Dis*. 2002; 39(Suppl):46-75.

Rule AD, Torres VE, Chapman AB, *et al*. Comparison of methods for determining renal function decline in early autosomal dominant polycystic kidney disease: the consortium of radiologic imaging studies of polycystic kidney disease cohort. *J Am Soc Nephrol*. 2006; 17(3):854-862 (GFR best predictor of kidney function).

Stevens LA, Coresh J, Greene T, Levey AS. Assessing kidney function—measured and estimated glomerular filtration rate. *N Engl J Med*. 2006; 354(23):2473-83.

Tsai JJ, Yeun JY, Kumar VA, Don BR. Comparison and interpretation of urinalysis performed by a nephrologist versus a hospital-based clinical laboratory. *Am J Kidney Dis*. 2005; 46(5):820-829 (nephrologist more likely to recognize urine abnormalities than lab).

VanderVelde M, Halbesma N, deCharro FT, *et al*. Screening for albuminuria identifies individuals at increased renal risk. *J Am Soc Nehrol*. 2009; 20(4):852-62 (39% not aware of CKD; 50% not treated).

Voswinckel P. A marvel of colors and ingredients: The story of urine test strips. *Kidney Int*. 1994; 46(Suppl):3-7.

Walter PD, Cavallo T, Bonsib SM. Ad Hoc Committee on Renal Biopsy Guidelines of the Renal Pathology Society: Practice guidelines for the renal biopsy. *Mod Pathol*. 2004; 17(12):1555-1563.

Weiner DE, Rifkin DE, *et al*. Kidney function and the risk of cardiovascular disease. *BMJ*. 2009; 338:b1307.

C. Early Detection

Chaudhary K, Phadke G, Nistala R, *et al*. The emerging role of biomarkers in diabetic and hypertensive chronic kidney disease. *Curr Diab Rep*. 2010; 10(1):37-42 (NGAL as a biomarker).

Kirby T. Screening for chronic kidney disease shows promise. *Lancet*. 2010; 375(9722):1240-1 (need to screen widely for CKD due to CVD relationship).

James MT, Hemmelgarn BR, Tonelli M. Early recognition and prevention of chronic kidney disease. *Lancet*. 2010; 375(9722):1296-309 (treating hypertension is mainstay in managing progression of CKD).

Vasseloti SA, Stevens LA, Levey AS. Testing for chronic kidney disease: a position statement from the National Kidney Foundation. *Am J Kidney Dis*. 2007; 50(2):169-80 (CKD can be detected with 2 simple tests: a urine test for proteinuria and a blood test for GFR).

Waley-Connell AT, Sowers JR, Stevens LA, *et al*. CKD in the United States: kidney early evaluation program (KEEP) and National Health and Nutrition Examination Survey (NHANES) 1999-2004. *Am J Kidney Dis*. 2008; 51(4 Suppl 2):513-20 (greater prevalence of CKD detected on KEEP screening than in NHANES data).

Chapter 9. Common Causes of Chronic Kidney Disease

A. Diabetes

American Diabetes Association. http:www.diabetes.org/diabetes-basics/diabetes-statistics/ (accessed February 2011)(diabetes statistics; data from National Diabetes Fact Sheet, 2011).

American Diabetes Association. Nephropathy screening and treatment. *Diabetes Care*. 2010; 33(Suppl 1):S34-6. (diabetes leading cause of CKD; glucose control reduces risk).

American Diabetes Association. Nutrition Recommendations and Interventions for Diabetes: A position statement of the American Diabetes Association. *Diabetes Care*. 2008; 31(Suppl 1):S61-S78.

American Diabetes Association. Standards of medical care in diabetes—2010. *Diabetes Care* 2010; 33(Suppl 1):S11-S61.

American Diabetes Association. Summary of Revisions for the 2010 Clinical Practice Recommendations. *Diabetes Care*. 2010; 33(Suppl 1):S3 (diagnosis of diabetes).

American Heart Association. Heart Disease and Stroke Statistics--2010 update at www.american heart.org/presenter.jhtm/?/identifier=3000090 (accessed September 5, 2010) (box info on glycemic control).

Centers for Disease Control and Prevention. http://www.cdc.gov/diabetes/statistics/index.htm (accessed February 2011)(diabetes statistics).

Cheng YI, Gregg EW, Geiss LS, *et al*. Association of A1C and fasting plasma glucose levels with diabetic retinopathy prevalence in the U.S. population: Implications for diabetes diagnostic thresholds. *Diabetes Care*. 2009; 32(11):2027-2032. (A1C of 5.5% for diabetes diagnosis).

Department of Health and Human Services Centers for Disease Control and Prevention, National Diabetes Fact Sheet 2007. www.cdc.gov/diabetes/subs/factsheet07.htm (accessed September, 2010)(statistics on diabetes).

Mazurek JA, Hailpern SM, Goring T, Nordin C. Prevalence of hemoglobin A1c greater than 6.5% and 7.0% among hospitalized patients without a known diagnosis of diabetes at an urban inner city hospital. *J Clin Endocrinol Metab*. 2010; 95(3):1344-1348 (Many diabetics undiagnosed but with high A1c levels).

Plantinga LC, Crews DC, Coresh J, *et al*. Prevalence of chronic kidney disease in U.S. adults with undiagnosed diabetes or prediabetes. *Clin J Am Soc Nephrol*. 2010; 5(4):673-82 (CDC study of diabetes and kidney disease, 80% diagnosed diabetics and 42% undiagnosed diabetics have CKD).

Saladin KS. *Anatomy & Physiology: The Unity of Form and Function*, The McGraw Hill Companies, Inc., 4th Ed., 2007; 919 (box information on sweet urine).

Skyler JS, Bergenstal R, Bonow RO, *et al.* Intensive glycemic control and the prevention of cardiovascular events: implications of the ACCORD, ADVANCE, and VA Diabetes Trials: a position statement of the American Diabetes Association and a Scientific Statement of the American College of Cardiology Foundation and the American Heart Association. *J Am Coll Cardiol.* 2009; 53(3):298-304.

United States Renal Data System: USRDS 2010 Annual Data Report: Atlas of Chronic Kidney Disease and End-Stage Renal Disease in the United States, National Institutes of Health, National Institute of Diabetes and Digestive and Kidney Diseases, Bethesda, Md. 2010; Vol 1, Ch. 1; Ch. 2 (all CKD statistics).

Wolf G, Sharma K, Ziyadeh FN. Pathphysiology and pathogenesis of diabetic nephropathy. In Alpern RJ, Hebert SC (eds): Seldin & Giebisch's *The Kidney.* 4ᵗʰ ed., Philadelphia, Elsevier/Academic Press, 2007; 2215-2233 (how nephropathy develops).

B. High Blood Pressure

American Heart Association. Heart Disease and Stroke Statistics--2010 update at www.american heart.org/presenter.jhtm/?/identifier=3000090 (accessed September 5, 2010) (statistics regarding hypertension).

Murphree DD, Thelen SM. Chronic kidney disease in primary care. *J Am Board Fam Med.* 2010; 23(4):542-50 (hypertension causes CKD and treatment slows progression of CKD).

Plantinga LC, Miller ER, Stevens LA, *et al.* Blood pressure control among persons without and with chronic kidney disease: U.S. trends and risk factors 1999-2006. *Hypertension.* 2009; 54(1):47-56. (uncontrolled high blood pressure a greater problem in people with CKD).

United States Renal Data System: USRDS 2010 Annual Data Report: Atlas of Chronic Kidney Disease and End-Stage Renal Disease in the United States, National Institutes of Health, National Institute of Diabetes and Digestive and Kidney Diseases, Bethesda, Md. 2010. Vol 1, Ch 1 and Ch 6 (all statistics relating to CKD).

Viazzi F, Leocini G, Conti M, *et al.* Microalbuminuria is a predictor of chronic renal insufficiency in patients without diabetes and with hypertension: the MAGIC Study. *Clin J Am Soc Nephrol.* 2010; 5:1099-1106.

C. Glomerular Diseases

Alexopoulos E, Papagianni A, Tsamelashvili M, *et al.* Induction and long-term treatment with cyclosporine in membranous nephropathy with the nephrotic syndrome. *Nephrol Dial Transplant.* 2006; 21(11):3127-3132.

Bartosik LP, Lajoie G, Sugar L, Cattran DC. Predicting progressions in IgA nephropathy. *Am J Kidney Dis.* 2001; 38(4):728-735.

Dussol B, Morange S, Barley S, *et al.* Mycophenolate mofeld monotherapy in membraneous nephropathy: a 1-year randomized and controlled trial. *Am J Kidney Dis.* 2008; 52(4):699-705 (treatment of MGN).

Genovese G, Tonna SJ, Knob AU, *et al.* A risk allele for focal segmental glomerulosclerosis in African Americans is located within a region containing APOL1 and MYH9. *Kidney Int.* 2010; 78(7):698-704.

Herlitz LC, Markowitz GS, Farris AB, *et al.* Development of focal segmental glomerulosclerosis after anabolic steroid abuse. *J Am Soc Nephrol.* 2010; 21(1):163-72 (bodybuilders and steroid use).

Hogg RJ, Lee J, Nardelli N, *et al.* Clinical trial to evaluate omega-3 fatty acids and alternate day prednisone in patients with IgA nephropathy: report from the Southwest Pediatric Nephrology Study Group. *Clin J Am Soc Nephrol.* 2006; 1(3):467-474.

Kistier AD, Poster D, Krauer F, *et al.* Increases in kidney volume in autosomal dominant polycystic kidney disease can be detected within 6 months. *Kidney Int.* 2009; 75(2):235-241.

Lesavre P, Davison AM. Infection related glomerulonephritis. Davison AM, Cameron JS, Grünfeld JP, *et al* (eds). *Oxford Textbook of Clinical Nephrology,* Vol 1, 3ʳᵈ ed. Oxford, Oxford University Press, 2005; pp. 601-623.

Meyrier A. An update on the treatment options for focal segmental glomerulosclerosis. *Expert Opin Pharmacother.* 2009;10(4):615-28.

Moroni G, Doria A, Ponticelli C. Cyclosporine (CsA) in lupus nephritis: assessing the evidence. *Nephrol Dial Transplant.* 2009; 24(1):15-20. (use of steroids in lupus)

NIH Publication No. 06-4358. National Kidney and Urologic Disease Information Clearinghouse, A Service of the National Institute of Diabetes and Kidney and Digestive Diseases.

Peyser A, MacHardy N, Tarapore F, *et al.* Follow-up of phase I trial of adalimumab and rosigistazone in FSGS: III. Report of the FONT Study Group. *BMC Nephrol.* 2010; 11:2 (FSGS and antifibrotic agents).

Troyanov S, Roasio L, Pandes M, *et al.* Renal pathology in idiopathic membranous nephropathy: A new perspective. *Kidney Int.* 2006; 69(9):1641-1648.

Turchin I, Bernatsky S, Clarke AE, *et al.* Cigarette smoking and cutaneous damage in systemic lupus erythematosus. *J Theumatol.* 2009; 36(12):2691-3.

Ushigome H, Suzuki T, Fujiki M, *et al.* Efficacy of tonsillectomy for patients with recurrence of IgA nephropathy after kidney transplantation. *Clin Transplant.* 2009; 23(Suppl 20):17-22.

United States Renal Data System: USRDS 2010 Annual Data Report: Atlas of Chronic Kidney Disease and End-Stage Renal Disease in the United States, National Institutes of Health, National Institute of Diabetes and Digestive and Kidney Diseases, Bethesda, Md. 2010; Ref. Table B7, Vol 2 (malignancy in MGN; statistics regarding incidence).

Weening JJ, D'Agati VD, Schwartz MM, *et al.* The classification of glomerulonephritis in systemic lupus erythematosus. *J Am Soc Nephrol.* 2004; 15(2):241-50; *Kidney Int.* 2004; 65(2):521-530.

Working group of the International IgA Nephropathy Network and the Renal Pathology Society. The Oxford IgA nephropathy clinicopathological classification is valid for children as well as adults. *Kidney Int.* 2010; 77(10):921-7.

Wyatt CM, Morgello S, Katz-Malamed R, *et al.* The spectrum of kidney disease in patients with AIDS in the era of antiretroviral therapy. *Kidney Int.* 2009; 75(4):428-34.

D. Inherited Diseases

Abanez L, Morlans M, Vidal X, *et al.* Case-control study of regular analgesic and nonsteroidal anti-inflammatory use and end-stage renal disease. *Kidney Int.* 2005; 67:2393-2398.

Baghrie-Lachidan M, McNeill H. What drives cyst formation in CKD? *J Am Soc Nephrol.* 2010; 21(2):200-2 (protein malfunction in PKD).

Gregory MC, Shamshirsam A, Kamgar M, Bekhernia MR. Alport's syndrome, Fabry's disease and nail-patella syndrome. In Schrier RW (ed): *Diseases of the Kidney*, 8th ed. Boston, Little, Brown. 2007: 540-569.

LeBleu V, Sugimoto H, Mundel TM, *et al.* Stem cell therapies benefit Alport syndrome. *J Am Soc Nephrol.* 2009; 20(11):2359-70.

McKie KT, Hanevold CD, Hernandez C, *et al.* Prevalence, prevention, and treatment of microalbuminuria and proteinuria in children with sickle cell disease. *J Pediatr Hematol Oncol.* 2007; 29(3):140-144.

Schillingford JM, Piontek KB, Germino GG, Weimbs T. Rapamycin ameliorates PKD resulting from conditional inactivation of PKD1. *J Am Soc Nephrol.* 2010; 21(3):489-97 (drug slowed PKD cyst growth).

Wüthrick RP, Serra AL, Kistler AD. Autosomal dominant polycystic kidney disease: new treatment options and how to test their efficacy. *Kidney Blood Press Res.* 2009; 32:380-87 (drugs currently used and also being developed to slow PKD).

E. Drugs / Poisons

Glaser J, Rolita L. Educating older adults in over-the-counter medication use. *Geriatric Aging.* 2009; 12(2):103-109. (elderly 2 to 7 times more likely to suffer drug side effects; 40% of hospitalizations from medication use)

Henrich WI, Clark RL, Kelly JP, *et al.* Non-contrast-enhanced computerized tomography and analgesic-related kidney disease: report of the national analgesic nephropathy study. *J Am Soc Nephrol.* 2006; 17(5):1472-1480.

Ibanez L, Morlans M, Vidal X, *et al.* Case-control study of regular analgesic and nonsteroidal anti-inflammatory use and end-stage renal disease. *Kidney Int.* 2005; 67(6):2393-2398.

Munar MY, Singh H. Drug dosing adjustments in patients with chronic kidney disease. *Am Fam Physician.* 2007; 75(10):1487-1496 (drug dosing errors are common in patients with renal impairment).

Schillingford JM, Piontek KB, Germino GG, Weimbs T. Rapamycin ameliorates PKD resulting from conditional inactivation of PKD1. *J Am Soc Nephrol.* 2010; 21(3):489-97 (drug slowed PKD cyst growth).

Solomon RJ, Mehran R, Natarajan MK, *et al.* Contrast-induced nephropathy and long-term adverse events: cause and effect? *Clin J Am Soc Nephrol.* 2009; 4(7):1162-9.

Spruill WJ, Wade WE, Cobb HH. Comparison of estimated glomerular filtration rate with estimated creatinine clearance in the dosing of drugs requiring adjustments in elderly patients with declining renal function. *Am J Geriatr Pharmacother.* 2008; 6(3):153-160.

Weisbord SD, Palevsky PM. Strategies for the prevention of contrast-induced acute kidney injury. *Curr Opin Nephrol Hypertens.* 2010; PMID:20625289.

Chapter 10.   Dialysis

A. Hemodialysis

Beddhu S, Samore MH, Roberts MS, *et al.* Impact of timing of initiation of dialysis on mortality. *J Am Soc Nephrol.* 2003; 14: 2305-2312.

Culleton BF, Walsh M, Klarenbach SW, *et al.* Effect of frequent nocturnal hemodialysis vs conventional hemodialysis on left ventricular mass and quality of life: A randomized controlled trial. *JAMA* 2007; 298:1291-1299.

Gura V, Macy AS, Beizai M, *et al.* Technical Breakthrough in the Wearable Artificial Kidney (WAK), *Clin J Am Soc Nephrol.* 2009; 4(9):1441-8.

Khan S, Xue J, Kazmi W, *et al.* Does predialysis nephrology care influence patient survival after initiation of dialysis? *Kidney Int.* 2005; 67:1038-1046.

Lacson Jr. E, Wang W, Lester K, *et al.* Outcomes associated with in-center nocturnal hemodialisys from a large multicenter program. *Clin J Am Nephrol.* 2010; 5(2):220-6.

Lee DK, Chertow G III, Zenios SA. Reexploring differences among for-profit and non-profit dialysis providers. *Health Serv. Res.* 2010; 45(3):633-46.

McClellan WM, Wasse H, McClellan HC, *et al.* Treatment center and geographic variability in pre-ESRD care associated with increased mortality. *J Am Soc Nephrol.* 2009; 20: 1079-1085 (late referral to nephrologist increases mortality of ESRD patients).

Mehrotta R, Agarwal R. End-stage renal disease and dialysis. *Neph SAP.* 2008; 7:374-441.

Pauley RP, Gill SS, Rose CL, *et al.* Survival among nocturnal home hemodialysis patients compared to kidney transplant recipients. *Nephrology Dialysis Transplantation* 2009; 24(9): 2915-2919.

Powell JR, Oluwaseun O, Woo YM, Padmanabhan N, *et al.* Ten years' experience of in-center thrice-weekly long overnight hemodialysis. *Clin J Am Soc Nephrol.* 2009; 4(6):1097-1101 (overnight dialysis and reduced death rate).

Renal Week 2010: American Society of Nephrology 43rd Annual Meeting. Presented Nov. 2010 (mortality in U.S. dialysis centers).

Rocco MV. Short daily and nocturnal hemodialysis: new therapies for a new century? *Saudi J Kidney Dis Transpl.* 2009; 20(1):1-11 (lengthy dialysis led to better blood pressure control and reduced phosphates).

Slinin Y, Guo H, Gilbertson DT, *et al.* Meeting K/DOQI Guideline goals at hemodialysis initiation and survival during the first year. *Clin J Am Soc Nephrol.* 2010; 5(9):1574-81.

Twardowski ZJ, Misra M. "Daily" dialysis--lessons from a randomized, controlled study. *N Engl J Med.* 2010; 363(24):2363-4.

United States Renal Data System: USRDS 2010 Annual Data Report. Atlas of Chronic Kidney Disease and End-Stage Renal Disease in the United States, National Institutes of Health, National Institute of Diabetes and Digestive and Kidney Diseases, Bethesda, Md. 2010; Vol. II, Intro: 200-222 and Ch. 1:253-66 (65% dialysis, AV fistula, graft, catheter); 213 (dialysis increase 35%: starting dialysis with catheter, infection rate higher; morbidity and mortality statistics for dialysis; dialysis and stroke risk).

B. Peritoneal Dialysis

Chiu Y-W, Teitelbaum I, Misra M, *et al.* Pill burden, adherence, hyperphosphatemia, and quality of life in maintenance dialysis patients. *Clin J Am Soc Nephrol.* 2009; 4:10891096 (box info regarding pill number).

Fenton SS, Schaubel DE, Desmeules M, *et al.* Hemodialysis versus peritoneal dialysis: A comparison of adjusted mortality rates. *Am J Kidney Dis.* 1997; 30:334-342.

Saxena R, West C. Peritoneal dialysis: a primary case perspective: pros and cons of peritoneal dialysis. *J Am Board Fam Med.* 2006; 19(4):280-9 (description of PD process and pros/cons).

National Kidney Foundation K/DOQI Clinical Practice Guidelines for Peritoneal Dialysis Adequacy: update 2006. Available at http://www.kidney.org/professional/KDOQI/guideline/htm (accessed September 2010).

United States Renal Data System: USRDS 2010 Annual Data Report. Atlas of Chronic Kidney Disease and End-Stage Renal Disease in the United States, National Institutes of Health, National Institute of Diabetes and Digestive and Kidney Diseases, Bethesda, Md. 2010; Ch. 1-6, Vol II.

C. How Much Dialysis is Enough

Argyropoulos C, Chang CH, Plantinga L, *et al. J Am Soc Nephrol.* 2009 20:20334-2043 (higher dialysis dosage correlates with better survival).

Chatoh DK, Golper TA, Gokal R. Morbidity and mortality in re-defining adequacy of peritoneal dialysis: A step beyond the National Kidney foundation Dialysis Outcomes Quality Initiative. *Am J Kidney Dis.* 1999; 33: 617-632.

Daugirdas JT, Depner TA, Greene T, *et al.* Standard Kt/V urea: a method of calculation that includes effects of fluid removal and residual kidney clearance. *Kidney Int.* 2010; 77(7):637-44.

Depner T, Daugirdas J, Greene T, *et al.* Hemodialysis Study Group: Dialysis dose and the effect of gender and body size on outcome in the HEMO Study. *Kidney Int.* 2004; 65:1386-1394.

K/DOQI Clinical Practice Guidelines and Clinical Practice Recommendations. 2006 Update: hemodialysis adequacy, peritoneal dialysis adequacy, and vascular access. *Am J Kidney Dis.* 2006; 48(Suppl 1).

National Kidney Foundation: NKF-K/DOQI Clinical Practice Guidelines for Hemodialysis Adequacy: Update 2006. Available at http://ww.kidnev.org/professionals/kdoqi/guideline_uphd_pd_va/index.htm (accessed September 2010).

D. Dialysis - Survival Facts

Baha I, Burnett-Bowie S-A, Ye J, *et al.* Clinical measures identify vitamin D deficiency in dialysis. *Clin J Am Soc Nephrol.* 2010; 5:460-7.

Beddhu S, Cheung AK, Larive B, *et al* and the HEMO Study Group. Inflammation and the inverse associations of body mass index and serum creatinine with mortality in hemodialysis patients. *J Ren Nutr.* 2007; 17:372-380.

Collins AJ, Foley RN, Herzog C, *et al.* Excerpts from the United States Renal Data System 2008 Annual Data Report. *Am J Kidney Dis.* 2009; 53 (Suppl 1):S1-S374.

DeJager DJ, Grootendorst DC, Jager KS, *et al.* Cardiovascular and noncardiovascular mortality among patients starting dialysis, *JAMA* 2009; 302(16):1782-1789. (CVD is 10-20 times higher in dialysis patients compared to general population; dialysis patients have increased risk of death unrelated to CVD).

DeLoach S, Mohler E. Peripheral arterial disease: a guide for nephrologists. *Clin J Am Soc Nephrol.* 2007; 2:839-846.

Jaar BG, Coresh J, Plantinga LC, *et al.* Comparing the risk for death with peritoneal dialysis and hemodialysis in a national cohort of patients with chronic kidney disease. *Ann Intern Med.* 2005;143:174-183.

Kalantar-Zadeh K, Abbott KC, Salahudeen AK, *et al.* Survival advantages of obesity in dialysis patients. *Am J Clin Nutrition.* 2005; 81: 543-554.

Katzir Z, Boaz M, Backshi I, *et al.* Medication apprehension and compliance among dialysis patients--a comprehensive guidance attitude. *Nephrol Clin Pract.* 2010; 114(2):c151-7.

Koyama H, Fukuda S, Shoji T, *et al.* Fatigue is a predictor for cardiovascular outcomes in patients undergoing hemodialysis. *Clin J Am Soc Nephrol.* 2010; 5(4):659-66.

Martin KJ, Gonzalez EA. Prevention and control of phosphate retention/hyperphosphotemia in CKD-MBD: What is normal, when to start, and how to treat? *Clin J Am Soc Nephrol.* 2011; 6(2):440-6 (dialysis patients need to limit phosphate and potassium).

Murphree DD, Thelen SM. Chronic Kidney Disease in primary care. *J Am Board Fam Med.* 2010; 23(4):542-550 (complications of CKD; potassium and phosphorus disruption).

Saliba W, El-Haddad B. Secondary Hyperparathyroidism: pathophysiology and treatment: calcium and phosphorus homeostasis. *J Am Board Fam Med.* 2009; 22(5): 574-81.

Singh AK, Szczech L, Tan KL, *et al.* Correction of anemia with epoetin alfa in chronic kidney disease. *N Engl J Med.* 2006; 355:2085-2098.

Suki WN, Zabaneh R, Cangiano JL, *et al.* Effects of sevelamer and calcium-based phosphate binders on mortality in hemodialysis patients. *Kidney Int.* 2007; 72:1130-1137.

United States Renal Data System: USRDS 2010 Annual Data Report. Atlas of Chronic Kidney Disease and End-Stage Renal Disease in the United States, National Institutes of Health, National Institute of Diabetes and Digestive and Kidney Diseases, Bethesda, Md. 2010; Vol. II, Ch. 6: 301-10.

Vonech EF, Snyder JJ, Foley RN, Collins AJ. Mortality studies comparing peritoneal dialysis and hemodialysis: What do they tell us? *Kidney Int Suppl.* 2006;103:S3-S11.

Winkelmayer WC, Liu S, Brookhart MA. Altitude and all-cause mortality in incident dialysis patients. *JAMA.* 2009;301(5):508-512.

Chapter 11. Deceased Donors and Waiting List

A. Transplant Waiting List

Devi SP, Kumar SS, Rao KS. Evaluation of kidney transplantation programs using system simulation. *J Med Syst.* 2010; PMID:20809253 (imbalance in donations among transplant centers).

Indiana Organ Procurement Organization, www.IOPO.org (accessed February 2011).

Kallab S, Bassil N, Esposito L, *et al.* Indications for and barriers to preemptive kidney transplantation: a review. *Transplant Proc.* 2010; 42(3):782-4 (preemptive transplant treatment of choice; related to better patient survival).

Ladner D, *et al.* The impact of physician years since graduation on patient referrals for preemptive living donor kidney transplantation. *Am Soc Nephrol.* 2009; Paper presented at American Society of Nephrology's 42nd annual Meeting and Scientific Exposition in San Diego.

National Organ Transplant Act of 1984, Pub. L. No. 98-507 (codified at 42 U.S.C. §§ 273-74) (requires hospitals to affiliate with OPOs).

Patzer RE, Amaral S, Wasse H, *et al.* Neighborhood poverty and racial disparities in kidney transplant waitlisting. *J Am Soc Nephrol.* 2009; 20(6):1330-40 (blacks from poor neighborhoods less likely than whites to be on waiting list).

Rosendale JD, Kauffman MH, McBride M, *et al.* Aggressive pharmacologic donor management results in more transplanted organs. *Transplantation.* 2003; 75(4):482-7 (preserving brain-dead donor organs with drugs).

Schold J, Srinivas TR, Sehgal AR, Meier-Kriesche HR. Half of kidney transplant candidates who are older than 60 years now placed on the waiting list will die before receiving a deceased-donor transplant. *Clin J Am Soc Nephrol.* 2009; 4(7):1239-45.

United Network for Organ Sharing (UNOS), www.unos.org (accessed February 2011).

United States Renal Data System, USRDS 2010 Annual Data Report. Atlas of Chronic Kidney Disease and End-Stage Renal Disease in the United States, National Institutes of Health, National Institute of Diabetes and Digestive and Kidney Diseases, Bethesda, Md. 2010; Vol. II, Ch 7:311-324 (transplant statistics, facts).

U.S. Department of Health and Human Services, Health Resources and Services Administration, Healthcare Sys. Bureau, Div. of Transplantation (HHS/HRSA/HSB/DOT), www.organdonor.gov (accessed February 2011).

B. Types of Deceased Donors

Delmonico FL, Burdick JF. Maximizing the success of transplantation with kidneys from older donors. *N Engl J Med.* 2006; 354(4):411-3.

Fraser SM, Rajasundaram R, Aldouri A, *et al.* Acceptable outcome after kidney transplantation using "expanded criteria donor" grafts. *Transplantation.* 2010; 89(1):88-96.

Kayler LK, Magliocca J, Kim RD, *et al.* Single kidney transplantation pediatric donors in the United States. *Am J Transplant.* 2009; 9(12):2745-51.

Leichtman AM, Cohen D, Keith D, *et al.* Kidney and pancreas transplantation in the United States, 1997-2006: the HRSA Breakthrough Collaborative and the 58 DSA Challenge. *Am J Transplant.* 2008; 8(4 Pt 2):946-57.

Locke JE, Segev DL, Warren DS, *et al.* Outcomes of kidneys from donors after cardiac death: implications for allocation and preservation. *Am J Transplant.* 2007; 7(7):1797-807.

Lucarelli G, Bettocchi C, Battaglia M, *et al.* Extended criteria donor kidney transplantation: comparative outcome analysis between single versus double kidney transplantation at 5 years. *Transplant Proc.* 2010; 42(4):1104-7.

Marks WH, Wagner D, Pearson TC, *et al.* Organ donation and utilization, 1995-2004: entering the collaborative era. *Am J Transplant.* 2006; 6(5 Pt 2):1101-1110.

McDiarmid S, Pruett T, Graham WK. The oversight of solid organ transplantation in the United States. *Am J Transplant.* 2008; 8(4):739-744.

Merion RM, Ashby VB, Wolfe RA, *et al.* Deceased-donor characteristics and the survival benefit of kidney transplantation. *JAMA.* 2005; 294(21):2726-33.

Miller FG, Truog RD, Brock DW. The dead donor rule: can it withstand critical scrutiny? *J Med Philos.* 2010; 35(3):299-312 (brain dead may not be dead; is it wrong to cause the death of a donor in some cases?).

O'Connor KJ, Delmonico FL. Increasing the supply of kidneys for transplantation. *Semin Dialysis.* 2005; 18(6):460-462.

Saidi RF, Elias N, Kawai T, *et al.* Outcome of kidney transplantation using expanded criteria donors and donation after cardiac death kidneys: realities and costs. *Am J Transplant.* 2007; 7(12):2769-74 (ECD and DCD provide more kidneys but graft survival rate lower, making use costly).

Snanoudj R, Rabant M, Timsit MO, *et al.* Donor-estimated GFR as an appropriate criterion for allocation of ECD kidneys into single or dual kidney transplantation. *Am J Transplant.* 2009; 9(11):2542-51 (ECD kidneys, single or double transplantation).

Steinbrook R. Organ donation after cardiac death. *N Engl J Med.* 2007; 357(3):209-213.

Sung RS, Galloway J, Tuttle-Newhall J, *et al.* Organ donation and utilization in the United States, 1997-2006. *Am J Transplant.* 2008; 8(4 Pt 2):922-34.

United States Renal Data System, USRDS 2010 Annual Data Report. Atlas of Chronic Kidney Disease and End-Stage Renal Disease in the United States, National Institutes of Health, National Institute of Diabetes and Digestive and Kidney Diseases, Bethesda, Md. 2010; Vol. II, Ch 7:311-324 (transplant statistics, facts).

Wijdicks EF, Varelas PN, Gronseth GS, *et al.* Evidence-based guideline update: determining brain dead in adults: report of the Quality Standards Subcommittee of the American Academy of Neurology. *Neurology.* 2010; 74(23):1911-8.

C. Becoming a Listed Candidate

Grubbs V, Gregorich SE, Perez-Stable FJ, Hsu CY. Health literacy and access to kidney transplantation. *Clin J Am Soc Nephrol.* 2009; 4(1):195-200.

Kutsogiannis A, Pagliarello G, Doig C, *et al.* Medical management to optimize donor organ potential: review of the literature. *Can J Anaesth.* 2006; 53(8):820-830.

Landin L, Rodriguez-Perez JC, Garcia-Bello MA, *et al.* Kidney transplants in HIV-positive recipients under HAART. A comprehensive review and meta-analysis of 12 series. *Nephrol Dial Transplant.* 2010; 25(9):3106-15.

Melancon JK, Kucirka LM, Boulware LE *et al.* Impact of Medicare coverage on disparities in access to simultaneous pancreas and kidney transplantation. *Am J Transplant.* 2009; 9(12):2785-2791 (greater percentage of whites registered than blacks/Hispanics).

Potluri K, Hou S. Obesity in kidney transplant recipients and candidates. *Am J Kidney Dis.* 2010; 56(1):143-56 (transplant complications in obese patients).

United States Renal Data System, USRDS 2010 Annual Data Report. Atlas of Chronic Kidney Disease and End-Stage Renal Disease in the United States, National Institutes of Health, National Institute of Diabetes and Digestive and Kidney Diseases, Bethesda, Md. 2010; Vol. II, Ch 7:311-324 (transplant statistics, facts).

D. What is a Match?

American Red Cross, www.redcrossblood.org (accessed September 2010) (Blood types and percentages).

Bielmann D, Hönger G, Lutz D, *et al.* Pretransplant risk assessment in renal allograft recipients using virtual crossmatching. *Am J Transplant.* 2007; 7(3):626-32.

Bray RA, Nolen JD, Larsen C, *et al.* Transplanting the highly sensitized patient: The emory algorithm. *Am J Transplant.* 2006; 6(10):2307-2315 (1/3 waitlist patients sensitized to HLA antigens).

Cai J, Terasaki PI, Mao Q, *et al.* Development of nondonor-specific HLA-DR antibodies in allograft recipients is associated with shared epitopes with mismatched donor DR antigens. *Am J Transplant.* 2006; 6(12):2947-2954.

Gebel HM, Bray RA, Nickerson P. Pre-transplant assessment of donor-reactive, HLA-specific antibodies in renal transplantation: contraindication vs. risk. *Am J Transplant.* 2003; 3(12):1488-1500.

Helman SW, Pollack MS. Interpretation of HLA typing results for entry into UNet implications for the OPTH/UNOS HLA Matching algorithm, prepared on behalf of the OPTN/UNOS histocompatibility committee 2003.

Ho EK, Vasilescu ER, Colovai AI, *et al.* Sensitivity, specificity and clinical relevance of different cross-matching assays in deceased-donor renal transplantation. *Transpl Immunol.* 2008; 20(1-2):61-7.

International Society of Blood Transfusion, www.ISBTweb.org. (accessed April 2010) (blood types and antigens).

Jordan SC, Vo AA, Peng A, Toyoda M, Tyan D. Intravenous gammaglobulin (IVIG): a novel approach to improve transplant rates and outcomes in highly HLA-sensitized patients. *Am J Transplant.* 2006; 6(3):459-66.

Mizutani K, Terasaki P, Hamdani E, *et al.* The importance of anti-HLA-specific antibody strength in monitoring kidney transplant patients. *Am J Transplant.* 2007; 7(4):1027-1031 (strong immune system leads to risk of graft failure).

Revised Uniform Anatomical Gift Act (2006)(last revised and amended in 2009) drafted by the National Conference of Commissioners on Uniform State Laws.

Vo AA, Lukovsky M, Toyoda M, *et al.* Rituximab and intravenous immune globulin for desensitization during renal transplantation. *N Engl J Med.* 2008; 359(3):242-51.

E. The Kidney Allocation Point System

Freeman R. Survival benefit: quality versus quantity and trade-offs in developing new renal allocation systems. *Am J Transplant.* 2007; 7(5):1043-1046.

Frei U, Noeldeke J, Machold-Fabrizii V, *et al.* Prospective age-matching in elderly kidney transplant recipients: a 5-year analysis of the Eurotransplant Senior Program. *Am J Transplant.* 2008; 8(1):50-7 (transporting kidneys lessens survival of organs).

Rao PS, Schaubel DE, Guidinger MK, *et al.* A comprehensive risk qualification score for deceased donor kidneys: the kidney donor risk index. *Transplantation.* 2009; 88(2):231-6 (14 donor factors associated with graft failure).

Scandling JD, Norman DJ. United network of organ sharing (UNOS) organ allocation policy and kidney utilization. *Am J Kidney Dis.* 2010; 56(1):7-9.

Schold JD, Sriniors TR, Guerra G, *et al.* A "weight-listing" paradox for candidates of renal transplantation? *Am J Transplant.* 2007; 7(3):550-559 (weight loss may not improve transplant survival rate).

Schold JD, Sriniors TR, Poggio ED, *et al.* Hidden selection bias deriving from donor organ characteristics does not affect performance evaluations of kidney transplant centers. *Clin J Am Soc Nephrol.* 2010; PMID:20813856 (multiple organ transplants with poor results).

United Network for Organ Sharing (UNOS), www.unos.org (accessed February 2011).

F. Deceased Organ Becomes Available

Hamilton TE. Improving organ transplantation in the United States--a regulatory perspective. *Am J Transplant.* 2008; 8(12):2503-5.

Kurtz SF, Strong CW, Gerasimow D. The 2006 Revised Uniform Anatomical Gift Act – A law to save lives. *Health Law Analysis*, February 2007: 44–9 (UAGA; box info).

G. Survival

United States Renal Data System, USRDS 2010 Annual Data Report. Atlas of Chronic Kidney Disease and End-Stage Renal Disease in the United States, National Institutes of Health, National Institute of Diabetes and Digestive and Kidney Diseases, Bethesda, Md. 2010; Vol. II, Ch 7:311-324 and Table F: 557 (transplant statistics, facts).

Chapter 12. Living Donor

A. Important Considerations

Davis CL, Delmonico FL. Living-donor kidney transplantation: a review of the current practices for the live donor. *J Am Soc Nephrol.* 2005; 16(7):2098-110.

Delmonico FL, Dew MA. Living donor kidney transplantation in a global environment. *Kidney Int.* 2007; 71(7):608-614.

Gibney EM, Doshi MD, Hartmann EL, *et al.* Health insurance status of U.S. living kidney donors. *Clin J Am Soc Nephrol.* 2010; 5(5):912-6.

Herring AA, Woolhandler S, Himmelstein, D. Insurance status of U.S. organ donors and transplant recipients: the uninsured give, but rarely receive. *Int J Health Serv.* 2008; 38(4):641-52.

Ibrahim HN, Akkins SK, Leister E, *et al.* Pregnancy outcomes after kidney donation. *Am J Transplant.* 2009; 9(4):825-34 (post- and pre-donation outcomes differed).

Josephson MA. Transplantation: pregnancy and kidney donation: more questions than answers. *Nat Rev Nephrol.* 2009; 5(9):495-7.

Nevis IF, Garg AX. Donor Nephrectomy Outcomes Research (DONOR) Network. Maternal and fetal outcomes after kidney donation. *Am J Transplantation.* 2009; 9(4):661-8.

The Patient Protection and Affordable Care Act. Pub. L. 111-48, 124 Stat. 119.

Reese PP, Huverserean A, Bloom RD. Pregnancy outcomes among live kidney donors. *Am J Transplant.* 2009; 9(8):1967 (pregnancy after donation does not harm kidney or mother).

United States Renal Data System, USRDS 2010 Annual Data Report. Atlas of Chronic Kidney Disease and End-Stage Renal Disease in the United States, National Institutes of Health, National Institute of Diabetes and Digestive and Kidney Diseases, Bethesda, Md. 2010; Vol. II, Ch 7:311-324 (transplant statistics, facts).

Witczak BJ, Leivestad T, Line PD. Experience from an active preemptive kidney transplantation program--809 cases revisited. *Transplantation.* 2009; 88(5):672-7.

Yang RC, Thiessen-Philbrook H, Klarenbach S, *et al.* Donor Nephrectomy Outcomes Research (DONOR) Network. Insurability of living donors: a systematic review. *Am J Transplant.* 2007; 7(6):1542-51.

B. About Living Donations

Congressional Subcommittee on Health and Environment hearings regarding H.R. 4080, Oct. 17, 1983 (exchange between Barry Jacobs and Al Gore).

Danovitch GM. From Helsinki to Istanbul: what can the transplant community learn from experience in clinical research? *Nephrol Dial Transplant.* 2008; 23(4):1089-92.

Danovitch GM, Delmonico FL. The prohibition of kidney sales and organ markets should remain. *Curr Opin Organ Transplant.* 2008; 13(4):386-94.

Delmonico FL. The implications of Istanbul Declaration on organ trafficking and transplant tourism. *Curr Opin Organ Transplant.* 2009; 14(2):116-9.

Delmonico FL, McBride M. Analysis of the wait list and deaths among candidates waiting for a kidney transplant. *Transplantation* 2008; 86(12):1678-83.

Educating CKD patient's family encourages kidney donation. *Renal Week.* 2009: American Society of Nephrology 2009 Annual Meeting; presented Oct. 29, 2009.

Gill J, Madhira B, Gjertson D, *et al.* Transplant tourism in the United States: a single-center experience. *Clin J Am Soc Nephrol.* 2008; 3:1820-8.

Gore JL, Danovitch GM, Litwin MS, Pham PT, Singer JS. Disparities in the utilization of live donor renal transplantation. *Am J Transplant.* 2009; 9(5):1124-9 (disparities in access to transplant).

Halpern SD, Raj A, Kohn R, *et al.* Regulated payments for living kidney donation: an empirical assessment of the ethical concerns. *Ann Intern Med.* 2010; 152(6):358-65 (promotes regulated payments for kidney donations).

Hippen B. Introduction: symposium on a regulated market in transplantable organs. *J Med Philos.* 2009; 24(6):541-51.

Hippen B, Matas A. Incentives for organ donation in the United States: feasible alternative or forthcoming apocalypse? *Curr Opin Organ Transplant.* 2009; 14(2):140-6.

Kok NF, Weimar W, Alwayn IP, *et al.* The current practice of live donor nephrectomy in Europe. *Transplantation.* 2006; 82:892-7.

Leider S, Roth AE. Kidneys for sale: who disapproves, and why? *Am J Transplant.* 2010; 10(5):1113-4 (Americans surveyed in favor of kidney markets).

Liem YS, Weimar W. Early living-donor kidney transplantation: a review of the associated survival benefit. *Transplantation.* 2009; 87(3):317-8.

Montgomery RM, Katznelson S, Bry WI, *et al.* Successful three-way kidney paired donation with cross-country live donor allograft transport. *Am J Transplant.* 2008; 8(10):2163-8 (paired kidney donation).

Petosky News, www.petoskynews.com/news/article_a61bb754-561d-5377-8b86-6e7d2f551b.html (accesssed September 8, 2010).

Rees MA, Kopke JE, Pelletier RP, *et al.* A nonsimultaneous, extended, altruistic-donor chain. *N Engl J Med.* 2009; 360(1):1096-101.

Roth AE, Sönmez T, Unver M, *et al.* Utilizing list exchange and nondirected donation through 'chain' paired kidney donations. *Am J Transplant.* 2006; 6(11):2694-705.

Tilney NL, Chapman JR, Delmonico FL. Debate on financial incentives is off the mark of national and international realities. *Transplantation.* 2010; 89(7):906-7 (buying kidneys).

United States Renal Data System, USRDS 2010 Annual Data Report. Atlas of Chronic Kidney Disease and End-Stage Renal Disease in the United States, National Institutes of Health, National Institute of Diabetes and Digestive and Kidney Diseases, Bethesda, Md. 2010; Vol. II, Ch 7:311-324 (graft survival rates).

U.S. Department of Health and Human Services, Organ Procurement and Transplantation Network. http://OPTN.transplant.hrsa.gov/policies and bylaws/policies (accessed June 2010).

U.S. Department of Health and Human Services, Organ Procurement and Transplantation Network. http://OPTN.transplant.hrsa.gov (accessed February, 2011)(statistics, donor characteristics).

C. Informed Consent

Adams P, Cohen DJ, Danovitch GM, *et al.* The nondirected live-kidney donor: ethical considerations and practice guidelines: a national conference report. *Transplantation.* 2002; 74(4):582-9 (non-related donors and need for informed consent).

Compelled medical procedures involving minors and incompetents and missapplication of the substituted judgment doctrine. *Journal of Law and Health,* Vol 7; 107-30(1992).

Danovitch GM. The doctor-patient relationship in living donor kidney transplantation. *Curr Opin Nephrol Hypertens.* 2007; 16(6):503-5.

Dew MA, Jacobs CL, Jowsy SG, *et al.* Guidelines for the psychosocial evaluation of living unrelated kidney donors in the United States. *Am J Transplant,* 2007; 7(15):1047-54.

The Federal Register, Vol. 72, No. 61. Rules and Regulations 15205 (independent donor advocate).

Friedman AL, Cheung K, Roman SA, Sosa JA. Early clinical and economic outcomes of patients undergoing living donor nephrectomy in the United States. *Arch Surg.* 2010; 145(4):356-62.

Pham PC, Wilkinson AH, Pham PT. Core Curriculum in nephrology: evaluation of the potential living kidney donor. *Am J Kidney Dis.* 2007; 50(6):1043-51.

Reese PP, Feldman HI, McBride MA, *et al.* Substantial variation in the acceptance of medically complex live kidney donors across US renal transplant centers. *Am J Transplant.* 2008; 8(10):2062-70.

Rodrigue JR, Pavlakis M, Danovitch GM, *et al.* Evaluating living kidney donors: relationship types, psychosocial criteria, and consent processes at US transplant programs. *Am J Transplant.* 2007; 7(10):2326-32.

Ross LF. What the medical excuse teaches us about the potential living donor as patient. *Am J Transplant.* 2010; 10(4):731-6 (donor's right to refuse donation).

Sharp J, McRae A, McNeill Y. Decision making and psychosocial outcomes among living kidney donors: a pilot program. *Prog Transplant.* 2010; 29(1):53-7.

D. Pre-Donation Testing

Dew MA, Jacobs CL, Jowsy SG, *et al.* Guidelines for the psychosocial evaluation of living unrelated kidney donors in the United States. *Am J Transplant.* 2007; 7(15):1047-54 (donor psychosocial evaluation guildelines).

Gaston RS. Might health literacy be a prerequisite for kidney transplantation? *Clin J Am Soc Nephrol.* 2009; 4(1):16-7 (health literacy and transplantation).

Mandelbrot DA, Pavlakis M, Danovich GM, *et al.* The medical evaluation of living kidney donors: a survey of U.S. transplant centers. *Am J Transplant.* 2007; 7(10):2333-43.

Pei Y, Obaji J, Dupuis A, *et al.* Unified criteria for ultrasonographic diagnosis of ADPKD. *J Am Soc Nephrol* 2009; 20(1):205-212.

Pham PC, Wilkinson AH, Pham PT. Evaluation of the potential living donor. *Am J Kidney Dis.* 2007; 50(6):1043-51.

Raman SS, Pojchamarnwiputh S, Muangsomboon K, *et al.* Surgically relevant normal and variant renal parenchymal and vascular anatomy in preoperative 16-MDCT evaluation of potential laparoscopic renal donors. *AJR Am J Roentgenol.* 2007; 188(1):105-14.

Raman SS, Pojchamarnwiputh S, Muangsomboon K, *et al.* Utility of 16-MDCT angiography for comprehensive preoperative vascular evaluation of laparoscopic renal donors. *J Roentgenol.* 2006; 186(6):1630-4.

Silva E, Alba A, Castro A, *et al.* Evaluation of HLA matchmaker compatibility as predictor of graft survival and presence of Anti-HLA antibodies. *Transplant Proc.* 2010; 42(1):266-9.

Steiner RW, Danovitch GM. The medical evaluation and risk estimation of end-stage renal disease for living kidney donors. In: Steiner RW, ed. Educating, Evaluating and Selecting living kidney donors. Philadelphia: Kluwer Academic Publishers, 2004:49.

E. The Surgery and Post-Surgery

Aboutaleb E, Herbert P, Crane J, Hakim N. Mini-incision donor nephrectomy techniques: a systematic review. *Exp Clin Transplant*. 2010; 8(3):189-95.

Allaf ME, Singer A, Shen W, *et al.* Laparoscopic live donor nephrectomy with vaginal extraction: initial report. *Am J Transplant*. 2010; 10(6):1473-7.

Boni L, Dionigi G, Rovera F, *et al.* Laparoscopic left nephrectomy for living donor kidney transplant. *Arch Surg.* 2010; 145(6):590-1.

Breda A, Bui MH, Liao JC, Schulam PG. Association of bowel rest and ketorolac analgesia with short hospital stay after laparoscopic donor nephrectomy. *Urology*. 2007; 69(5):828-31.

Breda A, Veale J, Liao J, Schulam PG. Complications of laparoscopic living donor nephrectomy and their management: the UCLA experience. *Urology*. 2007; 69(1):49-52.

Combined kidney and hematopoietic cell transplant indices thereon, presented at the American Transplant Congress, 2010. www.medscape.com/viewarticle 721476.

Davis CL, Cooper M. The state of U.S. living donors. *Clin J Am Soc Nephrol*. 2010; 5(10):1873-80 (need for donor registry).

Friedman AL, Peters TG, Ratner LE. Perioperational mortality and long-term survival following live kidney donation. *JAMA* 2010; 303(22):2248-9.

Santos L, Macario F, Alves R, *et al.* Risks of living donor nephrectomy. *Transplant Proc*. 2010; 42(5):1484-6.

Shokeir AA. Open versus laparoscopic live donor nephrectomy: a focus on the safety of donors and the need for a donor registry. *J Urol*. 2007; 178(5):1860-66.

F. Living with One Kidney

Chien CH, Wang HH, Chian YJ, *et al.* Quality of life after laparoscopic donor nephrectomy. *Transplant Proc*. 2010; 42(3):696-8.

Davis CL, Cooper M. Long-term consequences of kidney donation. *N Engl J Med*. 2009; 360(22):2370.

Davis CL, Cooper M. The state of U.S. living kidney donors. *Clin J Am Soc Nephrol*. 2010; 5(10):1873-80 (need for donor registry).

Delmonico F; Council of the Transplantation Society. A report of the Amsterdam Forum on the Care of the Live Kidney Donor: data and medical guidelines. *Transplantation*. 2005; 79(6 Suppl):S53-S56.

Fehrman-Ekholm I, Norden G, Lennerling A, *et al.* Incidence of end-stage renal disease among live kidney donors. *Transplantation*. 2006; 82(12):1646-1648.

Foley RN, Ibrahim HN. Long-term outcomes of kidney donors. *Curr Opin Nephrol Hypertens*. 2010; 19(2):129-33 (donation not a major threat to longevity).

Garg AX, Muirhead N, Knoll G *et al.* Donor Nephrectomy Outcomes Research (DONOR) Network. Proteinuria and reduced kidney function in living donors: A systematic review, meta-analysis and meta-regression. *Kidney Int*. 2006; 70:1801-10.

Garg AX, Muirhead N, Knoll G, *et al.* Proteinuria and reduced kidney function in living kidney donors: a systematic review, meta-analysis, and meta-regression. *Kidney Int*. 2006; 70(10):1801-10.

Garg AX, Prasad GV, Thiessen-Philbrook H, *et al.* Cardiovascular disease and hypertensionrisk in living kidney donors: an analysis of health administrative data in Ontario, Canada. *Transplantation*. 2008; 86(3):399-406 (CKD and CVD).

Ibrahim H, Foley R, Tan L, *et al.* Long-term consequences of kidney donation. *N Engl J Med*. 2009; 360(5):459-69 (criticism of lack of studies on living donor outcomes).

Levey AS, Eckardt KU, Tsukamoto Y, *et al.* Definition and classification of chronic kidney disease: A position statement from kidney disease: Improving global outcomes (KDIGO). *Kidney Int*. 2005; 67(6):2089-100.

Mjoen G, Midtvedt K, Holme I, *et al.* One- and five-year follow-ups on blood pressure and renal function in kidney donors. *Transpl Intl*. 2011; 24(a):73-7 (no evidence of decline in renal function beyond initial following surgery).

Mjoen G, Oyen O, Haldaas H, *et al.* Morbidity and mortality in 1022 consecutive living donor nephrectomies: benefits of a living donor registry. *Transplantation*. 2011; 24(1):73-7.

National Kidney Foundation-Kidney Disease Outcome Quality Initiative. Clinical practice guidelines for chronic kidney disease: Evaluation, classification and stratification. *Am J Kidney Dis*. 2002; 39(Suppl 1):S1-S266.

Parasuraman R, Venkat KK. Utility of estimated glomerular filtration rate in live kidney donation. *Clin J Am Soc Nephrol*. 2008; 3(6):1608-1609 (decrease in GFR after donation).

Saran R, Marshall SM, Madsen R, Keavey P, Tapson JS. Long-term follow-up of kidney donors: A longitudinal study. *Nephrol Dial Transplant*. 1997; 12(8):1615-21 (some increase in hypertension and protein post-donation).

Segev DL,. Muzaale AD, Caffo BS, *et al.* Perioperational mortality and long-term survival following a kidney donation. *JAMA*. 2010; 303:959-966 (surgical death risk, long-term risk to donors; donating a kidney does not shorten or lengthen life)

Tan JC, Chertow G. Cautious optimism concerning long-term safety of kidney donation. *N Engl J Med*. 2009; 360(5):522-3.

Wan RK, Spalding E, Winch D, Brown K, Geddes CC. Reduced kidney function in living donors. *Kidney Int*. 2007; 71(10):1077.

Young A, Nevis IF, Geddes C *et al.* Donor Nephrectomy Outcomes Research (DONOR) Network. Do biochemical measures change in living kidney donors? A systematic review. *Nephron Clin Pract*. 2007; 107(3):82-9 (slight increase in creatinine post donation).

G. Critical Reflections

Barri Y, Parker TF, Daoud Y, Glassock RJ. Definition of chronic kidney disease after uninephrectomy in living donors: What are the implications? *Transplantation.* 2010; 90(5):575-80.

Barri Y, Parker III T, Kaplan B, Glassock RJ. *Primum non nocere*: is chronic kidney disease staging appropriate in living kidney donors? *Am J Transplantation.* 2009; 9(4):657-660 (faulty labeling of donors as having CKD, few centers follow renal function of donors, little documented harm to donors).

http://www.abstracts2view.com/atc/view.php?nr=ATCook 1478 Mia H Marietta, *et al.* Are living kidney donors receiving adequate long-term medical followup? Presented at the American Transplant Congress, 2009.

http://www.organdonor.gov/research/acotnov2008 notes.htm.ACOT November 2008 meeting notes. (donors follow-up exams not covered after 1 year; 40% no health insurance)

McCune TR, Armata T, Mendez-Picon G, *et al.* The living organ donor network: a model registry for living kidney donors. *Clin Transplantation.* 2004; 18(Supp.12):33-38.

Mandelbrot DA, Paviakis M, Karp SJ, *et al.* Practices and barriers in long-term living kidney donor followup: a survey of U.S. transplant centers. *Transplantation.* 2009; 88(7):855-60 (significant changes required to improve donor follow-up by transplant centers).

National Kidney Foundation, Living Donor Council, www.livingdonor@kidney.org (launch of council at www.kidney.org/transplantation/living donors/index.cfm) (accessed September 2010).

Ommen ES, Winston JA, Murphy B. Medical risks in living kidney donors: absence of proofs is not proof of absence. *Clin J Am Soc Nephrol.* 2006; 1(4):885-95 (registration of living donors essential for better long-term studies).

Chapter 13. Kidney Transplantation

Introduction

United States Renal Data System: USRDS 2010 Annual Data Report. *Atlas of Chronic Kidney Disease and End-Stage Renal Disease in the United States,* National Institutes of Health, National Institute of Diabetes and Digestive and Kidney Diseases, Bethesda, Md. 2010; Vol. II, Ch 7:311-324.

U.S. Department of Health & Human Services, Organ Procurement and Transplantation Network. www.optn.transplant.hnsa.gov/data (accessed September 2010).

A. Transplantation, Generally

Fairhead T, Knoll G. Recurrent glomerular disease after kidney transplantation. *Curr Opin Nephrol Hypertens.* 2010; PMID: 20639758 (recurrence of glomerulonephritis is third leading cause of graft failure).

Leichtman A, Cohen D, Keith D, *et al.* Kidney and pancreas transplantation in the United States 1997-2006: the HRSA breakthrough collaborative and 58 DSA challenge. *Am J Transplant.* 2008; 8(4 Pt 2):946-57 (projected need for kidneys to transplant and challenges).

Sener A, Bella AJ, Nguan C, Luke PP, House AA. Focal segmental glomerular scleroses in renal transplant recipients: predicting earlier disease recurrence may prolong allograft function. *Clin Transplant.* 2009; 23(1):96-100.

United States Renal Data System: USRDS 2010 Annual Data Report. *Atlas of Chronic Kidney Disease and End-Stage Renal Disease in the United States,* National Institutes of Health, National Institute of Diabetes and Digestive and Kidney Diseases, Bethesda, Md. 2010; Vol. II, Ch 7:311-324.

U.S. Department of Health & Human Services, Organ Procurement and Transplantation Network. www.optn.transplant.hnsa.gov/data (accessed September 2010).

B. Evaluation for Transplant Surgery

Danovitch GM. A kidney for all ages. *Am J Transplant* 2006; 6:1267-1268.

Dobbels F, Skeans MA, Snyder JJ, *et al.* Depressive disorder in renal transplantation: an analysis of Medicare claims. *Am J Kidney Dis.* 2008; 51(5):819-828.

Hartman EL, Wu C. The evolving challenge of evaluating older renal transplant candidates. *Adv Chronic Kidney Dis.* 2010; 17(4):358-67.

Ivanyi B. A primer on recurrent and de novo glomerulonephritis in renal allografts. *Nat Clin Prac Nephrol.* 2008; 4(8):446-56 (prevalence of glomerulonephritis post transplant).

Kasiske BL, Cangro CB, Hariharan S, *et al.* The evaluation of renal transplant candidates: clinical practice guidelines. *Am J Transplant* 2002; 1(Supp 2):3-95.

Lentine KL, Hurst FP, Jindal RM, *et al.* Cardiovascular risk assessment among potential kidney transplant candidates: approaches and controversies. *Am J Kidney Dis.* 2010; 55(1): 152-67.

Meier-Kriesche HU, Scornik JC, Susskind B, Rehman S, Schnold JD. A lifetime versus a graft life approach redefines the importance of HLA matching in kidney transplant patients. *Transplantation.* 2009; 88(1):23-9.

Pilmore H. Cardiac assessment for renal transplantation. *Am J Transplant.* 2006; 6(4):659-65.

Potluri K, Hou S. Obesity in kidney transplant recipients and candidates. *Am J Kidney Dis.* 2010; 56(1):143-56 (transplant complications in obese patients).

Roland ME, Barin B, Carlson L, *et al.* HIV-infected liver and kidney transplant recipients: 1- and 3-year outcomes. *Am J Transplant.* 2008; 8(3):355-65.

Schold J, Srinivas TR, Sehgal AR, Meier-Kriesche HU. Half of kidney transplant candidates who are older than 60 years now placed on the waiting list will die before receiving a deceased-donor transplant. *Clin J Am Soc Nephrol.* 2009; 4(7):1239-45.

Steinman TI, Becker BN, Frost AE, *et al.* Guidelines for the referral and management of patients eligible for solid organ transplantation. *Transplantation.* 2001; 71(9):1189-1204 (guidelines proposed by Clinical Practice Committee of the American Society of Transplantation).

Surman OS, Cosimi AB, DiMartini A. Psychiatric care of patients undergoing organ transplantation. *Transplantation.* 2009; 87(12):1753-761 (transplant patients may require psychological assistance with transplant adjustments).

U.S. Department of Health & Human Services, Organ Procurement and Transplantation Network. www.optn.transplant.hrsa.gov/data (accessed February 2011).

United States Renal Data System: USRDS 2010 Annual Data Report. *Atlas of Chronic Kidney Disease and End-Stage Renal Disease in the United States,* National Institutes of Health, National Institute of Diabetes and Digestive and Kidney Diseases, Bethesda, Md. 2010; Vol II, Ch 7:311-324.

C. The Transplant Surgery

Bruno S, Remuzzi G, Ruggenenti P. Transplant renal artery stenosis. *J Am Soc Nephrol.* 2004; 15(1):134-141.

Mangus RS, Haag BW. Stented versus nonstented extravesical ureteroneocystostomy in renal transplantation: a meta-analysis. *Am J Transplant.* 2004; 4(11):1889.

Rouviere O, Berger P, Beziat C, *et al.* Acute thrombosis of renal transplant artery. *Transplantation.* 2002; 73(3):403-9.

Veale JL, Yew J, Gjertson DW, *et al.* Long-term comparative outcomes between 2 common ureteroneocystostomy techniques for renal transplantation. *J Urol.* 2007; 177(2):632-6.

D. Following Surgery

Abbud-Filho M, Adams PL, Alberu J, *et al.* A report of the Lisbon Conference on the Care of the Kidney Transplant Recipient. *Transplantation.* 2007; 83(8 Suppl):S1-22.

Chakkera HA, Knowler WC, Devarapalli Y, *et al.* Relationship between inpatient hyperglycemia and insulin treatment after kidney transplantation and future new onset diabetes mellitus. *Clin J Am Soc Nephrol.* 2010; 5(9):1669-75.

Chavalitdhamrong D, Danovitch GM, Bunnapradist, *et al.* Is there reversal of reverse epidemiology in renal transplant recipients? *Semin Dial.* 2007; 20(6):544-8 (lower risk of cardiovascular disease post-transplant).

Eckhard M, Schindler RA, Renner FC, *et al.* New-onset diabetes mellitus after renal transplantation. *Transplant Proc.* 2009; 41(6):2544-5.

Gordon EJ, Prohaska TR, Gallant MP, *et al.* Prevalence and determinants of physical activity and fluid intake in kidney transplant recipients. *Clin Transplant.* 2010;24(3):E69-81.

Gupta G, Unruh ML, Nolan TD, Hasley PM. Primary care of the renal transplant patient. *J Gen Intern Med.* 2010; 25(7):731-40.

Humar A, Matas AJ. Surgical complications after kidney transplantation. *Semin Dial.* 2005: 18(6):505-10.

Israni AK, Snyder JJ, Skeans MA, *et al.* Who is caring for kidney transplant patients?: Variation by region, transplant center, and patient characteristics. *Am J Nephrol.* 2009; 30(5):430-9.

Kasiske BL, Zeier MG, Chapman JR, *et al.* KDIQO Clinical Practice Guidelines for the care of kidney transplant recipients: a summary. *Kidney Int.* 2010; 77(4):299-311 (guidelines for care post-transplant).

Kurtkoti J, Sakhuja V, Sud K, *et al.* The utility of 1- and 3-month protocol biopsies on renal allograft function: a randomized controlled study. *Am J Transplant.* 2008; 8(2):317-23.

Montgomery R, Hardy M, Jordan S, *et al.* Consensus opinion from the antibody working group on the diagnosis, reporting, and risk assessment for antibody-mediated rejection and desensitization protocols. *Transplantation.* 2004; 78(2):181-5.

Mora PF. New-onset diabetes after renal transplantation. *J Investig Med.* 2010; 58(6):753-63 (tacrolimus use increases risk of new-onset diabetes after transplantation).

Moghani LM, Noorbala MH, Assari S. Causes of re-hospitalization in different post-kidney transplant periods. *Ann Transplant.* 2009; 14(4):14-9.

Naesens M, Kuypers D, Sarwal M. Calcineurin inhibitor nephrotoxicity. *Clin J Am Soc Nephrol.* 2009; 4(2):481-508.

Naesens M, Lerut E, Sarwal M, *et al.* Balancing efficacy and toxicity of kidney transplant immunosuppression. *Transplant Proc.* 2009; 41(8):3393-5.

Ozbay LA, Smidt K, Mortensen DM, *et al.* Cyclosporin and tacrolimus impair insulin secretion and transcriptional regulation in INS-1E beta cells. *Br J Pharmacol.* 2011; 162(1):136-46.

Randhawa P, Brennan DC. BK virus infection in transplant recipients: an overview and update. *Am J Transplant.* 2006; 6(9): 2000-5.

Roberts K. *The Complete Human Body,* DK Publishing, NY, NY, 2010; 366-369 (Ruth Tucker first kidney transplant 1957).

Schmid-Mohler G, Thut MP, Wüthrich RP, *et al.* Non-adherence to immunosuppressant medication in renal transplant recipients within the scope of the Integrative Model of Behavioral Prediction: a cross-sectional survey. *Clin Transplant.* 2010; 24(2):213-22 (intention to adhere to drug schedule is critical).

Srinivas TR, Schold JD, Guerra G, *et al.* Mycophenolate mofetil/sirolimus compared to other common immunosuppressive regimens in kidney transplantation. *Am J Transplant.* 2007; 7(3):586-74.

Starzl TE. Immunosuppressive therapy and tolerance of organ allografts. *N Engl J Med.* 2008; 358(4):407-11.

Trofe J, Hirsch HH, Ramos E. Polyomavirus-associated nephropathy: Update of clinical management in kidney transplant patients. *Transpl Infect Dis.* 2006; 8(2):76-85.

United States Renal Data System: USRDS 2010 Annual Data Report. *Atlas of Chronic Kidney Disease and End-Stage Renal Disease in the United States,* National Institutes of Health, National Institute of Diabetes and Digestive and Kidney Diseases, Bethesda, Md. 2010; Vol. II, Ch 7:311-324.

E. Long-Term Survival

Bataille S, Moal V, Gaudart J, *et al.* Cytomegalovirus risk factors in renal transplantation with modern immunosuppression. *Transpl Infect Dis.* 2010; 12(6):480-8.

Chabra D, Grafals M, Skaro A, *et al.* Impact of anemia on patient and graft survival and on rate of acute rejection. *Clin J Am Soc Nephrol.* 2008; 3(4):1168-74 (anemia post-transplant is associated with lower graft survival).

Djamali A, Samaniego M, Muth B, *et al.* Medical care of kidney transplant recipients after the first posttransplant year. *Clin J Am Soc Nephrol.* 2006; 1(4):623-40.

Fishman JA. Infection in organ transplantation: risk factors and evolving patterns of infection. *Infect Dis Clin North Am.* 2010; 24(2):273-83.

Fishman JA. Infections in organ-transplant recipients. *N Engl J Med.* 2007; 357(25):2601-14.

Gallagher MP, Kelly PJ, Jardine M, *et al.* Long-term cancer risk of immunosuppressive regimens after kidney transplant. *Am Soc Nephrol.* 2010; 21(5):852-8 (nearly 50% developed some form of cancer).

Ison MG, Hager J, Blumberg E, *et al.* Donor-derived disease transmission events in the United States: Data reviewed by the OPTN/UNOS Disease Transmission Advisory Committee. *Am J Transplant.* 2009; 9(8):1929-35 (diseases transmitted from donor to kidney recipient increasingly recognized as source of morbidity and mortality).

Mossad SB. Preventing CMV Viremia and disease 3-6 months after renal transplantation. *Am J Transplant.* 2010; PMID:20636458.

Rama I, Grinyo JM. Malignancy after renal transplantation: the role of immunosuppressants. *Nat Rev Nephrol.* 2010; 6(9):511-9.

Schena F, Pascoe M, Albaru J, *et al.* Conversion from calcineurin inhibitors to sirolimus maintenance therapy in renal allograft recipients: 24-month efficacy and safety results from the CONVERT trial. *Transplantation.* 2009; 87(2):233-42 (changing to sirolimus lowers cancer risk).

Shah T, Kasravi A, Huang E, *et al.* Risk factors for development of new-onset diabetes mellitus after kidney transplantation. *Transplantation.* 2006; 82(12):1673-6 (risk factors for developing diabetes post transplant are modifiable).

Solez K, Colvin RB, Racusen LC, *et al.* Banff of Classification of Renal Allograft Pathology: Updates and future direction. *Am J Transplant.* 2008; 8(4):753-60.

Strauss DC, Thomas JM. Transmission of donor melanoma by organ transplantation. *Lancet Oncol.* 2010; 11(8):790-6.

Tang IY, Meyer-Kriesche HU, Kaplan B. Immunosuppressive strategies to improve outcomes of kidney transplantation. *Semin Nephrol.* 2007; 27(4):377-92.

United States Renal Data System: USRDS 2010 Annual Data Report. *Atlas of Chronic Kidney Disease and End-Stage Renal Disease in the United States,* National Institutes of Health, National Institute of Diabetes and Digestive and Kidney Diseases, Bethesda, Md. 2010; Vol. II, Ch 7:311-324.

G. The Costs

United States Renal Data System: USRDS 2010 Annual Data Report. *Atlas of Chronic Kidney Disease and End-Stage Renal Disease in the United States,* National Institutes of Health, National Institute of Diabetes and Digestive and Kidney Diseases, Bethesda, Md. 2010; Vol. II, Intro: 213.

Chapter 14.   Taking Charge--The Obvious

A. Assume Responsibility for Your Own Care

Breidthardt T, Mebazea A, Mueller CE. Predicting progression in non-diabetic kidney disease: the importance of cardiorenal interactions. *Kidney Int.* 2009; 75(3):253-255.

Chodosh J, Morton SC, Mojica W, *et al.* Meta analysis: chronic disease self-management programs for older adults. *Ann Intern Med.* 2005; 143:427-38.

Fraenkel L, Peters E. Patient responsibility for medical decision-making and risky treatment options. *Arthritis Rheum.* 2009; 61(12):1674-6.

Harvey PW, Petkov JN, Misan G, *et al.* Self-management support and training for patients with chronic and complex conditions improves health-related behaviour and health outcomes. *Aust Health Rev.* 2008; 32(2):330-8 (self-management improves health).

King DE, Mainous AG, Carnemolia M, Everett CJ. Adherence to healthy lifestyle habits in U.S. adults, 1988-2006. *Am J Med.* 2009; 122(6). (self-management and lifestyle changes benefit health; 25% of adults smoke; only 8% of adults adhere to healthy lifestyle habits).

Lenz O, Nekala DP, Patel DV, *et al.* Barriers to successful care for chronic kidney disease. *BMC Nephrology.* 2005; 6:11.

Traynor K. Joint Commission updates National Patient Safety Goals for 2010. *Ann J Syst Pharm.* 2009; 66(23):2062-4 (Joint Commission's recommendations for improved health with patient involvement).

B. Partner with a Nephrologist

Consumer Reports National Research Center, www.consumerreports.org/health/conditions-and-treatment/type-2-diabetes/overview/index.htm (accessed September 2010).

Department of Health and Human Services, Centers for Disease Control and Prevention, Diabetes Data and Trends, http://apps.nccd.cdc.gov/DDTSTES/default.aspx (accessed September 2010) (diabetes sixth leading cause of death; number of Americans with pre-diabetes and diabetes).

DiNapoli A, Valle S, d'Adamo G, *et al.* Survey of determinants and effects of timing of referral to a nephrologist: the patient's point of view. *J Nephrol.* 2010; 23(5):603-13.

Israni RK, Shea JA, Joffe MM, Feldman HI. Physician characteristics and knowledge of CKD management. *Am J Kidney Dis.* 2009; 54(2):238-47 (need to improve CKD knowledge in primary care physicians).

Lenz O, Nekala DP, Patel DV, *et al.* Barriers to successful care for chronic kidney disease. *BMC Nephrology.* 2005; 6:11.

McClellan WM, Wasse H, McClellan AC, *et al.* Treatment center and geographic variability in pre-ESRD care associated with increased mortality. *J Am Soc Nephrol.* 2009; 20:1078-85.

National Kidney Foundation, K/DOQI Clinical Practice Guidelines for Chronic Kidney Disease Evaluation, Classification, and Stratification, www.kidney.org/professionals/kdoqi/ckd/pi_exec.htm (accessed September, 2010) (CKD is under diagnosed and undertreated).

Shin SJ, Kim HW, Chung S, *et al.* Late referral to a nephrologist increases the risk of uremia-related cardiac hypertrophy in patients on hemodialysis. *Nephron Clin Pract.* 2007; 107(4):c139-46.

United States Renal Data System: USRDS 2009 Annual Data Report. Atlas of Chronic Kidney Disease and End-Stage Renal Disease in the United States, National Institutes of Health, National Institute of Diabetes and Digestive and Kidney Diseases, Bethesda, Md. 2009.

C. Diabetes--the Key is Control

American Diabetes Association. *Diabetes Care.* 2003; 26:S5-S20 (risks for type 2 diabetes).

American Diabetes Association. *Diabetes Care.* 2003; 26:S106-S108.

American Diabetes Association. *Diabetes Care.* 2004; 27:1798-1811 (red flags for type 2 diabetes).

American Diabetes Association, Diagnosis and Classification of Diabetes Mellitus, *Diabetics Care.* 2006; 29:S43-S48 (fasting glucose levels).

Diabetes Prevention Program Research Group, Knowle WC, Fowler SE, *et al.* 10-year follow-up of diabetes incidence and weight loss in the Diabetes Prevention Program Outcomes Study. *Lancet.* 2009; 374(9702):1677-86.

Geiss LS, James C, Gregg EW, *et al.* Diabetes risk reduction behaviors among U.S. adults with prediabetes. *Am J Prev Med.* 2010; 38(4):403-9 (lack of awareness of prediabetes condition).

Hodson L, Hamden KE, Roberts R, *et al.* Does the DASH diet lower blood pressure by altering peripheral vascular function? *J Hum Hypertens.* 2010; 24(5):312-9 (DASH diet lowers blood pressure).

Kirby T. Screening for chronic kidney disease shows promise. *Lancet.* 2010; 375(R722):1240-1241.

Knowle WC, Burett-Connor E, Fowler SE, *et al.* Reduction in the incidence of type 2 diabetes with lifestyle intervention or metformin. *N Engl J Med* 2002; 346(6): 393-403 (Diabetes Prevention Program).

Lewis EJ, Hunsicker LG, Bain RP, *et al.* The effects of angiotensin-converting-enzyme inhibition on diabetic nephropathy. The Collaborative Study. *N Engl J Med.* 1993; 329(20):1456-62.

Misra A. Prevention of type 2 diabetes: the long and winding road. *Lancet.* 2009; 374(9702):1655-6.

Mozaffarian D, Kamineni A, Camethon M, *et al.* Lifestyle risk factors and new-onset diabetes mellitus in older adults: the cardiovascular health study. *Arch Intern Med* 2009; 169(8):798-807 (healthy habits cut diabetes risk 80%).

National Kidney Foundation K/DOQI Clinical Practice Guidelines and Clinical Practice Recommendations for Diabetes and Chronic Kidney Disease. www.kidney.org/professionals/ KDOQI/guideline_diabetes/cpr4.htm (accessed October 2010)(background, Clinical Practices Recommendation 4: behavioral self management in diabetes and CKD).

Ninomiya T, Perkovic V, deGolan BE, *et al.* Albuminuria and kidney function independently predict cardiovascular and renal outcomes in diabetes. *Am Soc Nephrol.* 2009; 20(8):1813-21.

Porterfield DS, Hinnant L, Stevens DM, *et al.* The diabetes primary prevention initiative interven-tions focus area: a case study and recommendations. *Am J Prev Med.* 2010; 39(3):235-42.

Thoenes M, Reil JC, Khan BV, *et al.* Abdominal obesity is associated with microalbuminuria and an elevated cardiovascular risk profile in patients with hypertension. *Vasc Health Risk Manag.* 2009; 5(4):577-85 (large waist doubles risk).

Walker DZ, O'Dea K, Gomez M, *et al.* Diet and exercise in prevention of diabetes. *J Hum Nutr Diet.* 2010;23(4):344-52.

United States Renal Data System: USRDS 2010 Annual Data Report. Atlas of Chronic Kidney Disease and End-Stage Renal Disease in the United States, National Institutes of Health, National Institute of Diabetes and Digestive and Kidney Diseases, Bethesda, Md. 2010.

D. Monitor and Control Blood Pressure

Chobanian AV, Bakris BJ, Black HR, *et al,* and the National High Blood Pressure Education Program Coordinating Committee. The Seventh Report of the Joint National Committee on Prevention, Detection, Evaluation, and Treatment of High Blood Pressure, *JAMA* 2003; 289(19):2560-72.

deGalan BE, Perkovic V, Ninomiya T, *et al.* Lowering blood pressure reduces renal events in type 2 diabetes. *J Am Soc Nephrol.* 2009; 20(4):883-92.

Hodson L, Hamden KE, Roberts R, *et al.* Does the DASH diet lower blood pressure by altering peripheral vascular function? *J Hum Hyperten.* 2010; 24(5):312-9 (DASH diet lowers blood pressure).

JNC 7 Express. The Seventh Report of the Joint National Committee on Prevention, Detection, Evaluation and Treatment of High Blood Pressure. *NIH Publication No. 03-5233.* December 2003.

Kalsitzidis RG, Bakris GL. Prehypertension: Is it relevant for nephrologists? *Kidney Int.* 2010; 77(3):194-200.

Paige J, Carson H. Examining the link between blood pressure and lifestyle. *U.S. Pharmacist.* 2010; 335(2):1-4 (1/3 U.S. adults have hypertension; lifestyle risk factors).

Pickering TG, Hall SE, Appel LS, *et al.* Recommendations for blood pressure measurements in humans: an AHA scientific statement from the council on high blood pressure research, professional and public education subcommittee. *Circulation.* 2005; 111(5):697-716.

Reboldi G, Gentile G, Angeli F, Verdecchia P. Choice of ACE inhibitor combinations in hypertensive patients with type 2 diabetes: update after recent clinical trials. *Vas Health Ris Manag.* 2009; 5(1):411-27.

Sanoski CA. Aliskiren: an oral direct rennin inhibitor for the treatment of hypertension. *Pharmacotherapy.* 2009; 29(2):193-212.

The Seventh Report of the Joint National Committee on Prevention, Detection, Evaluation and Treatment of High Blood Pressure. National High Blood Pressure Education Program. Bethesda, MD: National Heart, Lung, and Blood Institute (US); 2004 Aug.

United States Renal Data System: USRDS 2010 Annual Data Report. Atlas of Chronic Kidney Disease and End-Stage Renal Disease in the United States, National Institutes of Health, National Institute of Diabetes and Digestive and Kidney Diseases, Bethesda, Md. 2010.

E. Lose the Fat--It's Dangerous

Afshinnia F, Wilt TJ, Duval S, *et al.* Weight loss and proteinuria: systematic review of clinical trials and comparative cohorts. *Nephrol Dial Transplant.* 2010; 25(4):1173-1183 (weight loss reduces proteinuria).

Flegal KM, Carroll MD, Ogden CL, Curtis LR. Prevalence and trends in obesity among U.S. adults, 1999-2008. *JAMA.* 2010; 303(3):235-241.

Ford ES, Li C, Zhao G, Tsai J. Trends in obesity and abdominal obesity among adults in United States from 1999-2008. *Int J Obes.* 2010; Sept 7: PMID: 20820173.

Kramer H, Tuttle KR, Leehey DL, *et al.* Obesity management in adults with CKD. *Am J Kidney Dis.* 2009; 53(1):151-65.

Navaneethan S, Yehnert H, Moustarah, F, *et al.* Weight loss interventions in chronic kidney disease: a systematic review and meta-analysis. *Clin J Am Soc Nephrol.* 2009; 4(10):1565-74.

Pischon I, Boeing H, Hoffman K, *et al.* General and abdominal adiposity and risk of death in Europe. *N Engl J Med.* 2008; 359(20):2015-20 (large waist doubles risk of death).

F. Reduce your Cardiovascular Disease Risk to Increase Kidney Health

American Heart Association Heart Health Risk Assessment, Life's Simple 7. www.newsroom.heart.org/ index.php7S=43&item=931 (accessed September 2010).

James MT, Hemmelgarn BR, Tonelli M. Early recognition and prevention of chronic kidney disease. *Lancet.* 2010; 375(9722):1296-1309.

G. Lifestyle Changes

American Heart Association. Heart Disease and Stroke Statistics--2010 update at www.american heart.org/presenter.jhtm/?/identifier=3000090 (accessed September 5, 2010).

Beddhu S, Baird BC, Zitterkoph J, *et al.* Physical activity and mortality in chronic kidney disease (NHANES III). *Clin J Am Soc Nephrol.* 2009 Dec; 4(12):1901-6 (exercise gives survival benefit to CKD patients).

Buxton OM, Marcelli E. Short and long sleep are positively associated with obesity, diabetes, hypertension, and cardiovascular disease among adults in United States. *Soc Sci Med.* 2010; 71(5):1027-36.

Cianciaruso B, Pota A, Belizzi V, *et al.* Effect of a low-versus moderate-protein diet on progression of CKD: follow-up of a randomized controlled trial. *Am J Kidney Dis.* 2009; 54:1052-1061.

Knutson KL, VanCauter E, Rathouz PJ *et al.* Association between sleep and blood pressure in midlife: the CARDIA sleep study. *Arch Intern Med.* 2009; 169(11):1055-1061 (box info on sleeping less than 5 hours and increased blood pressure).

Pechter U, Otis M, Mesikepp S, *et al.* Beneficial effects of water-based exercise in patients with chronic kidney disease. *Int J Rehabil Res.* 2003; 26(2):153-6 (aquatic exercise resulted in 50% decrease in proteinuria).

Robinson ES, Fisher MD, Forman JP, Curhan GC. Physical activity and albuminuria. *Am J Epidemiol.* 2010; 171(5):515-521 (nurses health study; greater physical activity associated with lower albuminuria).

Sabonayagam C, Shankar A. Sleep duration and cardiovascular disease: results from the National Health Interview Survey. *Sleep.* 2010; 33(8):1037-42.

Chapter 15.   Control Internal Culprits
A. Monitor and Control Imbalances

American Heart Association. 2010. Daily Salt intake? www.americanheart.org (accessed September 2010) (1500 mg. recommendation).

American Heart Association. 2010. What is high blood pressure? www.americanheart.org (accessed August 2010).

Bhan I, Hewison M, Thadhani R. Dietary vitamin D intake in advanced CKD/ESRD. *Semin Dial.* 2010; 23(4):407-10.

Craig WJ, Mangels AR. American Dietetic Association, Position of the American Dietetic Association: vegetarian diets. *J Am Diet Assoc.* 2009; 109(7):1266-82.

deBristo-Ashurst I, Varagunam M, Raftery MJ, Yaqoob MM. Bicarbonate supplementation slows progression of CKD and improves nutritional status. *J Am Soc Nephrol.* 2009; 20(9):2075.84.

Dietary Guidelines for Americans. Overview and daily requirements for sodium, potassium, calcium, phosphorus. 2010. Available at www.health.gov/dietaryguidelines (accessed September 2010).

Guyton AC, Hall JE. Unit V: The body fluids and kidney. In Guyton AC, Hall JE: *Textbook of Medical Physiology*, 11ᵗʰ ed. Philadelphia, Elsevier, 2006.

He FJ, Marciniak M, Visagie E, *et al*. Effect of modest salt reduction on blood pressure, urinary albumin, and pulse wave velocity in white, black, and Asian mild hypertensives. *Hypertension*. 2009; 54(3):482-8.

Intermountain Medical Center. Inadequate levels of vitamin D may significantly increase risk of stroke, heart disease and death. 2009. http://www.sciencedaily.com/releases/2009/11/09111 6085038. htm (accessed August 2010).

Murphee DD, Thelen SM. Chronic kidney disease in primary care. *J Am Board Fam Med*. 2010; 23(4):542-50 (anemia, PTH, vitamin D, acidosis).

National Kidney Foundation K/DOQI Clinical Practice Guidelines for Bone Metabolism and Disease in Chronic Kidney Disease. www.kidney.org/professionals/KDOQI/guidelines_bone/index.htm (accessed October 2010) (guidelines regarding calcium, phosphorus, PTH).

Office of Dietary Supplements, DkI Dietary Reference, 2010. Intake: Calcium, Phosphorus, Magnesium, Vitamin D. Available at http://www.nap.edu/catalog.php?record_id=5776 (accessed September 2010). U.S. Department of Health and Human Services.

Pimenta E, Gaddam KK, Oparil S, *et al*. Effects of dietary sodium reduction on blood pressure in subjects with resistant hypertension: result from a randomized trial. *Hypertension*. 2009; 54(3):475-81 (salt restriction improved hypertension).

Quazi RA, Martin KJ. Vitamin D in kidney disease: pathophysiology and the utility of treatment. *Endocrinol Metab Clin North Am*. 2010; 39(2):355-63.

Ruggenenti P, Remuzzi C. Proteinuria: Is the ONTARGET renal subsidy actually off-target? *Nat Rev Nephrol*. 2009; 5:436-437 (use of ACE inhibitors and ARBs together increased risk in dialysis).

Smith-Spangler CM, Juusola JL, Enns EA, *et al*. Population strategies to decrease sodium intake and the burden of cardiovascular disease: a cost-effective analysis. *Ann Intern Med*. 2010; 152:481-7, W170-3 (sodium consumption increased blood pressure, increasing risk of heart attack, stroke, and CKD).

Stanton BA, Koeppen BM: The kidney. In Berne RM, Levy MN, Koeppen BM, Stanton BA (eds): *Physiology*, 5ᵗʰ ed. Section VII. St. Louis, CV Mosby, 2004, pp 621-716.

United States Renal Data System: USRDS 2010 Annual Data Report: Atlas of Chronic Kidney Disease and End-Stage Renal Disease in the United States, National Institutes of Health, National Institute of Diabetes and Digestive and Kidney Diseases, Bethesda, Md. 2010; Vol I, Ch. 1 & 4; Vol. II, Ch. 3 & 5).

U.S. Department of Health and Human Services, National Institutes of Health, National Institute of Diabetes and Digestive and Kidney Diseases. Anemia in Kidney Disease and Dialysis (anemia begins when person still has 20-50% kidney function; TSAT, EPO).

B. Keep Cholesterol in Check

American Heart Association. 2010. Cholesterol. www.heart.org/HEARTORG/conditions/cholesterol (accessed September 2010) (cholesterol levels and categories).

Bowden RG, JItomir J, Wilson RL, Gentile M. Effects of omega-e-fatty acids supplementation on lipid levels in end-state renal disease patients. *J Ren Nutr*. 2009; 19(4):259-66 (omega-3 supplementation increased HDLs in dialysis patients).

Fletcher B, Baira K, Ades P, *et al*. Managing abnormal blood lipids. *Circulation*. 2005; 112:3184-209 (AHA scientific statement--recommendations on treating abnormal blood lipids).

C. Revisiting Diabetes

American Diabetes Association. Diagnosis and Classification of Diabetes Mellitus. *Diabetes Care*. 2010; 33:S62-S69 (resulting health effects and testing).

American Diabetes Association. Standards of Medical Care in Diabetes--2010. *Diabetes Care*. 2010; 33:S11-S61.

Funnell MM, Brown TL, Childs BP, *et al*. National Standards for diabetes self-management education. *Diabetes Care*. 2010;33:S89-S96 (self-care important in diabetes).

Lorenzo C, Wagenknecht LE, Hanley A, *et al*. A1c between 5.7 and 6.4% as a marker for identifying diabetes, insulin sensitivity and secretion, and cardiovascular risk factors: the insulin resistance atherosclerosis study (IRAS). *Diabetes Care*. 2010; 33:2104-9.

Takahasi O, Farmer AJ, Shimbo T, *et al*. A1c to detect diabetes in healthy adults: when should we recheck? *Diabetes Care*. 2010; 33:2016-7 (in people with A1c less than 6%, rescreening 3 years later is appropriate).

Centers for Disease Control and Prevention. National Diabetes fact sheet: estimates of diabetes in the United States, 2007. Atlanta, GA: U.S. Department of Health and Human Services, Centers for Disease Control and Prevention, 2008 (estimates for impaired glucose levels).

Olsen DE, Rhee MK, Herrick K, *et al*. Screening for diabetes and prediabetes with proposed A1c-based diagnostic criteria. *Diabetes Care*. 2010, doi: 10. 2337/dc10-0433 (A1c test will not diagnose all with diabetes).

D. Anemia is a Common Problem

Centers for Disease Control and Prevention, MMWR. Recommendations to Prevent and Control Iron Deficiency in the United States, April 1998/47(RR-3);1-36 (iron deficiency most common in world).

Cusick SE, Mei Z, Freed DS, *et al*. Unexplained decline in the prevalence of anemia among U.S. children and women between 1988-1994 and 1999-2002. *Am J Clin Nutr*. 2008; 88(6):1611-7 (anemia rates declined but unrelated to iron or folate deficiency).

Lorber D, Reddan D. Clinical characteristics of chronic kidney disease patients with and without diabetes: a subanalysis of the PAER1 Study. *Clin Nephrol*. 2006; 66(1):11-6.

McClellan W, Aronoff SL, Bolton WK, *et al.* The prevalence of anemia in patients with chronic kidney disease. *Curr Med Res Opin.* 2004; 20(9):1501-10.

National Kidney Foundation. K/DOQI Clinical Practice Guidelines and Clinical Practice Recommendations for Anemia in Chronic Kidney Disease in Adults. www.kidney.org/professionals/kdoqi/guidelines_anemia 2006 Guidelines and 2007 update for testing and diagnosing anemia (accessed September 2010).

Patel AV, Singh AK. Anemia in chronic kidney disease: new advances. *Heart Fail Clin.* 2010; 6(3):347-57.

Singh AK. What is causing the mortality in treating the anemia of chronic kidney disease: erythropoetin dose or hemoglobin level? *Curr Opin Nephrol Hyperten.* 2010; 19(5):420-4 (correction of anemia levels should not be above normal).

United States Renal Data System: USRDS 2010 Annual Data Report: Atlas of Chronic Kidney Disease and End-Stage Renal Disease in the United States, National Institutes of Health, National Institute of Diabetes and Digestive and Kidney Diseases, Bethesda, Md. 2010; Vol. II, Ch. 3, 5, and 6 (prevalence of LVH).

World Health Organization, Worldwide Prevalence of Anaemia, 993-2005: WHO Global Database of Anaemia. Edited by deGenoist B, McLean E, Cogswell M.

E. Obtain Lab Results

Casalino LP, Dunham D, Chin MH, *et al.* Frequency of failure to inform patients of clinically significant outpatient test results. *Arch Intern Med.* 2009; 169(12):1123-9.

Chapter 16. Coping, Depression, Death

A. Coping with Chronic Disease

Cukor D, Rosenthal DS, Jindal RM, *et al.* Depression is an important contributor to low medication adherence in hemodialyzed patients and transplant recipients. *Kidney Int.* 2009; 75(11):1223-9.

Egnew TR. The meaning of healing: transcending suffering. *Ann Fam Med.* 2005; 3(3):255-62 (healing mechanisms personal, subjective).

Groves M, Muskin PR. Psychological responses to illness. In Levenson JL, ed. *The American Psychiatric Publishing Textbook of Psychosomatic Medicine.* Arlington, VA: American Psychiatric Publishing, 2005.

Herring MP, O'Connor PJ, Dishman RK. The effect of exercise training on anxiety symptoms among patients: a systematic review. *Arch Int Med.* 2010; 170(4):321-31.

National Council on Aging, NCOA Chronic Condition Survey. Available at www.ncoa.org/news-ncoa/news/ncoa-chronic-condition-survey.htm (accessed September 2010)(chronic disease accounts for 75% of nation's 2 trillion health care costs; 50% of people with a chronic disease are depressed).

Partnership for Solutions: Better Lives for People with Chronic Conditions, Robert Wood Johnson Foundation. www.rwjf.org/reports/nreports/betterlives.htm (accessed September 2010) (people with chronic conditions see numerous physicians and fill numerous prescriptions annually).

United States Renal Data System: USRDS 2010 Annual Data Report. *Atlas of Chronic Kidney Disease and End-Stage Renal Disease in the United States,* National Institutes of Health, National Institute of Diabetes and Digestive and Kidney Diseases, Bethesda, Md. 2010; Vol. I, Ch.2:52-64 (introduction boxes).

VanDijk S, *et al.* Patients' representations of their ESRD: relation with mortality. *Nephrol Dial Transplant.* 2009; 24(10):3183-5 (perceptions related to mortality rates).

Veale BM. Meeting the challenge of chronic illness in general practice. *Med J Aust.* 2003; 179(5):247-9 (depression, diabetes, and asthma are the 3 most common chronic conditions managed by general practitioners).

B. Depression in CKD

American Association of Kidney Patients, *Understanding Depression in Kidney Patients.* www.aakp.org/brochure/understanding-depression/index.cfm (accessed September 2010) (depression impacts 30 million).

Anderson RJ, Freedland KE, Clouse RE, Lustman PJ. The prevalence of comorbid depression in adults with diabetes: a meta-analysis. *Diabetes Care.* 2001; 24(6):1069-78.

Brown AD, Barton DA, Lambert GW. Cardiovascular abnormalities in patients with major depressive disorder: autonomic mechanisms and implications for treatment. *CNS Drugs.* 2009; 23(7):583-602 (link of depression to cardiovascular disease).

Centers for Medicare & Medicaid Services. www.cms.gov/center/CSRD.asp (accessed September 2010) (depression in CKD).

Chiu YW, Teitelbaum I, Misram, *et al.* Pill burden, adherence, hyperphosphotemia, and quality of life in maintenance dialysis patients. *Clin J Am Soc Nephrol.* 2009; 4(6)1089-96 (more pills, less quality of life for kidney patients).

deGroot M, Anderson R, Freedland KE, Clouse RE, Lustman PJ. Association of depression and diabetes complications: a meta-analysis. *Psychosom Med.* 2001; 63(4):619-30.

Depression Guideline Panel. Clinical Practice Guidelines No. 5: Depression in Primary Care, 1: Detection and diagnosis. Rockville, MD; U.S. Dept. of Health and Human Services, Agency for Healthcare Policy and Research; 1993. AHCPR Publication 93-1550 (physicians fail to address depression).

Dobbels F, Skeans MA, Snyder JJ, *et al.* Depressive disorder in renal transplantation: an analysis of Medicare claims. *Am J Kidney Dis.* 2008; 51(5):819-828 (depression associated with 2-fold greater risk of graft failure).

Goldberg D. The detection and treatment of depression in the physically ill. *World Psychiatry.* 2010; 9:16-20.

Hedayati SS, Bosworth HB, Briley LF, *et al.* Death or hospitalization of patients on chronic dialysis is associated with a physician-based diagnosis of depression. *Kidney Int.* 2008; 74:930-6 (80% of depressed dialysis patients died or were hospitalized).

Hedayati SS, Minhajuddin AT, Afshar M, *et al.* Association between major depressive episodes in patients with chronic kidney disease and initiation of dialysis, hospitalization, or death. *JAMA.* 2010; 303(19):1946-1953 (presence of depression increases poor outcome).

Hedayati SS, Minhajuddin AT, Toto RD, *et al.* Prevalence of major depressive episode in CKD. *Am J Kidney Dis.* 2009; 54(3):424-32 (depression in early CKD prevalent).

House A, Knapp P, Bamford J, Vail A. Mortality at 12 and 24 months after stroke may be associated with depressive symptoms at 1 month. *Stroke.* 2001; 32(3):696-701.

Luppino FS, deWit LM, Boury PF, *et al.* Overweight, obesity, and depression: a systematic review and meta-analysis of longitudinal studies. *Arch Gen Psychiatry.* 2010; 67(3):220-229 (depression and obesity linked).

Mykletun A, Bjerkeset O, Overland S, *et al.* Levels of anxiety and depression as predictions of mortality: the HUNT Study. *The Brit J of Psychiatry* 2009; 195(2):118-25 (depression risk factor for mortality).

National Kidney Foundation. *Understanding Depression,* www.kidney.org/kidneydisease/CKD/coping.cfm (accessed September 2010).

Nedayati SS, Minhajuddin AT, Toto RD. Prevalence of major depressive episodes in CKD. *Am J Kidney Dis.* 2009; 54(3):424-32 (depression impacts CKD; quality of life issues overlooked).

Ströhle A. Physical activity, exercise, depression and anxiety disorders. *J Neurol Transm.* 2009; 116(6):777-84.

United States Renal Data System: USRDS 2010 Annual Data Report. *Atlas of Chronic Kidney Disease and End-Stage Renal Disease in the United States,* National Institutes of Health, National Institute of Diabetes and Digestive and Kidney Diseases, Bethesda, Md. 2010; Vol. I, Ch 2:52-64 (comorbidities in CKD); Vol. II, Ref. Table C2:421 (patients working).

C. Death, A Choice

Bostwick JM, Cohen LM. Differentiating suicide from life-ending acts and end-of-life decisions: a model based on chronic kidney disease and dialysis. *Psychosom.* 2009; 50:1-7.

Cruz DN, Ricci Z, Bagshaw SM, *et al.* Renal replacement therapy in adult critically ill patients: when to begin and when to stop. *Contrib Nephrol.* 2010; 165:263-73.

Cukor D, Cohen SD, Peterson RA, Kimmel PL. Psychosocial aspects of chronic disease ESRD as a paradigmatic illness. *J Am Soc Nephrol.* 2007; 18(12):3042-55 (social interaction may reduce mortality).

Davison SN. End of life care preferences and needs: perceptions of patients with chronic kidney disease. *Clin J Am Soc Nephrol.* 2010; 5(2):195-204(61% of patients regret starting dialysis).

DelVecchio L, Locatelli F. Ethical issues in the elderly with renal disease. *Clin Geriatr Med.* 2009; 25(3):543-53.

Dobbels F, Skeans M, Snyder JJ, *et al.* Depressive disorder in renal transplantation: an analysis of Medicare claims. *Am J Kidney Dis.* 2008; 51(5):819-28 (depression is associated with a 2-fold greater risk of graft failure).

Germain MJ, Cohen LM, Davison SN. Withholding and withdrawing from dialysis: what we know about how our patients die. *Seminar in Dialysis* 2007; 20(3):195-9 (process of withdrawal from dialysis).

Griva K, Davenport A, Harrison M, Newman S. An evaluation of illness, treatment perceptions, and depression in hospital-U.S. home-based dialysis modalities. *J Psychosom Res.* 2010; 69(4):363-70.

Kurella TM, Corvinsky KE, Chertow GM, *et al.* Functional status of elderly adults before and after initiation of dialysis. *N Eng J Med.* 2009; 361(16):1539-47 (suffering caused by dialysis for nursing home seniors may outweigh its benefits).

Kurella TM, Kimmel PL, Young BS, *et al.* Suicide in the United States end-stage renal disease program. *J Am Soc Nephrol.* 2005; 16(3):774-81 (persons with ESRD more likely to commit suicide than general population).

Mailloux LU, Bellucci AG, Napolitano B, *et al.* Death by withdrawal from dialysis: a 20-year clinical experience. *J Am Soc Nephrol.* 1993; 3(9):1631-7.

National Kidney Foundation K/DOQI Guidelines, Withdrawal of Dialysis. www.kidney.org/professionals/kdoqi/guidelines_updates (accessed September 2010).

Noble H, Meyer J, Bridges J, *et al.* Patient experience of dialysis referral or withdrawal--a review of the literature. *J Ren Care.* 2008; 38(2):94-100.

Son YJ, Choi KS, Park YL, *et al.* Depression symptoms and quality of life in patients on hemodialysis for end-stage renal disease. *Am J Nephrol.* 2009; 29(1):36-42 (over 25% of dialysis patients depressed).

White AM, Philogene GS, Fine L, Sinha S. Social support and self-reported health status of older adults in the United States. *Am J Pub Health.* 2009; 99(10):1872-8 (social support associated with better self-reported health status).

Chapter 17.   Poor Nutrition Leads to Poor Health

America's Eating Habits: changes and consequences. Agriculture Information Bulletin No. (A1B750) May 1999 (changes in eating habits of U.S.).

American Diabetes Association. Standards of Medical Care in Diabetes--2010. *Diabetes Care.* 2010; 33(1):S11-S61.

American Heart Association, 2010. What is daily salt intake? Available at www.americanheart.org (accessed September 2010)(daily salt limit 1500 mg; sodium product labeling).

American Heart Association, High Blood Pressure Research Conference 2009, www.americanheart.org/presenter.jhtml?identifier=3062454 (accessed September 2010).

American Heart Association, www.heart.org/HEARTORG (accessed September 2010) (link to DASH diet; recommended sugar consumption, cutting sugar).

Appel LJ; American Society of Hypertension Writing Group. ASH position paper: dietary approaches to lower blood pressure. *J Clin Hyperten.* 2009;11(7): 358-68 (salt and hypertension; 1500 mg/daily; racial disparity).

Appel LJ; American Society of Hypertension Writing Group. ASH position paper: dietary approaches to lower blood pressure. *J Clin Hyperten.* 2009;11(7): 358-68 (salt and hypertension; 1500 mg/daily; racial disparity).

Azadbakht L, Ford NR, Karimi M, *et al.* Effects of dietary approaches to stop hypertension (DASH) eating plan and cardiovascular risks among type 2 diabetic patients: a randomized cross-over clinical trial. *Diabetes Care.* 2010; PMID:20843978.

Bernstein AM, Sun Q, Hu FB, *et al.* Major dietary protein sources and risk of coronary heart disease in women. *Circulation.* 2010; 122(9):876-83 (red meat intake increases risk of coronary heart disease).

Bibbins-Domingo K, Chertou GM, Coxson PG, *et al.* Projected effect of dietary salt reductions on future cardiovascular disease. *N Engl J Med.* 2010; 55(5):1102-9 (reducing salt to 1200 mg/day could reduce heart disease, heart attacks, stroke, deaths; AHA report in box).

Bleich SN, Wang YC, Wang Y, Gortmaker SL. Increasing consumption of sugar-sweetened beverages among U.S. adults: 1988-1994 to 1999-2004. *Am J Clin Nutr.* 2009; 89:372-381 (sugared drink consumption highest among people at greatest risk of obesity and diabetes).

Bodor JN, Rice JG, Farley TA, *et al.* The association between obesity and urban food environments. *J Urban Health.* 2010; 87(5):771-81.

Bomback AS, Derebail VK, Shoham DA, et al. Sugar-sweetened soda consumption, hyperuricemia, and kidney disease. *Kidney Int.* 2010; 77(7):609-16.

Centers for Disease Control and Prevention. www.cdc.gov/nchs/fastats/overwt.htm (accessed September 2010) (percent obese adults).

Chen L, Caballero B, Mitchell DC, *et al.* Reducing consumption of sugar-sweetened beverages is associated with reduced blood pressure: a prospective study among United States adults. *Circulation.* 2010; 121(22):2398-406 (sugared drinks raise blood pressure).

Chen ST, Maruthur NM, Appel LJ. The effect of dietary patterns on estimated coronary heart disease risk: results from the Dietary Approaches to Stop Hypertension (DASH) trial. *Circ Cardiovasc Qual Outcomes.* 2010; 3(5):484-9 (DASH lowered 10-year risk of heart attack, LDLs, and blood pressure).

deBrito-Ashurat I, Varagunam M, Raftery MJ, Yaqoob MM. Bicarbonate supplementation slows progression of CKD and improves nutritional status. *J Am Soc Nephrol.* 2009; 20(9):2075-84.

DeKoning L, Fung TT, Chiuve S, *et al.* Prudent diet scores and incident type 2 diabetes among men. 70th Scientific Sessions (2010); abstract number 48-LB (DASH beneficial in diabetics).

Fulgoni VL. Current protein intake in America: analysis of the National Health and Nutrition Examination Survey, 2003-2004. *Am J Clin Nut.* 2008; 87(5):1554S-1557S.

Garneata L, Mircescu G. Nutritional intervention in uremia—myth or reality? *J Ren Nutr.* 2010; 20(5 Suppl):S31-4.

Guarnieri G, Zanetti M, Vinci P, *et al.* Metabolic syndrome and chronic kidney disease. *J Renal Nutr.* 2010; 20(5 Suppl):S19-23 (metabolic syndrome increases risk of CKD).

Harsha DW, Lin P, Obarzanek E, *et al.* Dietary Approaches to Stop Hypertension: A Summary of Study Results. *J Am Diet Assoc.* 99(8 Suppl): S35-S39.

Ibrahim HN, Weber ML. Weight loss: a neglected intervention in the management of chronic kidney disease. *Curr Opin Nephrol Hypertens.* 2010; 19(6):534-8 (urinary protein excretion, blood pressure, and GFR improve with weight loss).

J Paige High Carson. Exploring the link between blood pressure and lifestyle. *U.S. Pharmacist.* 2010; 35(2):1-4 (1 out of 3 adults has hypertension; lifestyle factors causing hypertension; 10% U.S. children overweight; 2/3 high blood pressure attributed to obesity; effects of alcohol on blood pressure).

Jia Y, Hwang SY, House JD, *et al.* Long-term high intake of whole proteins results in renal damage in pigs. *J Nutr.* 2010; 140(9):1646-52 (high protein diet damages kidneys).

JNC 7 Express. The Seventh Report of the Joint National Committee on Prevention, Detection, Evaluation, and Treatment of High Blood Pressure. NIH Publication No. 03-5233. December 2003; Your Guide to Lowering your Blood Pressure with DASH. U.S. Department of Health and Human Services. NIH Publications No. 06-4082. Revised April 2006. www.nhlbi.nih.gov/health/public/heart/hbp/dash/new_dash.pdf (accessed August, 2010).

Johnson CM, Angell SY, Lederer A, *et al.* Sodium content of lunchtime fast food purchases at major U.S. chains. *Arch Intern Med.* 2010; 170(8):732-4.

Kopple JD. Obesity and chronic kidney disease. *J Ren Nutr.* 2010; 20(5 Suppl):S29-30.

Li F, Harmer P, Cardinal BJ, *et al.* Obesity and the built environment: does the density of neighborhood fast-food outlets matter? *Am J Health Promot.* 2009; 23(3):203-9.

Lin J, Fung TT, Hu FB, Curhan GC. Association of Dietary Patterns with Albuminuria and Kidney Function Decline in Older White Women: A subgroup analysis from the Nurses' Health Study. *Am J Kidney Dis.* 2011; 57:245-254.

Lin J, Hu FB, Curhan GC. Associations of diet with albuminuria and kidney function decline. *Clin J Am Soc Nephrol.* 2010; 5(5):836-43 (intake of red meat, animal protein, and animal fat increases proteinuria; high sodium intake leads to progression of CKD).

Lin J, Judd S, Lee A, *et al.* Association of dietary fat with albuminuria and kidney dysfunction. *Am J Clin Nutr.* 2010; 92(4):897-904 (saturated fat significantly associated with high albuminuria).

Lippi G, Franchini M, Favaloro EJ, Targher G. Moderate red wine consumption and cardiovascular risk: beyond the "French paradox". *Semin Thromb Hemost.* 2010; 36(1):59-70 (moderate red wine consumption benefits cardiovascular function).

378

Micha R, Wallace SK, Mozaffarian D. Red and processed meat consumption and risk of coronary heart disease, stroke, and diabetes mellitus: a systematic review and meta-analysis. *Circulation.* 2010; 121(21):2271-83 (sodium and processed meats).

Nakamura T, Fujiwara N, Sugaya T, *et al.* Effect of red wine on urinary protein, 8-hydroxydeoxy-guanosine, and liver-type fatty acid-binding protein excretion in patients with diabetic nephropathy. *Metabolism.* 2009; 58(8):1185-90.

National Institutes of Health, National Heart, Lung, and Blood Institute. Primary Prevention of Hypertension: Clinical and Public Health Advisory from the National Blood Pressure Education Program. Available at www.nhlbi.nih.gov/health/prof/heart/hbp/pphbp.pdf. (accessed September, 2010).

National Institutes of Health, National Heart, Lung, and Blood Institute. The DASH Eating Plan. Available at www.nhlbi.nih.gov/health/public/heart/hbp.dash. (accessed September, 2010).

National Institutes of Health, National Heart, Lung, and Blood Institute. The DASH Eating Plan. Available at www.nhlbi.nih.gov/health/public/heart/hbp.dash (accessed September, 2010).

National Kidney Foundation Kidney Disease Outcomes Quality Initiative (NKF-K/DOQI) Clinical Practice Guidelines for Nutrition in Chronic Kidney Disease. *Am J Kidney Dis.* 2000; 35(6)(Supp 2):S1-S140.

National Kidney Foundation, NKF KDOQI Clinical Practice Guidelines for Diabetes and Chronic Kidney Disease. 2007;29(2 Suppl 2):S38-S108 (protein in diet).

National Kidney Foundation: NKF-K/DOQI clinical practice guidelines for nutrition in chronic renal failure. *Am J Kidney.* 2000; 35(Suppl 2):S1-S140.

National Salt Reduction Initiative. www.nyc.gov/html/doh/html/cardio/cardio-salt-initiative.shtml (accessed September, 2010)

Nelson RG, Tuttle KR. The new KDOQI Clinical Practice Guidelines and clinical practice recommendations for diabetes and CKD. *Blood Purif.* 2007; 25(1):112-4.

Nowson CA, Patchett A, Wattanapenpaiboon N. The effects of a low-sodium base-producing diet including red meat compared with a high-carbohydrate, low-fat diet on bone turnover markers in women aged 45-74 years. *Br J Nutr.* 2009; 102(8):1161-70 (DASH lowers acidosis and preserves bone).

O'Donnell M, Xavier D, Diener C, *et al.* Rationale and design of INTERSTROKE: a global case-control study of risk factors for stroke. *Neuroepidemiology.* 2010; 35(1):36-44 (waist-to-hip ratio and heart disease).

Othman M, Kawar B, El Nahas AM. Influence of obesity on progression of non-diabetic chronic kidney disease: a retrospective cohort study. *Nephrol Clin Pract.* 2009; 113(1):C16-23 (BMI associated with CKD progression and obese progress to end stage twice as fast as normal weight CKD patients).

Sacks FM, Bray GA, Carey VJ, *et al.* Comparison of weight-loss diets with different compositions of fat, protein, and carbohydrates. *N Engl J Med.* 2009; 360:859-73 (calories and not type of diet count in losing weight).

Sanders PW. Dietary salt intake, salt sensitivity, and cardiovascular health. *Hypertension.* 2009; 53(3):442-5 (salt sensitivity).

Savica V, Gellinghieri G, Kopple JD. The effect of nutrition on blood pressure. *Ann Rev Nutr.* 2010; 30:365-401.

Savica V, Gellinghieri G, Kopple JD. The effect of nutrition on blood pressure. *Ann Rev Nutr.* 2010; 30:365-401.

Shoham DA, Durazo-Arvizu R, Kramen H, *et al.* Sugary soda consumption and albuminuria: results from the National Health and Nutrition Examination Survey, 1999-2004. *PLoS One.* 2008; 3(10):e3431 (soda consumption associated with kidney damage).

Stall S. Protein recommendations for individuals with CKD stages 1-4. *Nephrol Nurs J.* 2008; 35(3):279-82.

Stewart ST, Cutler DM, Rosen AB. Forecasting the effects of obesity and smoking on U.S. life expectancy. *N Engl J Med.* 2009; 361:2252-60 (increase in obesity over the years).

The United States Department of Health and Human Services, National Institute of Heart, Lung, and Blood, NIH Publication N006-4082. www.nhlbi.nih.gov/health/public/heart/hbp/dash/new_dash.pdf (accessed September 2010) (DASH eating plan).

Trapp C, Barnard N, Katcher H. A plant-based diet for type 2 diabetes: scientific support and practical strategies. *Diabetes Educ.* 2010; 36(1):33-48 (plant-based diet for diabetes).

U.S. Department of Agriculture www.usda.gov (accessed September 2010) (consuming high fructose corn syrup).

U.S. Department of Agriculture and U.S. Department of Health and Human Services. *Dietary Guidelines for Americans, 2010.* 7th Edition, Washington, D.C.; U.S. Government Printing Office, December 2010.

U.S. Food and Drug Administration, Salt in diet. www.fda.gov/ForConsumers/ConsumerUpdates/ucm181577.htm (accessed September 2010) (natural salt in food; added salt; salt labeling).

United States Renal Data System: USRDS 2010 Annual Data Report. Atlas of Chronic Kidney Disease and End-Stage Renal Disease in the United States, National Institutes of Health, National Institute of Diabetes and Digestive and Kidney Diseases, Bethesda, Md. 2010; Vol. 1 (CKD statistics; associated chronic diseases).

Welch JA, Sharma A, Abramson JL. Caloric sweetener consumption and dyslipidemia among U.S. adults. *JAMA.* 2010; 303(15):1490-7 (sugar intake related to cholesterol levels).

Wolongevicz DM, Brown LS, Millen BE. Nutrient database development: a historical perspective from the Framingham Nutrition Studies. *J Am Diet Assoc.* 2010; 110(6):898-903 (changes in America's eating habits).

Chapter 18.   Food -- How Much and What Kind

Babio N, Balanza R, Basulto J, *et al.* Dietary fibre: influence on body weight, glycemic control and plasma cholesterol profile. *Nutr Hosp.* 2010; 25(3):327-40 (dietary fiber has positive effect on control of diabetes and body weight).

379

Centers for Disease Control and Prevention. www.cdc.gov/nchs/fastats/lcod.htm (accessed March 2011)(leading causes of death).

Flint AJ, Hu FB, Glynn RJ, *et al.* Whole grains and incident hypertension in men. *Am J Clin Nutr.* 2009; 90(3):493-8.

International Food Information Council Foundation. 2010 International Food Information Foundation Food & Health Survey: Consumer attitudes towards food safety, nutrition, and health. www.foodinsight.org/content/3651/2010 FinalFullReport.pdf (accessed September, 2010).

Jafri H, Alsheikh-All AA, Karas RH. Baseline and on-treatment high-density lipoprotein cholesterol and the risk of cancer in randomized controlled trials of lipid-altering therapy. *J Am Coll Cardiol.* 2010; 55(25):2855-7 (high HDLs protect from cancer).

Kaluza J, Orsini N, Levitan EB, *et al.* Dietary calcium and magnesium intake and mortality: a prospective study of men. *Am J Epidemiol.* 2010; 171(7):801-7 (excess calcium intake reduces mortality risk).

Kerksick C, Thomas A, Campbill B, *et al.* Effects of a popular exercise and weight loss program on weight loss, body composition, energy expenditure, and health in obese women. *Nutr Metab.* 2009; 6:23.

National Heart, Lung and Blood Institute. www.nhibi.nih.gov/health/public/heart/chol/wyntk.htm (accessed September 2010) (optimal HDL level).

Neuhouser ML, Wasserthiel-Smoller S, Thomson C, *et al.* Multivitamin use and risk of cancer, and cardiovascular disease in the Women's Health Initiative cohorts. *Arch Intern Med.* 2009; 169(3):294-304 (vitamin supplements do not reduce health risks).

Pray WS. The health benefits of fiber: fiber's health benefits. www.medscape.com/viewarticle/540168 4 (accessed September 2010).

Roizen MF, Oz MC. You: The Owner's Manual. Harper Collins Publishers Inc. NY, NY 2005 p. 171 (the look of feces).

Sabate J, Oda K, Ros E. Nut consumption and blood lipid levels: a pooled analysis of 25 intervention trials. *Arch Intern Med,* 2010; 170(9):821-7 (nut consumption improves lipid levels).

Sinha R, Cross AJ, Graubardi BI, *et al.* Meat intake and mortality: a prospective study of over half a million people. *Arch Intern Med.* 2009; 169(6):562-71.

U.S. Department of Agriculture and U.S. Department of Health and Human Services, *Dietary Guidelines for Americans, 2010.* 7th Edition, Washington DC; U.S. Government Printing Office, December 2010.

Chapter 19. Now, Let's Eat

ABC News poll. www.abcnews.com.go.com/BMA/pollvault/story?id=762685 (accessed September 2010)(4 of 10 adults don't eat breakfast).

American Diabetes Association. http://www.diabetes.org/food-and-fitness/food/what-can-i-eat/carbohydrates.html (accessed October 2010) (fiber and carb counting).

Brooks L. Salt, Salt, Salt—Plus sleep and job stress: more data to share with your patients. *Medscape Cardiology.* www.medscape.com/viewarticle708291 (accessed June 2010)(ASH recommends DASH-like diet).

Carter P, Gray LJ, Troughton J, *et al.* Fruit and vegetable intake and incidence of type 2 diabetes mellitus: systematic review and meta-analysis. *BMJ.* 2010; 341:c4229.

Centers of Disease Control and Prevention. State-specific trends in fruit and vegetable consumption among adults--United States, 2000-2009. *MMWR Morb Mortal Wkly Rep.* 2010; 59(35):1125-30 (only 26.3% of adults eat 3 vegetables/day).

Clifton PM. Dietary treatment for obesity. *Nat Clin Pract Gastroenterol Hepatol.* 2008; 5(12):672-81 (breakfast important in weight-loss maintenance).

Cory S, Ussery-Hall A, Griffin-Blake S, *et al.* Prevalence of selected risk behaviors and chronic diseases and condition-steps communities, United States, 2006-2007. *MMWR Surveill Summ.* 2010; 59(8):1-37 (CDC survey of U.S. behaviors, including percent eating fruits/vegetables).

Epstein HA. Food for thought and skin. *Skinmed.* 2010; 8(1):50-1.

Farshchi HR, Taylor MA, Macdonald IA. Beneficial metabolic effects of regular meal frequency on dietary thermogenesis, insulin sensitivity, and fasting lipid profiles in healthy obese women. *Am J Clin Nutr.* 2005; 81(1):16-24.

Ferenczi EA, Asaria P, Hughes AD, *et al.* Can a statin neutralize the cardiovascular risk of unhealthy dietary choices? *Am J Cardiology.* 2010; 106:587-92.

Gonzalez CA, Riboli E. Diet and cancer prevention: contributions from the European Prospective Investigation into Cancer and Nutrition (EPIC). *Eur J Cancer.* 2010; 46(14):2555-62.

Lam TK, Ruczinski I, Helzinouer KJ, *et al.* Cruciferous vegetable intake and lung cancer risk: a nested case-control study matched on cigarette smoking. *Cancer Epidemiol Biomarkers Prev.* 2010; 14:PMID: 20841387.

The National Weight Control Registry, Brown Medical School/The Miriam Hospital Weight Control & Diabetes Research Center.

USDA National Nutrient Database. www.nat.usda.gov/fnic/foodcomp/search (accessed March 2011).

Williams BM, O'Nell CE, Keast DR, *et al.* Ready-to-eat cereal breakfasts are associated with improved nutritional intake and dietary adequacy but not body mass index in black adolescents. *Am J Lifestyle Med.* 2009; 3(6):500-8.

Woodruff SJ, Hanning RM, McGoldrick K, Brown KS. Healthy eating index-C is positively associated with family dinner frequency among students in grades 6-8 from Southern Ontario, Canada. *Eur J Clin Nutr.* 2010; 64(5):456-60.

Chapter 20.   Staying Alive Means Staying Active

A. Exercise - Medicine for the Kidneys

2010 Shape the Nation Report: Status of Physical Education in the USA. National Association for Sports and Physical Education (NASPE) and the American Heart Association. www.aahperd.org/NASPE (accessed September 2010).

Adams GR, Vaziri HD. Skeletal muscle dysfunction in chronic renal failure: effects of exercise. *Am J Physiol Renal Physiol.* 2006; 290(4):F753-F761.

Afshinnia F, Wilt TJ, Duval S. Weight loss and proteinuria: systematic review of clinical trials and comparative cohorts. *Nephrol Dial Transplant.* 2010; 25(4):1173-83.

Beddhu S, *et al.* Physical activity and mortality in chronic kidney disease (NHANES III). *Clin J Am Soc Nephrol.* 2009; 4(12):1901-6 (active people are 56% less likely to die).

Chan M, Cheema BSB, Singh MAF. Progressive resistance training and nutrition in renal failure. *J Ren Nutr.* 2007; 17(1):84-7 (exercise helps dialysis patients).

Chobanian AV, Bakras GL, Black HR, *et al.* The Seventh Report of the Joint National Committee on Prevention, Detection, Evaluation, and Treatment of High Blood Pressure: the GNC 7 Report. *JAMA.* 2003; 289(19):2560-72.

Delgado C, Johansen KL. Deficient counseling on physical activity among nephrologists. *Nephron Clin Pract.* 2010; 116(4):c330-c336.

Exercise and type 2 diabetes: American College of Sports Medicine and the American Diabetes Association joint position statement. Exercise and Diabetes. American College of Sports Medicine; American Diabetes Association. *Med Sci Sports Exerc.* 2010; 42:2282-303 (exercise guidelines for diabetics).

Johansen KL, Sakkas GK, Doyle R, *et al.* Exercise counseling practices among nephrologists caring for patients on dialysis. *Am J Kidney Dis.* 2003; 41(1):171-8 (nephrologists fail to counsel patients on exercise).

Moinuddin L, Leekey DJ. A comparison of aerobic exercise and resistance training in patients with and without chronic kidney disease. *Adv Chronic Kidney Dis.* 2008; 15(1):83-96 (weight-lifting during maintenance dialysis counteracts muscle wasting).

Navaneethen S, Yehnert H, Moustah F, *et al.* Weight loss interventions in chronic kidney disease: a systematic review and meta-analysis. *Clin J Am Soc Nephrol.* 2009; 4(10):1565-74 (weight loss in obese improves kidney function).

Odden MC. Physical functioning in elderly persons with kidney disease. *Adv Chronic Kidney Dis.* 2010 Jul; 17(4):348-57.

Pate RR. A national physical activity plan for the United States. *J Phys Act Health.* 2009; 6 Suppl 2:S157-8 (National Physical Activity Plan, initiated and implemented by the CDC and directed by the National Coalition for Promoting Physical Activity).

Robinson-Cohen C, Katy R, Mozaffarian D, *et al.* Physical activity and rapid decline in kidney function among older adults. *Arch Intern Med.* 2009; 169(22):2116-23, 2124-7 (physical activity slows kidney function decline). (This study was supported by the National Institutes of Health; the National Heart, Lung, and Blood Institute; the National Institute of Neurological Disorders and Strokes; and, the National Institutes on Aging).

Robinson FS, Fisher ND, Forman JP, *et al.* Physical activity and albuminuria. *Am J Epidemiol.* 2010; 171(5):515-521 (exercise improves albuminuria).

Takhreem M. The effectiveness of intradialytic exercise prescription in quality of life in patients with chronic kidney disease. *Medscape J Med.* 2008; 10(10):226 (exercise not routinely prescribed for CKD patients but is beneficial).

U.S. Department of Health and Human Services. The Surgeon General's Vision for a Healthy and Fit Nation. Rockville, MO: USD of HHS, Office of the Surgeon General, January 2010 (accessed September 2010) (healthcare providers should counsel patients on exercise).

Whelton SP, Chin A, Xin X, He J. Effect of aerobic exercise on blood pressure: a meta-analysis of randomized, controlled trials. *Ann Intern Med.* 2002; 136(7):493-503 (sedentary adults who then exercised decreased blood pressure).

B. Exercise - Medicine for the Whole Body

American College of Sports Medicine, Exercising With Hypertension: Prescription for Health. www.medscape.com/viewarticle/719396 (accessed August 2010).

Annesi JJ, Gorjala S. Association of reduction in waist circumference with normalization of mood in obese women initiating exercise supported by the Coach Approach protocol. *South Med J.* 2010; 103(6):517-521.

Auchincloss AH, Diez Roux AV, Mujahid MS, *et al.* Neighborhood resources for physical activity and healthy foods and incidence of type 2 diabetes mellitus: the multi-ethnic study of atherosclerosis. *Arch Intern Med.* 2009; 169(18):1698-1704.

Beddhu S, Baird BC, Zitterkoph J, *et al.* Physical activity and mortality in chronic kidney disease (NHANES III). *Clin J Am Soc Nephrol.* 2009 Dec; 4(12):1901-6.

Bureau of Labor Statistics, Economic News Release, American Time Use Survey Summary, June 22, 2010 www.bls.gov/news.release/atus.nro.htm (accessed September 2010)(percent of people engaging in sports; sedentary statistics).

Carnethon MR, Evans HS, Church TS, *et al.* Joint associations of physical activity and aerobic fitness on the development of incident hypertension. Coronary artery risk development in young adults (CARDIA) *Hypertension.* 2010; 56(1):49-55 (young adults most physically active have decreased risk of developing hypertension).

Dunstan DW, Barr ELM, Healy GN, Salmon J, *et al.* Television viewing time and mortality: the Australian Diabetes, Obesity, and Lifestyle Study (AusDiab). *Circulation.* 2010; 121(3):384-91.

Etgen T, Sander D, Huntgeburth U, *et al.* Physical activity and incident cognitive impairment in elderly persons: the INVADE Study. *Arch Intern Med.* 2010; 170(2):186-193 (physical activity preserves cognitive function).

Fatone C, Guescimi M, Balducci S, *et al.* Two weekly sessions of combined aerobic and resistance exercise are sufficient to provide beneficial effects in subjects with type 2 diabetes mellitus and metabolic syndrome. *J Endocrinol Invest.* 2010; 33(7):489-95.

Ford ES, Bergmann MM, Kroger J, *et al.* Healthy living is the best revenge: findings from the European Prospective Investigation into Cancer and Nutrition--Potsdam Study. *Arch Intern Med.* 2009; 169(15):1355-1362 (exercise and 80% reduction in chronic illness).

Goldstein, LB. Physical activity and risk of stroke. *Expert Rev Neurother.* 2010; 10(8):1263-5 (women's health study and stroke reduction through exercise).

Kidney Disease Outcomes Quality Initiative (K/DOQI). K/DOQI Clinical Practice Guidelines on Hypertension and Anti-hypertensive Agents in Chronic Kidney Disease. *Am J Kidney Dis.* 2004; 43(5)(Suppl 1):S1-S290.

Kemmler W, vonStengel S, Engelke K, *et al.* Exercise effects on bone mineral density, falls, coronary risk factors, and health care costs, in older women: the randomized controlled senior fitness and prevention (SEFIP) study. *Arch Intern Med.* 2010; 170(2):179-185 (exercise builds bone).

Laaksonen DE, Lindström J, Lakka TA, *et al.* Physical activity in the prevention of type 2 diabetes: the Finnish diabetes prevention study. *Diabetes.* 2005; 54(1):158-65.

Lee, I-M. Physical activity and cardiac protection. *Curr Sports Med Rep.* 2010; 9(4):214-219 (active people of all types have lower rates of disease than inactive people).

Lindström J, Llanne-Parikka P, Peltonen M, *et al.* Sustained reduction in the incidence of Type 2 diabetes by lifestyle intervention: followup to Finnish Diabetes Prevention Study. *Lancet.* 2006; 368(9548):1673-9.

Liu-Ambrose T, Nagamatsu LS, Graf P, *et al.* Resistance training and executive functions: a 12-month randomized controlled trial. *Arch Intern Med.* 2010; 170(2):170-8 (exercise benefits cognitive function).

Meyerhardt JA, Giovannucci EL, Ogino S, *et al.* Physical activity and male colorectal cancer survival. *Arch Intern Med.* 2009; 169(22):2102-2108 (lowers risk of death by 49%).

Monda KL, Ballantyne CM, North KE. Longitudinal impact of physical activity on lipid profiles in middle-aged adults: the Atherosclerosis Risk in Communities Studies. *J Lipid Res.* 2009; 50(8):1685-91 (exercise improves blood lipid levels).

Owen N, Healy GN, Matthews CE, Dunstar DW. Too much sitting: the population health science of sedentary behavior. *Exer Sport Sci Rev.* 2010; 38(3):105-113. (TV watching and riding in car increase death rate)

Peters TM, Moore SC, Gierach GL, *et al.* Intensity and timing of physical activity in relation to postmenopausal breast cancer risk: the perspective NIH-AARP diet and health study. *BMC Cancer.* 2009; 9:349 (exercise prevents cancer).

Progressive resistance training enhances mobility in seniors: 121 studies show older adults can maintain daily activities and independence through some form of PRT. *Duke Med Health News.* 2009; 15(10):1-2.

Rector RS, Rogers R, Ruebel M, *et al.* Lean body mass and weight-bearing activity in the prediction of bone mineral density in physically active men. *J Strength Cond Res.* 2009; 23(2):427-35.

Stessman J, Hammerman-Rozenberg R, Cohen A, *et al.* Physical activity, function and longevity among the very old. *Arch Intern Med.* 2009; 169(16):1476-83 (exercise extends life in people in 70's and 80's).

Sun Q, Townsend MK, Okereke OI, *et al.* Physical activity at midlife in relation to successful survival in women at age 70 years or older. *Arch Intern Med.* 2010; 170(2):124-5 (exercise associated with improved overall health).

Willey JZ, Moon YP, Paik MC, *et al.* Physical activity and risk of ischemic stroke in the Northern Manhattan Study. *Neurology.* 2009; 73(21):1774-9 (exercise reduces stroke risk in men).

C. Physical Activity Basics

Coblac LJ, Vos T, Barendregt JJ. Cost-effectiveness of interventions to promote physical activity: a modeling study. *PLoS Med.* 2009; 6(7):e1000110 (pedometers promote exercise).

Hashell WL, Lee I-M, Pate RR, *et al.* Physical activity and public health: updated recommendations for adults from the American College of Sports Medicine and the American Heart Association. *Circulation.* 2007; 116:1081-1093 (physical activity guidelines).

Hsia J, Larson JC, Ockene JK, *et al.* Resting heart rate as a low-tech predictor of coronary events in women: prospective cohort study. *BMJ.* 2009; 338:b219.dol: 10.1136/bmj.b219 (higher resting pulse rate, more likely to have heart attack).

International Food Information Council Foundation. 2010 International Food Information Foundation Food & Health Survey: Consumer attitudes towards food safety, nutrition, and health. www.foodinsight.org/content/3651/2010FinalFullReport.pdf (accessed September 2010) (77 percent of Americans fail to meet physical activity guidelines).

Nelson ME, Rejeski WJ, Blair SN, *et al.* Physical activity and public health in older adults: recommendations from the American College of Sports Medicine and the American Heart Association. *Circulation.* 2007; 116(9):1094-105 (recommendations for older adults; 0 to 10 exertion rating).

Progressive resistance training enhances mobility in seniors. 121 studies show older adults can maintain daily activities and independence through some form of PRT. *Duke Med Health News.* 2009; 15(10):1-2 (no author given).

Williamson J, Pahor M. Evidence regarding the benefits of physical exercise. *Arch Intern Med.* 2010; 170(2):124-5.

Yamamoto K, Kawano H, Gando Y, *et al.* Poor trunk flexibility is associated with arterial stiffening. *Am J Physical Heart Circ Physiol.* 2009; 297(4):H1314-8 (reach for toes test for artery health).

Chapter 21. Learning to Move It

American College of Sports Medicine; American Diabetes Association. Exercise and type 2 diabetes: American College of Sports Medicine and the American Diabetes Association's Joint Position Statement on Exercise and Diabetes. *Med Sci Sports Exerc.* 2010; 42:2282-2303 (exercise guidelines for diabetics).

Andersen LL, Andersen JL, Suetta C, *et al.* Effect of contrasting physical exercise interventions on rapid force capacity of chronically painful muscles. *J App Physio.* 2009; 107(5):1413 (strength exercises relieve shoulder pain).

Auchincloss AH, Roux AV, Mujahid MS *et al.* Neighborhood resources for physical activity and healthy foods and incidence of type 2 diabetes mellitus: the Multi-Ethnic Study of Atherosclerosis. *Arch Intern Med.* 2009; 169(18):1698-704.

Johnson RA, Meadows RL. Dog-walking: motivation for adherence to a walking program. *Clin Nurs Res.* 2010; PMID: 20651066.

Centers for Disease Control and Prevention. www.cdc.gov/homeandrecreationalsafety/falls/adultfalls.htm (accessed August 2010).

Cobiac LJ, Vos T, Barendregt JJ. Cost-effectiveness of interventions to promote physical activity: a modeling study. *PLoS Med.* 2009; 6(7):e1000110 DOI: 10.1371/journal.pmed.1000110 (pedometers effective in encouraging exercise).

Josse AR, Tang JE, Tamopolski MA, Phillips SM. Body composition and strength changes in women with milk and resistance exercise. *Med Sci Sports Exer.* 2010; 42(6)]1122-30.

Karst GM, Willett GM. Effects of specific exercise instructions on abdominal muscle activity during trunk curl exercises. *J Orthop Sports Phys Ther.* 2004; 34(1):4-12.

Nowicki M, Murlikiewicz K, Jagodzinska M. Pedometers as a means to increase spontaneous activity in chronic hemodialysis patients. *J Nephrol.* 2010; 23(3):297-305.

Patel AV, Berstein L, Deka A, *et al.* Leisure time spend sitting in relation to total mortality in a prospective cohort of U.S. adults. *Am J Epidemiol.* 2010; 172(4):419-29.

Sunkaria RT, Kumar V, Saxena SC. A comparative study on spectral parameters of HRV in yogic and non-yogic practitioners. *Int J Med Eng Informat.* 2010; 2(1):1-14 (yoga helps the heart).

Chapter 22. Kick It Up a Notch

Ades PA, Savage PD, Toth MJ, *et al.* High-calorie-expenditure exercise. A new approach to cardio rehabilitation for overweight coronary patients. *Circulation* 2009; DOI:10.1161/CIRCULATION HA.108.834184 (walking faster to lose more weight).

Arena R, Myers J, Guazzi M. The clinical significance of aerobic exercise testing and prescription: from apparently healthy to confirmed cardiovascular disease. *Am J Lifestyle Med.* 2008; 2(6):519-36.

Centers for Disease Control and Prevention. www.cdc.gov/healthyweight/tools/index.html (accessed September 2010) (weight loss occurs because of decreased calories; physical activity necessary to maintain weight loss).

Donnelly JE, Blair SN, Jakicic JM, *et al.* Appropriate physical activity intervention strategies for weight loss and prevention of weight regain for adults. American College of Sports Medicine. *Med Sci Sports Exerc.* 2009 Feb; 41(2):459-71. Erratum in *Med Sci Sports Exerc.* 2009 Jul; 41(7):1532.

Larson-Meyer DE, Redman L, Heilbronn LK, *et al.* Caloric restriction with or without exercise: the fitness versus fatness debate. *Med Sci Sports Exerc.* 2010; 42(1):152-9 (improve metabolic fitness of exercise while diet).

Lee IM, Djoussé L, Sesso HD, *et al.* Physical activity and weight gain prevention. *JAMA.* 2010; 303(12):1173-9.

Moholdt TT, Amundsen BH, Rustad LA, *et al.* Aerobic interval training versus continuous moderate exercise after coronary artery bypass surgery: a randomized study of cardiovascular effects and quality of life. *Am Heart J.* 2009; 158(6):1031-7.

Tabet JY, Driss AB, Weber H, *et al.* Benefits of exercise training in chronic heart failure. *Arch Cardiovasc Dis.* 2009; 102(10): 721-30.

Tjonna AE, Lee SJ, Rognmo O, *et al.* Aerobic interval training versus continuous moderate exercise as a treatment for the metabolic syndrome: a pilot study. *Circulation.* 2008; 118(4):346-54.

www.ingramcontent.com/pod-product-compliance
Lightning Source LLC
Chambersburg PA
CBHW071354170526
45165CB00001B/42